# Understanding Drugs Markets

Drawing on anthropology, historical sociology and social-epidemiology, this multidisciplinary book investigates how pharmaceuticals are produced, distributed, prescribed, consumed and regulated in order to construct a comprehensive understanding of the issues that drive pharmaceutical markets in the Global South today.

Based on primary research conducted in Benin and Ghana, and additional data collected in Cambodia and the Ivory Coast, this volume uses artemisinin-based combination therapies (ACTs) against malaria as a central case study. It highlights the influence of the countries' colonial and postcolonial history on their models for state regulation, production and distribution, explores the determining role transnational actors as well as industries from the North but also and increasingly from the South play in influencing local pharmaceutical markets and looks at the behaviour of healthcare professionals and individuals. Stepping back, the authors then unpick the pharmaceuticalization process and the multiple regulations at stake by looking at the workings of, and linkages between, (biomedical health) pharmaceutical systems, (representatives of companies) industries, actors in private and public distribution and consumer practices.

Providing a thorough comparative analysis of the advantages and disadvantages of different pharmaceutical systems, it is an important contribution to the literature on pharmaceuticalization and the governance of medication. It is of interest to students, researchers and policymakers interested in medical anthropology, the sociology of health and illness, global health, healthcare management and pharmacy.

**Carine Baxerres** is a researcher in anthropology at the French National Research Institute for Sustainable Development (IRD), in the research unit MERIT (IRD-University of Paris) and LPED (IRD-Aix-Marseille University). Her research interests are global and local pharmaceuticals markets in West Africa and more recently in Southeast Asia, and health-seeking behaviours.

**Maurice Cassier** is currently a senior researcher at the French National Center for Scientific Research (CNRS, CERMES3, Paris). He has published extensively on the tensions between exclusive intellectual property rights on medicines and the right to health and has developed a research programme on the new geographies of the pharmaceutical industries in the Souths. He is currently working on new models of innovation and local production of health products, based on the categories of public goods and commons.

## Routledge Studies in the Sociology of Health and Illness




For more information about this series, please visit: https://www.routledge.com/Routledge-Studies-in-the-Sociology-of-Health-and-Illness/book-series/RSSHI

# Understanding Drugs Markets

## An Analysis of Medicines, Regulations and Pharmaceutical Systems in the Global South

**Edited by Carine Baxerres and Maurice Cassier**

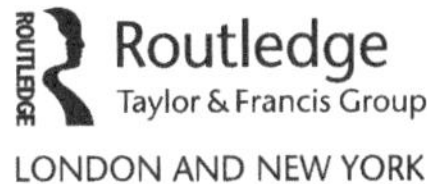


LONDON AND NEW YORK

First published 2022
by Routledge
2 Park Square, Milton Park, Abingdon, Oxon OX14 4RN

and by Routledge
605 Third Avenue, New York, NY 10158

*Routledge is an imprint of the Taylor & Francis Group, an informa business*

© 2022 selection and editorial matter, **Carine Baxerres and Maurice Cassier**; individual chapters, the contributors

The right of **Carine Baxerres and Maurice Cassier** to be identified as the authors of the editorial material, and of the authors for their individual chapters, has been asserted in accordance with sections 77 and 78 of the Copyright, Designs and Patents Act 1988.

All rights reserved. No part of this book may be reprinted or reproduced or utilised in any form or by any electronic, mechanical, or other means, now known or hereafter invented, including photocopying and recording, or in any information storage or retrieval system, without permission in writing from the publishers.

*Trademark notice*: Product or corporate names may be trademarks or registered trademarks, and are used only for identification and explanation without intent to infringe.

*British Library Cataloguing-in-Publication Data*
A catalogue record for this book is available from the British Library
*Library of Congress Cataloging-in-Publication Data*
A catalog record has been requested for this book

ISBN: 978-0-367-35067-3 (hbk)
ISBN: 978-1-032-04313-5 (pbk)
ISBN: 978-0-429-32951-7 (ebk)

Typeset in Goudy
by KnowledgeWorks Global Ltd.

I dedicate this work to Adèle, Rubin and Benjamin, who followed me to Benin and Ghana, on this beautiful coastal road that connects the two countries, to the lively streets of Adabraka and the overcrowded stores of the Okaishie market (Carine Baxerres).

I dedicate this work to all the participants of the Ouidah conference in March 2018, which was so rich for our exchanges on pharmaceutical markets in the Global South (Maurice Cassier).

# Contents

## PART II
## Global and local markets of new antimalarials



## PART III
## Pharmaceuticalization: Medicines at the heart of health systems and societies

# List of figures

# List of tables

# List of contributors

**Daniel Kojo Arhinful** is a Senior Research Fellow and past Head of the Epidemiology Department at the Noguchi Memorial Institute for Medical Research (NMIMR), University of Ghana. He holds a Ph.D. in Social Sciences with a speciality in Medical Anthropology from the University of Amsterdam. His key areas of research specialization are access to medicines, social health insurance and social security, maternal and child health, infectious and non-communicable diseases.

**Eve Bureau-Point** is anthropologist at the French National Center for Scientific Research (CNRS, Centre Norbert Elias, Marseille). She conducts researches in France and Southeast Asia on the social lives of chemical substances.

**Claudie Haxaire** is a pharmacist, ethnopharmacologist and medical anthropologist conducting research on medicines and pharmaceuticals. Being assistant in the pharmacy school in Abidjan, from 1979 to 1984, she is nowadays in collaboration with the laboratory of pharmacognosia. She is associated member of the CERMES3 (CNRS–INSERM–EHESS–Université de Paris).

**Roch Appolinaire Houngnihin** is a medical anthropologist at the University of Abomey-Calavi (Benin) and current head of the Laboratory of Applied Medical Anthropology (LAMA). His researches cover various topics including public policies and health systems in Africa: access to care, logic of caregivers, patient practices, therapeutic routes, etc.

**Adolphe Codjo Kpatchavi** is a professor of sociology and medical anthropology at the University of Abomey-Calavi in Benin. His main research topics are policies and governance of health systems, access to healthcare, malaria and drugs in the informal sector in Africa.

**Jean-Yves Le Hesran** is a medical epidemiologist and director of research at the French National Research Institute for Sustainable Development (IRD), in the research unit MERIT (IRD-University of Paris). His main research topics are malaria and access to healthcare and to medicines in Africa. His research fields are Benin, Ghana and Senegal.

**Stéphanie Mahamé** is a Ph.D. student in Sociology-Anthropology at the University of Abomey-Calavi (Benin) and at EHESS (Ecole des Hautes Etudes en Sciences Sociales) Paris (France). Her work focuses on health in Africa, and since 2014 she has been studying the drug markets in Benin and West Africa.

**Maxima Missodey** is Principal Research Assistant – Noguchi Memorial Institute for Medical Research, University of Ghana. She will defend her Ph.D. on Standardized Herbal Medicines in Ghana in 2021. Her research interests are pharmaceutical anthropology, medical sociology, health research.

**Jessica Pourraz** holds a Ph.D. in Sociology (2019) from the Ecole des Hautes Etudes en Sciences Sociales (EHESS) in Paris. She is a postdoctoral research fellow with IFRIS (Institute For Research and Innovation in Society), in the research unit CEPED (IRD-Paris Descartes). Her research interests focus on issues related to science, biomedicine, environment and health.

**Kelley Sams** is a postdoctoral researcher with the French National Research Institute for Sustainable Development (IRD), in the research unit LPED (IRD-Aix-Marseille University). She is also Contributing Faculty at Walden University (USA). Her research interests include infectious disease response, visual health communication and medication use.

# Foreword

Throughout the history, man's interaction with the environment has led him evolved survival mechanisms to cope with ill health, diseases and natural calamities. Through try and error with herbs and mineral resources, man developed appetite and need to consume remedies to remain healthy. Therefore, the focus of medicines or drugs to humans has been its usage for curative, preventive or health promotional purposes or effect.

Beyond this purpose, medicines have been realized over time to constitute significant connection of social-economic and cultural processes including knowledge, symbols and beliefs, politics, profit-making, trust and conflict.

The anthropology of medicines has once again been presented to us a unique opportunity to elucidate the role played by medicines in the lives of various societies and communities. Carine Baxerres and others, in this book, have presented to us using Artemisinin-based combination therapies (ACTs) as a "marker" to elucidate this kaleidoscopic picture. The choice of a pharmaceutical product in this study emphasizes the fact that drugs are not just any ordinary article of commerce. Indeed drugs or pharmaceuticals go through phases of conception, gestation, birth, production, distribution, growth, decline and death with consequential effects even after its demise. In each of these phases, drugs transcend through various man-made and artificial elements of the environmental ecosystem.

Again, the use of ACTs as a "unique drug identity" for their multi-state studies allows us to appreciate and affirm the uniqueness about most pharmaceutical drugs. Notwithstanding their curative or therapeutic intentions in health, pharmaceutical drugs and their associated activities are viewed differently and ascribed different values across different cultures and societies as they permeate variety of social, commercial and political systems. These features have been succinctly amplified in the book.

Drugs or pharmaceutical drugs have been demonstrated and proven in this book to have journeyed through various natural or artificial courses in a multi-level fashion, a concept suggested by a medical anthropological researcher. Van der Geest and other researchers in 1990 carried this assertion which was premised on the assumption that developments at various levels of social organization are interlinked. Also the characteristic features of these linkages have to be studied in order to understand what takes place at one specific level. Indeed Carine and other authors in this book, through their meticulous and painstaking studies have affirmed this proposition and enriched the intellectual world with their findings and conclusions.

The authors have also clearly articulated in this book that movement of drugs and the "rational" knowledge associated with them across cultural and physical borders is best understood in the broad and diverse context of mobility associated with globalization, and its social and cultural consequences in particular localities such as in Ghana, Benin, Côte d'Ivoire and Cambodia. In their well-researched book, they have thrown the spotlight on the way medicines are used and interpreted at the international, national, healthcare institution and household levels. The book also traced the basis for the crucial misunderstandings and conflicts that lead to inequality in access to medicines and to erratic drug policies experienced in some developing countries including Ghana, Benin and Cambodia.

Viewed against the background of multilevel approaches, the Carine and associated authors indeed threw more light into the processes in which political and commercial power and individuals play key significant roles in Ghana, Benin, Côte d'Ivoire and Cambodia. The leading idea is that actors at various levels seek to pursue their personal or group interests and thus steer the processes of importation, production, marketing, distribution and consumption of pharmaceuticals.

The choice of these countries for the studies has also revealed the British and French ambivalence of geopolitical philosophies that informed the developmental strategies and agenda for their colonies. It is a subject that will be of keen interest to students and scholars of development, sociology, anthropology, politics and economics.

Pharmacy practice can be viewed as a business or a health professional practice. The political dilemma has always been whether or not to confer the monopoly of business and professional practice of pharmacy on pharmacists as exclusive privilege. This dichotomy in model has been amplified in the book with historical antecedents traced to the colonialists' perspectives and experiences over the past hundreds of years in Europe. Ghana's model has been borrowed from the apparent flexible model of practice from the British experience where professional practice is the pharmacists' preserve and delinked from the business ownership. The converse holds true for francophone countries of West Africa where the pharmacists hold monopoly over practice and business. One of the dire implications is that there appears to be a role conflict on the part of pharmacists which arguably may lead to lowered ethical standards. It will take curious minds to explore further the demerits and demerits of this model as espoused in this book.

The new terminologies such as "pharmaceuticalization and de-pharmaceuticalization" have been introduced by the authors and the impact of these phenomena in the countries investigated. Cambodia is of special interest, and readers are encouraged to explore the impact of turbulent political transitions on the pharmaceutical practice and industry of that country. The experiences of pharmaceuticalization have unpacked the new reality in society's quest for acquisition of new values, utilization of economic and business opportunities and health-seeking behaviours. The newly acquired dependence on pharmaceutical drugs is evidently phenomenal to this effect.

The well-researched studies across different countries in this book have provided glimpses of some rationale, drivers, motivation and prioritization of specific agendas behind the colonization enterprise.

One of rational approaches to ensure that medicines are safe, efficacious and of right quality is the presence of effective regulation with the appropriate institutional framework in place. However, key revelation in these multiple states studies is the evolution of drug policies, medicines legislation and pharmaceutical regulation which, albeit alien, had become foist on the local societies with different values and beliefs systems. The interplay of conflicts and tensions, resulting from the introduction of such novel policies, legislations and regulation, especially on drugs and health practitioners, has unexpectedly produced outcomes not only geared towards the promotion of rational health and pharmaceutical industries but also the emergence of licit and illicit practices out of which emerged indigenous pharmaceutical entrepreneurs. The challenges and opportunities presented are well articulated for reference and worth reading in this book.

Overall, the insights provided by Carine and other authors in this book are evidently rich and insightful more importantly for its multilevel approaches, perspectives from different countries with varying colonial experiences and different economic and political systems. It is a masterpiece from world-class scholars, academicians, researchers and practitioners who collectively have wealth of experiences. I strongly recommend this book to policymakers, regulators, academicians, pharmacists, industrialists, anthropologists, researchers and political economists.

*By Pharm. Joseph Kodjo Nsiah Nyoagbe*
*B. Pharm. (Hons) KNUST Ghana; M.Sc. Bradford, UK; MBA (GIMPA); FPCPharm; FGCPharm; FPSGH*
*Fmr Registrar, Ghana Pharmacy Council and Current President of Ghana College of Pharmacists*

# Acknowledgments

The Globalmed research programme (2014–2019) entitled "Artemisinin-based combination therapy: an illustration of the global pharmaceutical drug market in Asia and Africa," supervised by Carine Baxerres, joins teams from the IRD (MERIT) and CNRS (CERMES3) in France, the University of Abomey-Calavi in Benin (CERPAGE and LAMA), the Noguchi Memorial Institute for Medical Research of the Legon University of Ghana and the University of Health Sciences of Cambodia. It has received funding from the European Research Council under the European Union's Seventh Framework Programme (FP7/2007–2013)/ERC grant agreement no. 337372. We are very grateful for this public-funding institution and thus to all the European citizens who, through their fiscal contributions, have made it possible to conduct this research.

Our thanks then extend to all the actors of the pharmaceutical markets we ethnographied and with whom we have communicated at length: producers, importers, wholesalers, retailers, pharmacists, chemists, doctors, midwives, nurses, care assistants, handlers, delivery people, pharmaceutical representatives, informal salesmen and woman, medical counter assistants whether they are graduates or not, OTC medicine sellers, telephonists, porters, order pickers, invoicers, checkers, accountants, packers etc.

We also thank the mothers and fathers, grandmothers and grandfathers, aunts and uncles, older sisters and brothers whom we interviewed regularly in Benin, Ghana and Cambodia over several months.

We do not forget the women and men, mainly pharmacists, who maintain or have maintained the regulatory authorities and health institution in the countries; to name but a few: Idrissou Abdoulaye, Prosper Ahonlonsou, Corneille Cakpo, Habib Ganfon, Benoit Hounkpevi, Carmelle Hounnou, Dorothée Kindé Gazard, Marina and Achille Massoubodji, Al-Fattah Onifade and Christophe Rochigneux in Benin; Vivian Aubyn, Constance Bart Plange, Samuel Asante Boateng, Ben Botwe, Theophilus Corquaye, Delese Mimi Darko, Nanaa Frempong, James Fripong, Martha Gwansa Lutterodt, Eric Karikari Boateng, Hudu Mogtari, Joseph Nyoagbe, Brenda Opong, Mercy Owusu-Asante and Seth Seaneke in Ghana; Serges Amari, Charles Boguifo, Assane Coulibaly, Rachel Duncan, Dieneba Kone-Bamba, Guillaume Loukou, Mahama Ouattara, Anglade Malan, Christophe Rochigneux, Olivier Yayo in Côte d'Ivoire; and Youk Lin Taing and Didier Fontenille in Cambodia. May they all be warmly thanked here.

Special thanks should be given to Pascal Millet, Jean-René Kiechel, Jean-François Corty, Luc Grislain, Tina Kauss, Jean-Marie Kindermans, Catherine Lacaze, Piero Olliaro and Jacques Pilloy, who agreed to describe to us the innovation process of the artesunate-amodiaquine combination coordinated by MSF and the DND*i* Foundation. Valérie Faillat Proux and François Bompart from Sanofi allowed us to visit the Sanofi-Maphar industrial site in Casablanca. Our thanks also go to the WHO archivist Reynald Erard, who facilitated our inquiry to study the trajectory of artemisinin-based drugs, and to Bright Botwe, archivist at the Public Records and Archives Administration Department in Ghana, who assisted us in our research within the archives of the Ministry of Industry.

We would also like to thank all the people working for international organizations and global health programmes in Ghana and Benin, as well as in the Geneva headquarters, who took the time to answer our questions and contribute to our reflections.

Beyond our research units, we would like to thank our fellow researchers and scholars who have nourished our reflections and supported us in this long-term work. While there is not space to name them all, we would like to thank in particular Artadji Attoumane, Doris Bonnet, Alila Brossard Antonielli, Claire Beaudevin, Laurent Brutus, Andrea Butcher, Fanny Chabrol, Nitsan Chorev, Marilena Correa, Akosua Darkwah, Alice Desclaux, Dorothée Dussy, Fred Eboko, Marc Egrot, Sylvie Fainzang, Jean-Paul Gaudillière, Bénédicte Gastineau, Nils Graber, Véronique Guienne, Rory Horner, Abou-Bakari Imorou, Koichi Kameda, Catherine Le Galès, Charlie Marquis, Andrew McDowell, Caroline Meier zu Biesen, Jean-Pierre Olivier de Sardan, Kris Peterson, Boris Petric, Laurent Pordié, Mathieu Quet, Charlie Marquis, Sandrine Musso, Christelle Rabier, Clémence Schantz, Kojo Senah, Marlee Tichenor and German Velasquez.

Finally, we would like to thank the following persons for their involvement in the data collection. They are not authors of the book, but they all contributed greatly to carrying out the field studies. For the qualitative data collection, we thank Anani Agossou, Emilienne Anago, Moïse Djralah, Audrey Hémadou and Aubierge Kpatinvoh in Benin; Emelia Agblevor, Eunice Ayimbila, the late Sandra Serwah Bredu,[1] Grace Kumi Kyeremeh and William Sackey in Ghana; and Malinda To in Cambodia. For the quantitative data collection, we thank Edwige Apetoh, Anani Agossou, Ines Boko, Ruth Boko, Moïse Djralah, Audrey Hemadou, Bernadette Kokoye and Aubierge Kpatinvoh in Benin; and William Sackey, Salomey Pomaah Adjani, Alberta Addo, Emmanuel Andam, Esther Appiah, Derrick Frimpong, Raymond Lamptey, Eric Nartey and Ohene Sakyi in Ghana. We thank Eunice Ayimbila and Aubierge Kpatinvoh for the qualitative data analysis and Hajar Ahachad, Edwige Apetoh, Georgia Damien, Arnaud Gbenou, Michael Addo Preko Ntiri and Marina Tilly for the quantitative data analysis.

Last but not least, we would like to warmly thank Michèle Hansen and Sharon Calandra of Global Health Language Services for their translation of the book from French into English.

1 Sandra Serwah passed away during the Globalmed programme following an illness. We pay tribute to her and her family here.

# List of abbreviations

| | |
|---|---|
| **ABRP** | Agence Béninoise de Régulation Pharmaceutique [Beninese Agency for Pharmaceutical Regulation] |
| **ACAME** | Association africaine des Centrales d'Achat de Médicaments Essentiels génériques [African Association of Central Medicine Stores for Generic Essential Drugs] |
| **ACCSQ** | ASEAN Consultative Committee for Standards and Quality |
| **ACT** | artemisinin-based combination therapy |
| **AFD** | Agence Française de Développement [French Development Agency] |
| **AFTA** | ASEAN Free Trade Area |
| **AIRP** | Autorité Ivoirienne de Régulation Pharmaceutique [Ivorian Pharmaceutical Regulatory Agency] |
| **AL** | artemether-lumefantrine |
| **AMFm** | Affordable Medicines Facility-malaria |
| **AMRH** | African Medicines Regulatory Harmonization |
| **AREPI** | Association of Representatives of Ethical Pharmaceutical Industries |
| **ARV** | antiretroviral |
| **ASAQ** | artesunate-amodiaquine |
| **ASEAN** | Association of Southeast Asian Nations |
| **ASMQ** | artesunate-mefloquine |
| **ASSP** | artesunate-sulfadoxine-pyrimethamine |
| **CAME** | Centrale d'Achat de Médicaments Essentiels et consommables médicaux [Central Purchasing Office for Essential Medicines and Medical Consumables] |
| **CAMEG** | Centrale d'Achat de Médicaments Essentiels génériques consommables médicaux [Central Purchasing Office for Essential Medicines and Generics] |
| **CEPICI** | Center for the Promotion of Investments in Côte d'Ivoire |
| **CERMES** | *Centre* de recherche médicale et sanitaire [Center for medical and health research] |
| **CFA franc** | Communauté Financière Africaine [African currency] |

**CHEMAL** Working Group on the Chemotherapy of Malaria
**CHPS** community-based health planning and services
**CITIC** China International Trust and Investment Corporation
**CMS** central medical store
**CNHU** Centre National Hospitalier Universitaire [National University Hospital Center]
**COPOB** Coopérative des Pharmaciens d'Officine du Bénin [Cooperative of Private Pharmacists in Benin]
**CTD** common technical document
**DDF** Department of Drugs and Food
**DES** Diplôme d'Études Spécialisées [post-graduate degree in a medical specialty]
**DGP** Direction Générale des Pharmacies [General Directorate of Pharmacies]
**DGS** Directorate General of Health Services
**DHPP** dihydroartemisinin-piperaquine
**DND*i*** Drugs for Neglected Diseases initiative
**DNDWG** Drugs for Neglected Diseases Working Group
**DPCI** Distribution Pharmaceutique de Côte d'Ivoire [Côte d'Ivoire Pharmaceutical Distribution]
**DPED** Direction des Pharmacies et des Explorations Diagnostiques [Directorate of Pharmacies and Diagnostic Investigations]
**DPM** Direction des Pharmacies et du Médicament [Directorate of Pharmacies and Medicines]
**DPMED** Direction des Pharmacies, du Médicament et des Explorations Diagnostiques [Directorate of Pharmacies, Medicine, and Diagnostic Investigations]
**DPML** Direction de la Pharmacie et du Médicament et des Laboratoires [Directorate of Pharmacy, Medicine, and Laboratories]
**DSP** Direction des Services Pharmaceutiques [Directorate of Pharmaceutical Services]
**ECOWAS** Economic Community of West African States
**EGM** essential generic medicines
**EHESS** Ecole des Hautes Etudes en Sciences Sociales
**EML** essential medicines list
**EPA** Établissement Publique à caractère Administratif [Public Establishment of an Administrative Nature]
**EPIC** Etablissement Public à Caractère Industriel et Commercial [Public Institution of an Industrial and Commercial Nature]
**ERPP** ECOWAS Regional Pharmaceutical Plan
**FACT** fixed-dose artesunate combination therapies
**FAPMA** Federation of African Pharmaceutical Manufacturers Associations
**FDA** Food and Drug Administration (US); Food and Drugs Authority (Ghana)

| | |
|---|---|
| **FDB** | Food and Drugs Board |
| **GAPOB** | Groupement d'Achat des Pharmaciens d'Officine du Bénin [Private Pharmacist Purchasing Association of Benin] |
| **GIHOC** | Ghana Industrial Holding Corporation |
| **GHC** | Ghanaian cedi (currency) |
| **GMP** | good manufacturing practice |
| **GOMPCI** | Groupement Pharmaceutique de Côte d'Ivoire [Pharmaceutical Group of Côte d'Ivoire] |
| **GPBN** | Groupement des Pharmaciens Bénin-Niger [Benin-Niger Pharmacist Group] |
| **IFPMA** | International Federation of Pharmaceutical Manufacturers Associations |
| **IMF** | International Monetary Fund |
| **INN** | International Nonproprietary Name |
| **KPF** | Kunming Pharmaceutical Factory |
| **LNCQ** | Laboratoire Nationale de Contrôle de Qualité [National Quality Control Laboratory] |
| **LNSP** | Laboratoire National de Santé Publique [National Laboratory of Public Health] |
| **LPCI** | Laboratoire Pharmaceutique de Côte d'Ivoire [Pharmaceutical Laboratory of Côte d'Ivoire] |
| **MA** | marketing authorization |
| **MMV** | Medicines for Malaria Venture |
| **MSF** | Médecins Sans Frontières [Doctors Without Borders] |
| **NAMCO** | Netherlands African Manufacturing Company |
| **NEPAD** | New Partnership for Africa's Development |
| **NGO** | nongovernmental organization |
| **NHIS** | National Health Insurance Scheme |
| **ONP** | Office National des Pharmacies du Bénin [Benin National Office of Pharmacies] |
| **OTC** | over-the-counter |
| **PARSSI** | Projet d'Appui à la Redynamisation du Secteur de la Santé en Côte d'Ivoire [Project to Support the Revitalization of Côte d'Ivoire's Health Sector] |
| **PMI** | President's Malaria Initiative |
| **PNDAP** | Programme National de Développement de l'Activité Pharmaceutique [National Program for the Development of Pharmaceutical Activity] |
| **PNLS** | Programme Nationale de Lutte contre le SIDA [National AIDS Control Program] |
| **PPWG** | Pharmaceutical Product Working Group |
| **PRAAD** | Public Records and Archives Administration Department |
| **PSCM** | Private Sector Copayment Mechanism |
| **PSP** | Pharmacie de la Santé Publique [Pharmacy of Public Health] |

| | |
|---|---|
| **PSPCI** | Pharmacie de la Santé Publique de Côte d'Ivoire [Côte d'Ivoire Pharmacy of Public Health] |
| **RAMU** | Régime d'Assurance Maladie Universelle [National Health Insurance Scheme] |
| **RBM** | Roll Back Malaria |
| **SCOA** | Société Commerciale d'Afrique de l'Ouest [West Africa Trading Company] |
| **SoBAPS** | Société Béninoise pour l'Approvisionnement en Produits de Santé [Beninese Society for Health Product Supply] |
| **SP** | sulfadoxine-pyrimethamine |
| **TAC** | Treatment Access Campaign |
| **TDR** | Tropical Disease Research |
| **UBPHAR** | Union Béninoise des Pharmaciens [Beninese Union of Pharmacists] |
| **UEMOA** | Union Économique et Monétaire Ouest Africaine [West African Economic and Monetary Union] |
| **UGPS** | Unité de Gestion des Programmes Spécifiques [Specific Program Management Unit] |
| **UNDP** | United Nations Development Programme |
| **UNICEF** | United Nations Children's Fund |
| **UNIDO** | United Nations Industrial Development Organization |
| **UNTAC** | United Nations Transitional Authority in Cambodia |
| **USAID** | United States Agency for International Development |
| **USP** | United States Pharmacopeia |
| **WAEMU** | West African Economic and Monetary Union |
| **WHO** | World Health Organization |
| **WTO** | World Trade Organization |

# Introduction

## Pharmaceutical markets in the Global South: Shaped by history and multiple regulations

*Carine Baxerres and Maurice Cassier*

Pharmaceutical specialties provide an ideal window into studying contemporary societies and understanding how and why they change. With dimensions that are simultaneously scientific, technical, therapeutic, popular, and commercial, these drugs are central to the health, economic, political, and social issues in play, both on a global and local scales. This economic sector is one of the most active and lucrative on the planet today (Hauray, 2006; Montalban, 2011).

When organic chemistry began to play a role in drug development, these new types of remedies were first produced industrially in Europe in the mid-19th century, and later in the United States. Their development was driven principally by their commercial potential (Faure, 2005). At the time of their emergence, they were poorly suited to the legislation then in place and were subjected to the most unrestrained rules of competition. Firms gradually began to establish "industry" regulations (standardization, increased number of biological trials, systematic control of raw materials and products, formalization of manufacturing protocols, etc.), the primary objective of which was scientific legitimacy for marketing needs (Gaudillière, 2005) before national legislation took over (Borchers, Hagie, Keen, & Gershwin, 2007; Marks, 1997). The goal of our book is to report on and analyze the construction and regulation of pharmaceutical markets in the Global South using case studies from Benin, Ghana, Côte d'Ivoire, and Cambodia.

### Recent shifts in the globalization of medicines in the Global South

The globalization of drug markets in the Global South is as old as the history of commercial drug products themselves. Historiography on the expansion of drug markets in Latin America has shown proliferation of imports by private traders, copying of drugs by local pharmacists who set up small firms in the early decades of the 20th century (Garcia, 2020, on Colombia), or commercial strategies by large firms from the Global North to establish themselves in these markets (Cramer, 2010, for Bayer in Latin America between the two world wars). Here we are more directly interested in the regions of Africa and Southeast Asia, which borrowed several market devices to distribute pharmaceuticals. For example, Myriam Mertens (2014) describes, in the context of Belgian

Congo, how procurement contracts from colonial administrations were used by their pharmaceutical industries back home to develop and market new therapies for tropical diseases, as early as the beginning of the 20th century and at a time when these diseases were a leading sector of pharmaceutical innovation. Laurence Monnais studied the circulation and use of medicines in Vietnam in the first half of the 20th century, first through the Indigenous Medical Assistance system and then through a handful of French pharmacies established in cities accessible to wealthy Vietnamese and European customers (Monnais, 2014). French pharmacies were also established in some cities in West and Central Africa; Jean Mazuet, for example, launched in several countries the wholesale companies we mention in the first section of this book. Historians and anthropologists alike have shown how medicines are promulgated in West and Central Africa: distributed free of charge through public health services and by religious missionaries (Vaughan, 1991), occasionally through forced preventive treatment campaigns (Lachenal, 2014), or by establishing commercial entities that create pharmaceutical depots. Some of these French distribution companies remain quite active in West Africa to this day (Baxerres, 2013).

Although our book addresses colonial legacies, it focuses on modern-day cycles of globalization with a concentration on three major shifts since the 1970s. The first is the new geography of the pharmaceutical industry, created when India and Brazil abandoned pharmaceutical patents in 1970–1971 (Cassier & Correa, 2003; Chaudhuri, 2005), at a time when China's model was the public ownership of inventions. Sudip Chaudhuri has clearly laid out the growth of the generics industry in India and the significance of Indian imports into the African countries where he focused his research, Ghana and Tanzania. World Health Organization (WHO) archives on the essential drugs policy advocated since 1977 show that Indian firms sometimes directly approach the WHO to supply that program.[1] This is the story of the expansion of generic drugs, defined as those either manufactured without patents in many countries of the Global South before the World Trade Organization (WTO) TRIPS (Trade-Related Aspects of Intellectual Property Rights) agreements were established in 1994, or after patents have expired.[2] On the African continent, we find national and regional markets based on local production centers being organized beginning in the 1980s and 1990s (Ghana, Kenya, Nigeria, South Africa, Tanzania, etc.) (Chorev, 2020; Mackintosh et al., 2016; Peterson, 2014; Pourraz, 2019). This is discussed in Chapter 1 in the countries of Benin, Côte d'Ivoire, and Ghana. Note, however, that nearly all African industries, with very few exceptions, are heavily dependent on imports of pharmaceutical raw materials from Asia, including in the most industrialized countries such as South Africa (Pelletan, 2019).

The second shift we examine is how the trajectories of market flows have changed. Although the countries studied here—Benin, Ghana, Côte d'Ivoire, and Cambodia—have been heavily influenced since independence by branded pharmaceuticals imported from their colonizers' firms and wholesalers (Baxerres, 2013 for Benin; Pourraz, 2019 for Ghana), the flow of generic imports from Asia now gives them stiff competition. We have witnessed the growth of South-South trade since the 1970s (Horner & Murphy, 2018), not only in imports of final products and raw materials, but of experts and even direct investments from Indian and Chinese firms as well. Our fields of research have led us to concentrate on movements between Asia and Africa and the agents that underpin them (wholesalers, pharmaceutical representatives, regulatory authorities, foundations, international organizations, etc.), employing a transregional approach in social sciences that is still under construction and lies between cultural areas and global studies (Canzler, Kaufmann, & Kesselring, 2008). To understand these movements, we paid particular attention to the social and professional backgrounds and education of the people we met.

The third major shift began in the 2000s with the appearance of global donor groups that fund large vertical programs to provide pharmaceutical treatments on a mass scale as part of the Global Health framework, such as the Global Fund to Fight AIDS, Tuberculosis and Malaria (Baxerres & Eboko, 2019; Gaudillière, Beaudevin, Gradmann, Lovell, & Pordié, 2020; Leon, 2015). Here again, Indian generics manufacturers have stepped into a predominant role, providing more than 90% of the antiretroviral drugs to treat AIDS in recipient countries. More recently they have begun supplying artemisinin-based combination therapies (ACTs) to combat malaria, a topic we cover in depth in this book, in the process replacing the Swiss multinational Novartis and the French company Sanofi, who had marketed the first ACTs. This third recent transformation of pharmaceutical markets in the Global South requires us to carefully consider the rationales, motivations, and practices of what we will call "transnational" actors[3] who provide subsidized medicines to countries primarily for infectious diseases and maternal and child health issues. They have a profound impact on these markets, putting the products they promote in often unfair competition with the products available in public and private markets (see the Global Fund's Affordable Medicine Facility–malaria initiative, AMFm, discussed in Chapter 6). The negotiated terms these transnational actors impose on the States of the Global South regarding their pharmaceutical and health policies were also central to our observations. Our findings question the "aid regime" under which many countries live (Lavigne Delville, 2010) even as we are experiencing a "return of the State" (Baxerres & Eboko, 2019). Certain transnational actors sometimes offer aid that achieves cross purposes, all the while supporting pharmaceutical import policies, and then also intervene in initiatives to develop local production.

In this book, we analyze the product hierarchy that results from these three historical changes: between innovative drugs and generics, between brand-name and generic drugs marketed under INNs (International Nonproprietary Names), and between different standards for copies. This hierarchy is objectified by norms governing intellectual property and standards, such as those defined by the WHO or the International Conference on Harmonisation of Technical Requirements for the Registration of Pharmaceuticals for Human Use (ICH).[4] Research on "similars" or generic drugs in South America and Africa has noted the dissemination of increasingly high standards of equivalence (Chorev, 2020; Correa, Cassier, & Loyola, 2019; Hayden, 2013), especially through the implementation in the early

2000s of the WHO prequalification program (Lantenois & Coriat, 2014). This hierarchy is also subjectified in the imaginaries of consumption that mix colonial and postcolonial legacies, the new dominance of Asian medicines, and the ascendency of Global Health.

## Multiple markets and regulations

A true understanding of pharmaceutical markets requires an interest in the history of pharmaceutical regulation as well as in the history of the tensions between market rules and the emergence of pharmacy policy and marketing authorizations (MAs) to protect population health. Historians have provided key contributions here, though until recently their work was largely focused on the markets of the industrialized and innovative countries of the Global North since the early 1800s. Olivier Faure's work on pharmacists and the dynamism of the drug market in 19th-century France contains a wealth of information on pharmacists' involvement in commercial and industrial logics (Faure, 1996) and on how the "dominant logic of commerce" incessantly spilled over into pharmacy-related frameworks and laws, including by pharmacists (Faure, 1993). Harry Marks' work on the history of pharmaceutical regulation in the United States highlights the role of distrust, particularly toward pharmaceutical companies, involved in the adoption of new standards for clinical research (Marks, 2000). The "adverse health events" associated with the use of therapeutic agents are used to justify strengthening the rules governing drug MAs (Bonah & Gaudillière, 2007; Chauveau, 2008).

The book edited by Jean-Paul Gaudillière and Volker Hess (2013) on the ways of medicine regulation proposes a synthetic model to explain the variety of regulatory tools deployed during the 20th century: professional, administrative, industrial, public, and legal. Regulation of pharmaceutical markets extends beyond the actions of the State, mobilizing professional pharmacist and physician organizations, and to a significant extent, academies of medicine, government committees and agencies, companies and industrial associations, consumer and patient associations, and the legal professions. An equally impressive array of knowledge and instruments is applied to cover procedures developed by professionals, drug patents, MAs, quality standards, post-marketing surveillance, clinical trials, and case law. This model is heuristic for analyzing pharmaceutical regulations in the Global South, as it was primarily developed from the history of pharmaceutical markets in the industrial and innovative countries of the Global North, with the exception of public and citizen regulation of patents during the AIDS crises in Brazil and India (Cassier, 2013). However, the research published here, which focuses on the sociology and anthropology of regulations from independence to recent cycles of globalization, reveals a history and modes of regulation that are somewhat different.[5]

The "professional" mode, primarily represented by pharmacists, is influential in Ghana, Benin, and Côte d'Ivoire (see Chapters 1–3), even though the creation of Orders and Faculties of Pharmacy is quite recent,[6] whereas this profession was for a time decimated in Cambodia (Chapter 4). One of the most urgent challenges faced by all four countries is the limited number of pharmacists who can be trained to populate the regulatory authorities, industrial firms, and distribution system that are part of the large market sector.

The "administrative" mode is characterized by the legacies of colonial pharmaceutical legislation, in this context from the United Kingdom and France (Chapters 1 and 3). Drug agencies are a relatively recent creation: in the late 1990s in Ghana, where the pharmacy board was established in 1961; in 2017 in Côte d'Ivoire; and not until 2020 in Benin, where the drug agencies replaced a Ministry of Health Directorate that was created at independence in 1960 and where they are still fairly incomplete. These agencies can foment strong tensions. More generally, the pharmaceutical policies of the countries studied are in turmoil, torn between public health needs and economic and industrial interests, and between the legacy they inherited and their desire for reform. The situation in Benin particularly illustrates these tensions. A period of major reforms in the pharmaceutical sector began in 2017 just as our research was ending there, following the election of President Patrice Talon. Reforms continue to this day and are discussed in this volume (see in particular Chapters 2 and 3).

The "industrial" mode of regulation operates through the foreign firms, mainly Western and Asian, that distribute their products in the countries we study, but also through local manufacturers. Industrial firms are unevenly distributed in these countries, except in Ghana, where the State has encouraged direct investments by multinational firms since independence along with the formation of an industry supported by national capital. We show that establishing local production tends to stimulate administrative regulation (Chapter 1). Industrial standards are hierarchical: local products that cannot access international certifications from WHO or industrialized countries' agencies are certified by the drug agencies of Ghana or Nigeria. Ghana's Food and Drugs Authority (FDA) assists local firms in adopting Good Manufacturing Practices (GMP).

Although pharmaceutical manufacturing is relatively modest in the countries we discuss herein, except in Ghana and to a lesser extent in Côte d'Ivoire and Cambodia, occupations associated with drug distribution form a large and influential economic sector. These include traders, formal and informal salespeople and resellers involved in wholesale and retail distribution, and pharmaceutical representatives whose activities extend beyond the pharmaceutical marketing of the Global North (Greffion, 2014; Ravelli, 2015). One of the original features of our book is the depth and breadth of information on the market regulations at play in the distribution sector, which is primordial in the contexts of the Global South, as shown by Kristin Peterson (2014) in Nigeria and Mathieu Quet (2018) in the links he studies between India and Kenya. The framework of practices and codes of conduct for professions and market activities presupposes pharmaceutical regulatory mechanisms, which are currently undergoing reforms in the countries studied and which give rise to bitter conflicts, as mentioned above in Benin.

Jessica Pourraz's work in Benin and Ghana, conducted as part of our project, has highlighted the need for another mode of regulation: the "global mode," which "overlaps and weakens the most traditional form of medicine regulation by States" (Pourraz, 2019, p. 58). This is discussed in the second part of the book devoted to ACTs, which lead us into our analysis of pharmaceutical markets in the Global South (see Chapters 5–7). Jessica Pourraz, who focused on national and transnational regulations as well as local production of ACTs in Benin and Ghana, describes three distinct regulation methods that are juxtaposed to and may either strengthen or oppose each other: administrative State methods, industrial rules (in Ghana only), and regulation led by transnational Global Health actors. This latter form of pharmaceutical market regulation is the focus of Nitsan Chorev's recent book (2020) on what she calls "developmental foreign aid" in East Africa, in which she shows the actual impact of foreign aid on the growth of the local pharmaceutical industry in Kenya, Tanzania, and Uganda.

Jean-Paul Gaudillière and Volker Hess characterize a model of citizen or public regulation that appears in specific circumstances, such as during health crises linked to drug-related adverse events (e.g., thalidomide) to supplement and reinforce MA standards; during a treatment-access crisis (e.g., AIDS); or to adapt patent law (Krikorian, 2014; Cassier, 2013). This citizen regulation does not feature in our work since this research was mainly focused on malaria, an acute pathology that has not seen patient-driven collective organization despite its severity and prevalence. We do, however, observe a form of regulation shaped by consumers, which we characterize as "popular" (see Chapters 4, 7, 8, 10, and 11). More fluid than other forms, this type of regulation is transmitted from one person to another and is exercised through the subjectivities forged by people's perceptions of their bodies, health, illness, and their health-care and treatment experiences. It is also limited by the availability of medical consultations and products and, more broadly, by local contexts. This popular regulation refers to a part of the disciplinary corpus of medical anthropology forged in both the Global South and North, which emphasizes both universalisms and particularisms that are observed locally (Benoist, 1996; Saillant & Genest, 2005), individual agency and vulnerability to social structures (Fassin, 1996; Scheper-Hughes, 1992), and the intimate and socialized processes involved in health (Fabrega, 1974; Kleinman, 1988). It falls under the umbrella of "pharmaceuticalization," a concept used by medical anthropologists since the late 1990s to describe the realities they observe as pharmaceuticals spread through many facets of social life.[7]

Mathieu Quet and his colleagues use the example of Southeast Asia to expand the concept of regulation, without describing each one in detail, to think symmetrically about the standards and laws that govern official markets and those that organize unofficial markets, since these latter are particularly extensive in the countries they study: "As we will show in the case of pharmaceutical regulation in Southeast Asia, the gravitating forces are as much located within as outside the control of central powers" (Quet et al., 2018, p. 2). In this, they converge with the anthropology of informal markets studied in Cameroon by Sjaak Van der Geest (1987), in Benin by us (Baxerres, 2013), and in Madagascar by Chiarella Mattern (2017). More generally, pharmaceutical anthropology, which investigates pharmaceutical systems, broadens the concept of these systems beyond the health institutions-based definition by associating them with all of the medicine supplies and services available in a given territory. This means focusing on both formal (public and private) and informal (Desclaux & Lévy, 2003), not just State pharmaceutical supply and distribution processes. It is a comprehensive approach to regulation, from the laws and guidelines of the medical professions to the practices and codes of conduct of sellers in formal and informal markets, and from commercial treaties to illicit cross-border transactions. Mathieu Quet and his colleagues are careful to capture these rules in the course of "social practices." This approach is able to highlight several pharmaceutical orders or regimes, as well as any friction, interaction, or harmonization between them. One of the harmonization processes studied by these authors is the State-run training for informal sellers observed by Laurent Pordié in Cambodia. Also in Cambodia, in Chapter 4, Eve Bureau-Point describes her research on forms of State supervision of the informal market, which since 1999 has granted licenses to "blue pharmacies" after training informal vendors. These processes are also described in Chapter 3 regarding the activity of Ghanaian wholesalers, which allows us to grasp the permeability of informal and formal practices and how they shift from one to the other, particularly businesses that are launched and formed within a capitalist system (Baxerres, 2018). The harmonization of rules presupposes specific investments by the State, in this case training programs for informal vendors and a system of special licenses.

Anthropologists have analyzed how drug markets continually challenge the limits of health controls in terms of "commodification" (Nichter, 1996). Sjaak Van der Geest uses this term to describe the disconnect between therapeutic value—assessed and controlled by registration and surveillance rules—and market value, as well as the gradually increasing importance of the latter over the former. However, that author considers the commodification created by informal markets to be a "lesser evil" since it gives patients access to therapies (Van der Geest, 2017). We have shown that drug distribution-related commodification processes were not specific to the informal markets of the Global South and that they are active in countries in the Global North as well, outside (or through the loopholes) of standards and laws (Baxerres, 2014).

Thus, the pharmaceutical markets we study are at the mercy of the numerous types of regulations described above: administrative, professional, industrial, commercial, global, and popular. The histories of each of the four countries we examine here and their regional industrial and political contexts determine the differences in how these various regulations are deployed.

## From the social lives of medicines to the making of pharmaceutical markets

To understand the links that bind the societies of the Global South to pharmaceuticals, we must go back to colonial times and unravel the thread of history to the present day, pausing to examine various time periods and the actors—economic, political, local, national, and international—who have affected it along the way. The countries we discuss—Benin, Ghana, Côte d'Ivoire, and

Cambodia—have different pharmaceutical supply and distribution processes in place. The form these processes take is influenced by historical elements: the colonial power and its pharmaceutical legislation, the conflicts and political regimes that the countries subsequently experienced (such as the Khmer Rouge period in Cambodia), and the economic zone of influence to which they belong (language, currency, and economic community, such as the Commonwealth). These various elements determine the extent of support for production activities, the diversity of import sources, and whether wholesale and retail distribution are broadly supervised by the State or left to the dynamism of economic actors. Our research questioned the impact of these structural elements (presented primarily in the first section of the book) on pharmaceutical consumption practices and how people use commercial drug products (elucidated in the third section of the book). Our main comparison is between Benin and Ghana, two West African countries, one formerly colonized by France and francophone, the other formerly colonized by the United Kingdom and anglophone. This comparison comprises 7 of the 11 chapters of the book. Côte d'Ivoire (one chapter) and Cambodia (two chapters), both former French colonies, provide perspective on the analyses of Benin and Ghana and enrich the understanding of the issues surrounding medicines in Global South societies. The prominent French-speaking perspective of our research constitutes one of the originalities of our work, as these contexts are less comprehensively described in the international social science literature on medicines, particularly with regard to the African continent. Another originality is the comparison between two "models" for medicines, one French-speaking, the other English-speaking, that we propose.[8]

A strength of our research is that it can compare and contrast a variety of regulatory mechanisms and hierarchies in pharmaceutical markets. It proposes an integrated consideration of all the social levels—and the categories of actors that come into play—involved in pharmaceutical markets within the studied Southern context: production, distribution (wholesalers and retailers), prescription, consumption, and uses.[9] This contribution is made possible by our multidisciplinary approach that combines the anthropology of drug distribution and use with the sociology of innovation and pharmaceutical regulation, which include an historical sociology approach and social epidemiology. We employ a cross-section of specific research methods from these disciplines, detailed below, which synergistically complemented each other. This approach allows us to go beyond conceptualization in terms of "social life of medicine" and "biographical stages of the drug" (Whyte et al., 2002), which is now classic and very didactic in the social sciences. As Desclaux and Egrot (2015) have rightly pointed out, this approach was undeniably valuable when first proposed: it sought to highlight the tensions or synergies associated with transitions from one stage to another, encourage monographs in the early stages of their research, introduce the political dimension, examine North and South with the same theoretical approach, conjugate theories of globalization and medical anthropology, and offer a reading list to order the work. Nevertheless, as with any model, its weaknesses lie in its strengths so it can lead to flattening social realities by presenting them in too linear a manner.

Our goal in this book is to focus on the confrontation and superposition of the challenges, actors, and processes generated by commercial drug specialties in the contexts we studied. We have found an intimate link between pharmaceutical distribution and consumption; drug production and use; local production and distribution since the same actors may be involved, particularly in Ghana; and local production and the strengthening of State mechanisms. The different chapters and sections of the book articulate these levels of social realities to reflect their complexity, both with regard to antimalarial treatments—their development, circulation, competition, and the attachments they generate (discussed in Part 2)—and more generally with regard to production and distribution practices and their impact on State sovereignty, formal and informal economies, the individual health of consumers, and public health (Part 1); and finally with regard to the activity of pharmaceutical representatives, the diversity of medicine supply and biomedical services, and their influence on how people manage their health and on their imaginaries of pharmaceutical consumption (Part 3).

This book covers the institution and regulation of pharmaceutical markets in several countries of the Global South. These markets are not free-standing entities, supported through the spontaneous intersection of supply and demand, but are supported by a set of institutions, rules, policies, calculations, and values: hence the interest in studying "the laws of the marketplace" or "trade arrangements" that bolster them, as Michel Callon invites us to do in his work (Callon, 1998, 2017). We pay close attention to the actors who establish, maintain, and develop these markets, from private wholesalers to pharmacists, from central purchasing offices to health centers (public or private, for-profit, or mission), from industrialists to pharmaceutical representatives, from experts in drug agencies or departments to ministers of health or industry, to the self-medication practices of consumers and patients, who have unequal access to care when it comes to paying for essential drugs, even if these are subsidized per the cost recovery principle adopted in Bamako in 1987 (Ridde, 2005). In addition to the plurality of regulations and market laws, we are careful to consider the asymmetries of actors' resources and power, such as when the World Bank influenced the creation of Benin's Essential Drugs Purchasing Office in the late 1980s. The imbalances and points of friction in these markets were also considered, such as when local producers in Ghana were excluded from the ACT market, unable to compete with the prices of subsidized drugs distributed in the country by the Global Fund in the early 2010s. Similarly, we analyze the economic sovereignty strategies used in Côte d'Ivoire with the constitution of a holding company owned by a group of pharmacists.

Several factors lead us to understand these markets as dynamic, open, and conflicting systems. These factors include the situated and historicized analysis, the numerous regulations, the interactions and circulation of humans and capital between distribution and production, various financial flows that support the purchase of medicines from international financiers to end users, and the frictions and imbalances that run through these markets. It is important to understand how they function in order to propose possible avenues for reflection to reform and "change" them, as Michel Callon invites us to do. We attempt this in the conclusion of the book.

## A multidisciplinary methodology using an ethnographic, socio-historical, and population-based approach

The data collection methodology we used mixes extended and in-depth observation with open and semi-structured interviews, archive consultation, and questionnaires given to representative samples of the population. It illustrates the richness produced by drawing from a variety of approaches and disciplines. Essentially qualitative, our method uses tools from ethnography that overlap with techniques used in history where the qualitative intersects with the quantitative, as well as some purely quantitative aspects.

To support the aspects discussed in this book, we believe it is imperative to precisely describe the data we collected and the methods used to do so. These form the basis of our contributions and support the credibility of our work. We decided to present them in three study packages: the first one is mainly ethnographic, the second socio-historical, and the third is epidemiological.[10]

### *The study of medicine distribution, circulation, and uses in Benin, Ghana, and Cambodia*

These studies were mainly conducted between 2014 and 2017, both in the economic or administrative capitals of the countries (Cotonou, Accra, and Phnom Penh) and in semirural areas: the Mono department in Benin, located between 50 and 80 km northwest of Cotonou; Breman Asikuma and the surrounding areas of Jamra, Ayipey, and Kuntanase in Ghana, about 150 km northwest of Accra; and the Battambang province in the northwestern part of Cambodia, about 250 km from Phnom Penh (see Figures 0.1, 0.2, and 0.4).

An ethnography of various wholesalers and retailers lasting 4–6 months was conducted in Benin and Ghana. Some of the retailers were exclusively distributors, while others also provided health-care services. In Benin, Anani Agossou, Moïse Djralah, Aubierge Kpatinvoh, and Stéphanie Mahamé, all master's degree students or research assistants at the time, conducted ethnographies with two wholesalers, three community pharmacies, two pharmaceutical warehouses, five informal vendors, four public health centers at different levels of the national health pyramid, two mission health centers, and three private health centers. In Ghana, Eunice Ayimbila, the late Sandra Serwah Bredu,[11] and Grace Kumi Kyeremeh, who had the same status as their counterparts in Benin, carried out ethnographies in three private pharmacies, six over-the-counter (OTC) medicine shops, one mission hospital, three public health centers at different levels, and one private health center.[12] During these ethnographies, many open-ended interviews were conducted with as many actors as possible, distributors as well as buyers and suppliers. At the intersection of qualitative and quantitative approaches, information was also systematically collected about the products sold, their name, price,

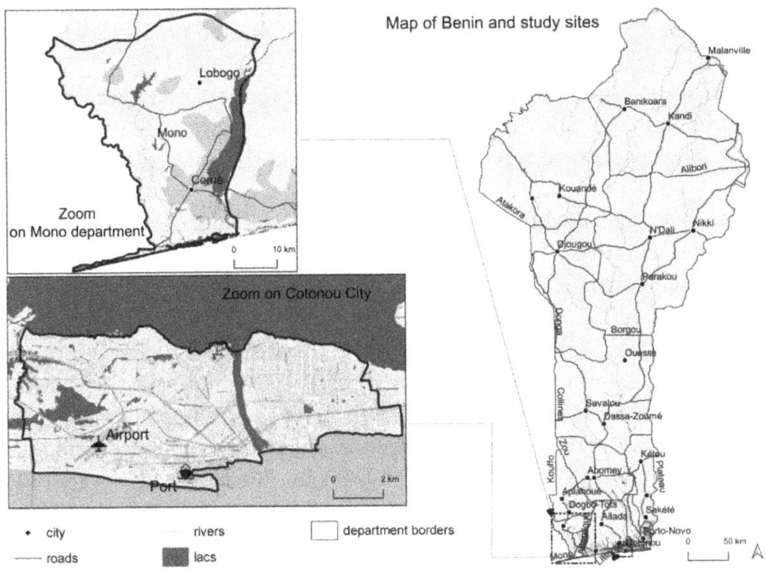


*Figure 0.1* Map of Benin and study sites.

Source: Data available for free on the Web and work of Artadji Attoumane (IRD, LPED)

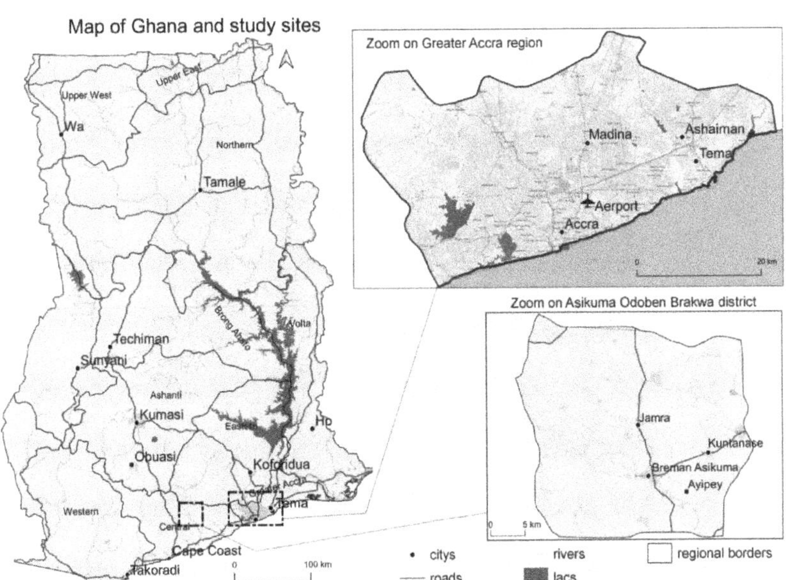


*Figure 0.2* Map of Ghana and study sites.

Source: Available for free on the Web and worked by colleagues and work of Artadji Attoumane (IRD, LPED)

quantity, and how they were purchased (upon presentation of a prescription, by asking for advice, or spontaneously specifying the desired product). These data, recorded in Excel files, enabled the quantifications contained herein. At the end of each of these ethnographies, semi-structured interviews were conducted with between 10 and 20 people carefully chosen for their category (facility staff, clients, suppliers, pharmaceutical representatives, etc.) and the interest they brought to the study.

In Ghana, Carine Baxerres led the study of wholesale distribution and pharmaceutical representatives. This study was generally conducted around the Okaishie market in Accra, which plays an important role as the center of pharmaceutical wholesale distribution in Ghana.[13] The ethnography of two private wholesalers was conducted over eight 15-day research trips between 2014 and 2016. Some 40 semi-structured interviews were held with retailers (whom she then accompanied when they made their pharmaceutical purchases), directors or representatives working for both small and large private wholesalers and for pharmaceutical firms, informal actors operating in the Okaishie market, and institutional and transnational actors.

In Benin, Stéphanie Mahamé followed up the 2014–2016 data collection on wholesale distribution with a study of pharmaceutical representatives from 2017 to 2020 as part of her sociology-anthropology PhD.[14] Data were collected over

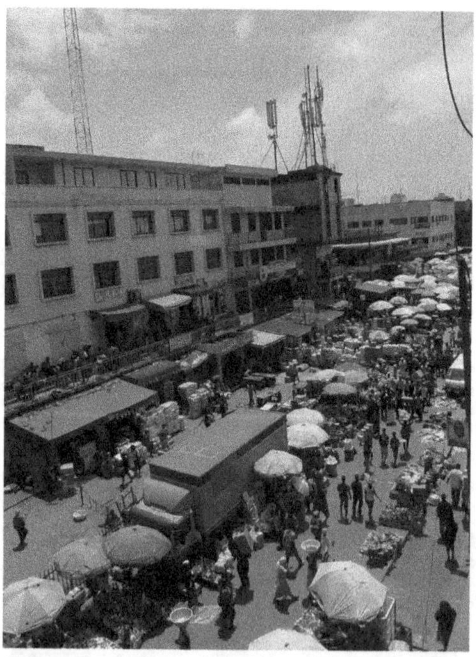

*Figure 0.3* Overlooking the drug lane sector of Accra's Okaishie market.

Source: © IRD/Carine Baxerres, Accra, August 2014

20 months of ethnography and included observations in a mission health center and a private clinic and shadowing of three pharmaceutical representatives during their daily activities. The ethnography was also interspersed with semi-structured interviews with drug reps, health workers, and State actors. Overall, 52 interviews were conducted in Benin. Several questions were examined more extensively during a subsequent 15-day research trip to Côte d'Ivoire through nine interviews with pharmaceutical representatives and pharmacists from the Pharmacy Directorate.

To investigate how medicines are used, two teams—Anani Agossou, Emilienne Anago, and Audrey Hémadou in Benin; and Emelia Agblevor and William Sackey in Ghana—conducted semi-structured interviews with the parent (usually the mother) and/or a grandmother of 30 families in Benin and 30 families in Ghana. Participating families were selected based on their socioeconomic status (income, housing, vehicle ownership, employment activities, and education level) to ensure representation across a broad range of the existing situations in the urban and semirural contexts studied.[15] The graduate students and research assistants in both countries used their survey observations to classify families as "wealthy," "middle-class," or "poor." Each family had to include at least one child under the age of five. Following the interviews and again combining qualitative with quantitative data collection, family members' medicine consumption was tracked bimonthly for 4–8 months based on their availability.

Eve Bureau-Point led the study in Cambodia, conducted between January 2015 and June 2016 with Malinda To, research assistant. Semi-structured and open-ended interviews were also held with 30 retailers (in pharmacies and pharmaceutical warehouses), 8 private medical practice proprietors (doctor, nurse, midwife), 10 semi-wholesalers, 7 public health center staff members, 3 informal vendors, 3 medical sales representatives, 5 representatives from "pharmaceutical companies," and 15 members of Ministry of Health staff.[16] Direct observations were made on site with these various distribution actors of the modes of interaction between sellers and buyers. The same qualitative-quantitative data collection tool used previously in Benin and Ghana was employed here to collect systematic information from 270 purchases in Phnom Penh and 121 in Battambang on the products sold and the modes of purchase. Semi-structured interviews were conducted with 24 mothers from diverse socioeconomic backgrounds to assess medicine use.[17] Once again we tracked these families' medicine consumption bimonthly for an average duration of three and a half months.

Finally, Maxima Missodey, doctoral student working with Globalmed, led the study of the contextual issues surrounding the standardization of herbal medicines in Ghana. Her ethnographic study employed participant observations and interviews. The observations were carried out in two OTC medicine shops in Breman Asikuma in the Central Region and an herbal medicine shop and pharmacy in the Greater Accra Region. The observations were carried out over a period of 8 months between 2016 and 2017. The interviews were conducted with 14 manufacturers and 10 distributors of manufactured herbal medicines. Additionally, exit interviews were conducted with willing customers who came to

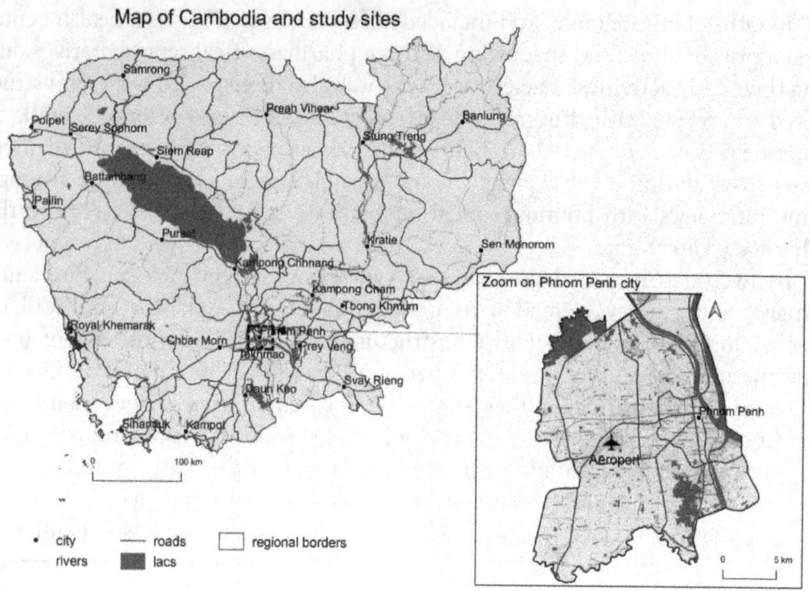


*Figure 0.4* Map of Cambodia and study sites.

Source: Available for free on the Web and worked by colleagues and work of Artadji Attoumane (IRD, LPED)

buy from the medicine outlets (30 customers from the herbal medicine shop and 7 from the pharmacy in Greater Accra Region). The exit interviews focused on the medicines purchased and general information on the consumption of herbal medicines.

These studies were supervised by Carine Baxerres, who partnered with Adolphe Codjo Kpatchavi in Benin, Daniel Kojo Arhinful in Ghana, and Eve Bureau-Point in Cambodia. The same data collection tools (observation checklists, interview guides, family medicine consumption tracking sheets, and drug purchase data collection sheets) were used in all three countries. Eunice Ayimbila, Carine Baxerres, Aubierge Kpatinvoh, Stéphanie Mahamé, Maxima Missodey, and Kelley Sams were responsible for analyzing the data collected in Benin and Ghana. Eve Bureau-Point was responsible for data collected in Cambodia.

### *ACT: An exploration of the Asia-Africa trajectory, local production, and national and transnational regulations in Benin, Ghana, and Côte d'Ivoire*

Mainly performed in Benin, Ghana, and Côte d'Ivoire, this series of studies involved travel to various innovation and manufacturing sites as well as to the headquarters of international organizations throughout Europe and Africa.

Maurice Cassier examined the trajectory of ACTs between 2008 and 2019, drawing on multiple sources to do so. He studied the accounts of Chinese inventors who discovered artemisinin and invented combination therapies, including of their collaborations with the WHO and multinational companies.[18] He also consulted the archives of the Tropical Disease Research (TDR) group, the WHO, and Roll Back Malaria in Geneva, including industry agreements on R&D,[19] industrialization, and distribution. He hunted through the archives of patents filed for single-tablet fixed-dose combinations, especially for artemether-lumefantrine. Finally, he used materials from a detailed investigation on the invention and industrialization of the artesunate-amodiaquine combination (ASAQ), during two periods of research, the first in 2008–2009 (under a contract with the French National Research Agency Pharmasud) and second in 2016–2019. He conducted semi-structured interviews with personnel from the universities and start-ups that developed the fixed-dose combination of ASAQ and from the Sanofi company that mass produced it, and with the organizations MSF (Médecins sans Frontières or Doctors Without Borders) and DND*i* (Drugs for Neglected Diseases Initiative) that governed this system. This investigation took Maurice Cassier from the

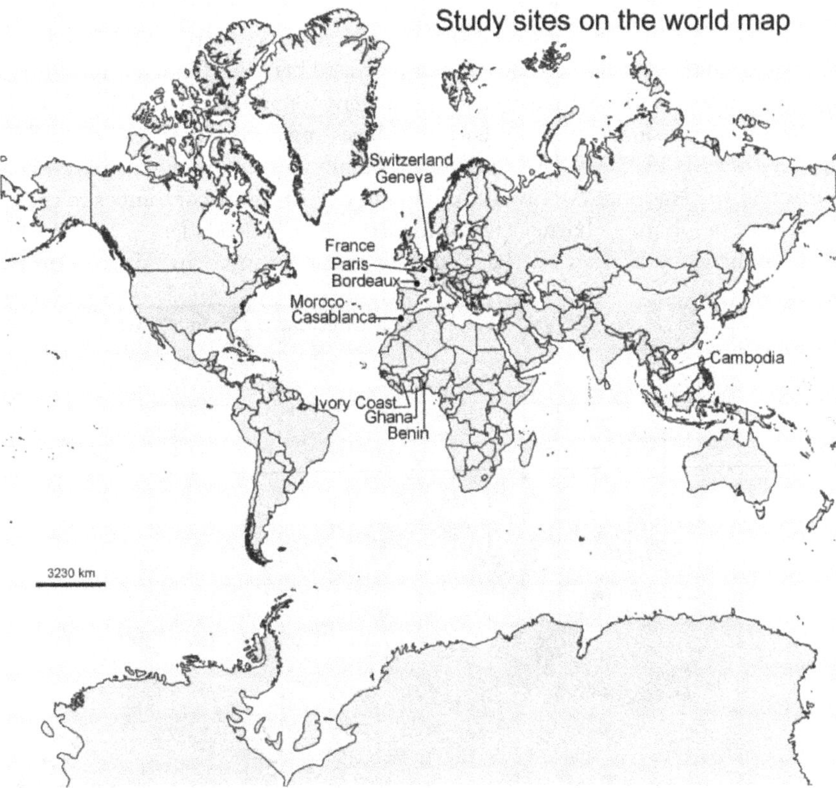


*Figure 0.5* Study sites on the world map.

Source: Available for free on the Web and work of Artadji Attoumane (IRD, LPED).

French city of Bordeaux to Sanofi's factories in Casablanca, Morocco, with stops along the way in Geneva, Switzerland, and Sanofi's headquarters in Paris. He also directed and coordinated the research on local production conducted in Ghana, Benin, and Côte d'Ivoire.

Jessica Pourraz conducted her research as part of a sociology PhD (Pourraz, 2019) at EHESS. The empirical data were collected over 14 months between August 2014 and May 2017 in Cotonou, Accra, Geneva, and Paris. She conducted semi-structured interviews and observations with various actors involved, such as national pharmaceutical regulatory authorities (the Directorate of Pharmacies, Medicine, and Diagnostic Investigations or DPMED in Benin and the FDA in Ghana), transnational actors that fund ACTs (United States Agency for International Development [USAID], President's Malaria Initiative, Global Fund, UNICEF, and the World Bank), the WHO, national malaria control programs, ministries of health in Benin and Ghana, and pharmaceutical industries and the associated union in Ghana. In total, Jessica Pourraz held nearly 100 interviews (32 in Cotonou, 58 in Accra, 5 in Geneva, and 2 in Paris). She also conducted observations at a pharmaceutical company producing ACTs in Accra, at the DPMED, and at Ghana's FDA during meetings of the technical committees that issue pharmaceutical MAs. She also observed working meetings between national malaria control programs and their international partners, between Ghanaian industry and the United Nations Industrial Development Organization (UNIDO), and at a training session on pharmaceutical policies organized for African regulatory pharmacists by the WHO in Geneva. Finally, Jessica conducted extensive research at the National Archives of Ghana to collect historical sources to trace the history of Ghana's pharmaceutical industry since independence, and at the WHO archives in Geneva on the history of malaria control in Africa. Daniel

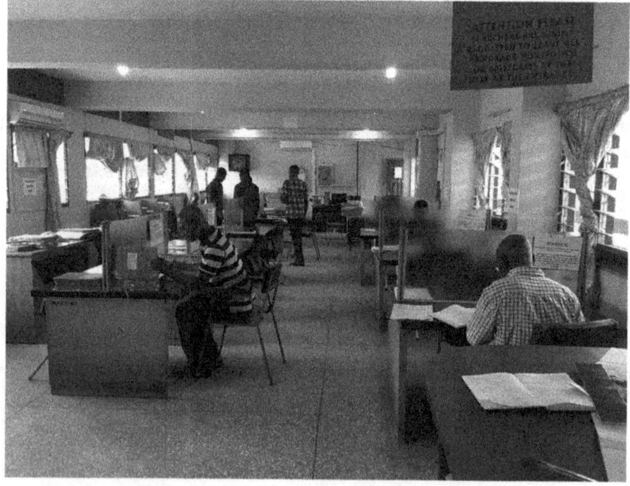

*Figure* 0.6 Consultation room of the National Archives in Accra.

Source: © IRD/Carine Baxerres, Accra, October 2019

Kojo Arhinful in Ghana and Adolphe Codjo Kpatchavi in Benin provided instrumental support to her investigations by introducing her to various actors in the ministries of health and sharing their extensive knowledge of the health system in their countries.

Claudie Haxaire studied in Côte d'Ivoire some of the aspects that Jessica Pourraz worked on in Benin and Ghana. Both a pharmacist and anthropologist, she taught at the Faculty of Pharmacy in Abidjan from 1979 to 1984 and regularly visited the country thereafter for ethno-pharmacological research missions. Between 2014 and 2017, this gave her the opportunity to participate in observations and informal meetings with the country's pharmaceutical stakeholders. These guided the semi-structured interviews she conducted and facilitated more targeted participant observations (visits to three manufacturing units, the public health pharmacy, and the analysis laboratory; and participation in a meeting of the technical committee regarding issuing an MA). This methodology also included participation in several symposia, including SympoINDUS19 in Abidjan in February 2019 for pharmaceutical industrialization and manufacturing in West Africa and the workshop to develop Côte d'Ivoire's new public health code for medicines. Her analysis of gray literature and information collected from the Internet and specialized journals led to the identification of companies listed as ACT manufacturers (four out of eight such firms in that country), wholesale distributors (initially three companies, then four), the central purchasing office, the national public health laboratory, the Directorate of Pharmacy, Medicine, and Laboratories (DPML; Direction de la Pharmacie et du Médicament et des Laboratoires), and the National Program for the Development of Pharmaceutical Activity (PNDAP; Programme National de Développement de l'Activité Pharmaceutique). On the basis of this information, she held 45 semi-structured interviews with the identified actors (experts who authored the reports, directors and deputy directors of state structures, pharmacists in charge of private manufacturing units or wholesale distributors, manufacturing unit directors to discuss financial aspects, commercial representatives, and international experts). The term of this project overlapped with the reform of the regulatory authority (DPML) into an agency. Claudie Haxaire followed this long process, staying in contact with the experts who were in charge of submitting legal texts and application decrees involved in founding the drug agency in Côte d'Ivoire. She collected the various actors' opinions on this ongoing issue.

Throughout our research and in addition to interviews, we stayed in close contact with the national actors responsible for pharmacy and medicine regulations, both during and predating our investigations. One example is Joseph Nyoagbe, head of the Pharmacy Council in Ghana from 2005 to 2016, who wrote the preface to this book.[20] We shared our results with health authorities and pharmaceutical system actors in Benin, Ghana, and Cambodia in 2016, 2017, and 2018. In March 2018, we organized an international colloquium on current issues regarding medicines in Africa in Ouidah, Benin, the final round table of which was illustrative of the bridges that we sought to create throughout this joint research between the academic, State, and transnational sectors, between researchers and

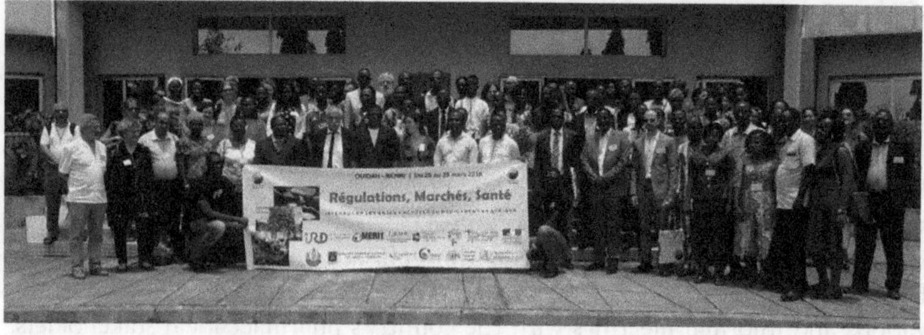


*Figure 0.7* Participants at the Globalmed symposium in Ouidah, Benin.
Source: © IRD/Charlie Marquis, Ouidah, March 2018

students in social sciences and pharmacy, and with national and regional political actors (Baxerres & Marquis, 2018). Roch Appolinaire Houngnihin, professor of socio-anthropology in Benin, was key to the success of this scientific event, which was a testimony to the action-–research character of our work.

### *The study of pharmaceutical consumption in Benin and Ghana*

This consisted of a series of quantitative surveys of the general population in the urban areas of Cotonou and Accra and in the same rural areas as the qualitative studies described above. We wanted to survey more remote rural areas than those studied in the qualitative research, which we qualified above as semirural. The surveys were conducted in the commune of Lobogo in Benin's Mono department and in the Kuntanase village of Breman Asikuma in Ghana's Central Region in Ghana (see Figures 0.1 and 0.2).

To ensure the sample population surveyed would be representative, households were randomly selected based on their GPS coordinates (Apetoh, 2020). The same methodology was applied in Cotonou, Madina (a neighborhood in Accra), and Lobogo. We first defined the study area in each of the survey areas based on administrative divisions. In Benin, we considered the entire city of Cotonou (13 districts, nearly 800,000 inhabitants) to be one study area and the rural Lobogo (17,000 inhabitants) in the Mono department to be another. In Ghana, our urban study area was Accra's eastern suburb Madina (nearly 140,000 inhabitants), which has a diversity of socioeconomic status comparable to the composition of the city of Cotonou.[21] To obtain sufficient power in the statistical tests, we calculated the number of families needed using Schwartz's formula (Schwartz, 1996), which gave us a minimum of 600 families to survey.[22] Kuntanase, a municipality located in the Breman Asikuma district, was an exception: given the size of this village, we decided to conduct an exhaustive survey, visiting all of the families (n = 853). To constitute our sample in the other three areas, we randomly selected a sufficient number of GPS points in the defined spaces using the Google Earth Pro™ application and the Geomidpoint.com website to generate the points (Apetoh, 2020;

Damien, Baxerres, Apetoh, & Le Hesran, 2020). We identified the building closest to each GPS coordinate point, and socio-anthropological investigators visited each one. If the building housed only one family, the family was included in the study after obtaining informed consent from a head of the household.[23] If there were several families in the building, one was selected at random and included in the study. The responsible adult in each family was questioned about the family's socioeconomic characteristics and their usual health-care practices, especially if malaria was suspected.

To study the health problems encountered, health-care practices, and medication use, we randomly selected one adult (≥18 years) and one child (<12 years). The adult and the child's caregiver were queried by questionnaire using two approaches. First, they were asked about any "health events"[24] experienced in the week prior to the interviewer's visit. They were asked to describe the symptoms presented, treatment decisions, and modalities (self-medication, consultation, advice from family or friends), therapy(ies) used, and where these were purchased. Secondly, if there had been no health event in the previous week, they were asked when was the last time they took a medicine, what it was, for what reason (symptoms, illnesses), for what purpose (preventive, curative, health maintenance), whether or not the drug was prescribed, and where it was purchased.

These quantitative data were collected by Edwige Apetoh in Benin as part of her epidemiology PhD (Apetoh, 2020), and in Ghana by William Sackey, a research assistant also involved in qualitative studies. They were under the supervision of Jean-Yves Le Hesran in both countries, who worked with Daniel Kojo Arhinful in Ghana. They were assisted in both Benin and Ghana by socio-anthropological investigators, some of whom were also involved in the qualitative studies: Anani Agossou, Ines Boko, Ruth Boko, Moïse Djralah, Audrey Hemadou, Bernadette Kokoye, and Aubierge Kpatinvoh in Benin; and Salomey Pomaah Adjani, Alberta Addo, Emmanuel Andam, Esther Appiah, Derrick Frimpong, Raymond Lamptey, Eric Nartey, and Ohene Sakyi in Ghana. They did a remarkable job, employing patience and pedagogy to create exceptional contact with the people surveyed and collect high-quality data. The data were analyzed by Georgia Damien, Michael Addo Preko Ntiri, Edwige Apetoh as part of her PhD; and Marina Tilly, Arnaud Gbenou, and Hajar Ahachad as part of their master's degree in public health (Ahachad, 2020; Gbenou, 2017; Tilly, 2017).

## Notes

1. WHO archives: E19372_2 –J5 – collaboration with industry.
2. Generics were included in U.S. legislation as early as the 1960s to reduce treatment costs (Greene, 2014) and in some Latin American countries (Colombia),and were later supported by the WHO's Essential Medicines Policy (Borchers, Hagie, Keen, & Gershwin, 2007; Whyte, Van der Geest, & Hardon, 2002). Numerous historical (Greene, 2014 for the United States; Garcia, 2000 for Colombia), anthropological (Hayden, 2013 for Mexico), sociological (Cassier & Correa, 2019 for Brazil; Nouguez, 2017 for France), and other studies have examined how generics' equivalence with originator drugs is regulated.

3. The expression "transnational actors" combines different types of extra-national actors currently involved in a country's public health issues: bilateral institutions (the various international aid agencies) and multilaterals (World Bank, Global Fund), nongovernmental organizations, foundations, and public-private partnerships that are sometimes aligned with the pharmaceutical industry.
4. The WHO Prequalification of Medicines Programme (PQP) was first applied in 2001 to antiretrovirals for AIDS, then to antimalarials and tuberculosis drugs, and gradually from 2006 on to contraceptives, antivirals for flu, and treatments for acute diarrhea and neglected tropical diseases. The ICH was founded in 1990 and is made up of pharmaceutical regulatory authorities and industry associations from the European Union, the United States, and Japan (Pourraz, 2019).
5. Moreover, Jean-Paul Gaudillière and Volker Hess state that the "ways of regulating" they identify at the end of their historical investigations do not constitute a fixed model, but that they are themselves socio-historical entities.
6. Although relatively recent, these organizations differ between the countries discussed. Pharmacy education began as early as 1921 in Ghana, where the first university department opened in the 1950s. In Côte d'Ivoire, the Faculty of Pharmacy began teaching in 1977, whereas in Benin, it began in 1999 and the first class of pharmacists graduated in 2006.
7. "Pharmaceuticalization" is the process by which social, behavioral, or physical conditions are treated with drugs or considered to require drug treatment by patients, physicians, or both. Developed in sociology, this concept is widely used in anthropology (Collin & David, 2016; Desclaux & Egrot, 2015; Nichter, 1996). It extends beyond the influence of biomedicine alone, also reflecting the autonomy of individuals who may use medicines outside of health-care relationships and facilities.
8. At the beginning of this research program, we conceived of two pharmaceutical models in West Africa, one "administered" in francophone areas and the other "liberal and market based" in anglophone areas (Baxerres, 2013). The various studies we report in this book have allowed us to expand and add complexity to this initial modeling, which is overly binary and reductive. While the more or less liberal character of pharmaceutical distribution models between English-speaking and French-speaking countries is globally relevant (see Chapter 3), the work on the "administrative" and "industrial" modes of regulation highlights the importance not only of institutional and historical legacies, but also of the degree of State political and financial autonomy, medication supply (imported and/or locally produced), and market structures and connections to Asian manufacturers. Rather than two models, these aspects show there are many possible scenarios in and between French-speaking and English-speaking countries, and that within the same country approaches may coexist that are quite liberal in some ways (distribution) yet highly administered or supervised in others (production, prescription), as is the case in Ghana.
9. However, we did not study the economics of clinical trials, which is an important and growing issue in the Global South (Sunder Rajan, 2012).
10. Research authorizations were obtained from national ethics committees in Ghana (May 10, 2014, GHS-ERC), Benin (No. 30 dated December 3, 2013, CER-ISBA), Cambodia (466, NECHR), and France (December 10–11, /2013, CCDE).
11. Sandra Serwah passed away during the Globalmed program following an illness. We pay tribute to her here.
12. Because different laws govern the pharmaceutical systems in Benin and Ghana, each category of actors plays a different role in pharmaceutical distribution. OTC medicine sellers in Ghana are private actors authorized to sell OTC drugs that require no medical prescription. They do not have a pharmacy degree. In Benin, drug warehouses, located only in rural areas, are businesses run by non-pharmacists

who are restricted to a limited list of drugs for distribution and must be supervised by the pharmacist in the closest pharmacy. Informal vendors in Benin distribute drugs outside of the formal circuits prescribed by the State: in markets, in shops, door to door, at home, in public transport hubs, etc. We encounter these categories of actors throughout the book.

13. The Druglane sector of the Okaishie market in Accra specializes in the sale of medicines and acts as the center of pharmaceutical wholesale distribution in Ghana. It consists of seven private buildings that are home to more than a hundred companies that invest in the medicines trade (Baxerres, 2018). Carine Baxerres has an upcoming book about Ghanaian medicine traders, much of which will be dedicated to this sector of the Okaishie market.
14. This thesis is being jointly supervised by the University of Abomey-Calavi in Benin and the Ecole des Hautes Etudes en Sciences Sociales (EHESS) in Paris, France. It is entitled "Pharmaceutical representatives and their activities in Benin. Contribution to the study of the social construction of drug markets in Africa" and will be defended in 2021.
15. By family, we mean people who live in a residential unit and share meals that have been prepared or purchased for all of them.
16. The categories of actors involved in drug distribution in Cambodia, according to the current laws, differ from those working in Benin and Ghana. Drug warehouses operating in Cambodia are run by health professionals (assistant pharmacists or retired doctors, nurses, or midwives) and are found in both rural and urban areas. Informal vendors work in unregistered pharmacies, in small grocery shops, or directly in the street. In local use, the term "pharmaceutical company" refers both to local medicine manufacturing firms and medicine import-export and distribution companies. Semi-wholesalers purchase their supply from "pharmaceutical companies," sell wholesale or retail, and have a pharmacy license. They are not authorized to import. Sometimes they run an import company alongside their pharmacy.
17. 3 living on <USD 100 per month, 10 on USD 100–400 per month, 8 on USD 400–2000 per month, and 3 on >USD 2000 per month.
18. Tu Youyou, discoverer of artemisinin; Zhou Yiqing, inventor of the artemether and lumefantrine combination; Li Guoqiao, inventor of the dihydroartemisinin and piperazine combination; as well as Jianfang's (2013) book.
19. R&D: this abbreviation refers here to the research and development activities for commercial drug specialties performed within pharmaceutical companies or in smaller organizations (university laboratories, start-ups, etc.).
20. This book will also be published in French, and the preface of that volume will be written by a major pharmacy actor in Benin.
21. The city of Accra is composed of numerous dissimilar neighborhoods (some quite posh, others very working class). Because it is much larger than Cotonou, working across the entire city would have required stratifying the neighborhoods. We chose to focus on the Madina neighborhood because its working- and middle-class population is closest to that of Cotonou, which we studied in Benin.
22. Here we use the same definition of family as in the qualitative studies, i.e., a unit of residence and shared meals.
23. An adult responsible for the family who was present at the time of the interviewers' visit and who was able to answer questions about family characteristics and health care practices. In most cases this was the mother.
24. We created this "health notion" in social epidemiology for the purposes of this study. The idea was to ask families about broader issues than just the "health problems" defined by biomedicine. By using the term "health event," we can include all the reasons why people use medication.

## Reference list

Ahachad, H. (2020). *Besoin de soins et gestion des problèmes de santé en population urbaine au Ghana [The need for care and management of urban health problems in Ghana]*. Unpublished master's thesis, Université de Paris, France.

Apetoh, E. (2020). *Pratiques thérapeutiques et consommation des médicaments pharmaceutiques dans les ménages à Cotonou, Bénin : Entre faible fréquentation des structures sanitaires et large recours aux circuits informels [Therapeutic practices and pharmaceutical drug consumption in households in Cotonou, Benin: Between low health structure attendance and wide use of informal circuits]*. Unpublished doctoral dissertation, Université Paris Diderot, Paris, France.

Baxerres, C. (2013). *Du médicament informel au médicament libéralisé : Une anthropologie du médicament pharmaceutique au Bénin [From informal to liberalized drugs: An anthropology of pharmaceutical drugs in Benin]*. Paris, France: Les Éditions des Archives Contemporaines.

Baxerres, C. (2014). La marchandisation du médicament au Bénin [The commodification of drugs in Benin]. *Journal des anthropologues*, 138–139, 113–136.

Baxerres, C. (2018). D'intermédiaire informel, devenir détaillant, grossiste puis producteur pharmaceutique : Les trajectoires « vertueuses » des hommes d'affaires du médicament au Ghana [From informal intermediary to becoming a retailer, wholesaler, and then pharmaceutical producer: The "virtuous" trajectories of drug businessmen in Ghana]. In C. Baxerres, & C. Marquis (Eds.), *Regulations, markets, health: Questioning current stakes of pharmaceuticals in Africa* (pp. 30–40). (Conference proceedings). HAL, Ouidah, Benin. https://hal.archives-ouvertes.fr/hal-01988227.

Baxerres, C., & Eboko, F. (Eds.). (2019). Global health: Et la santé ? [Global health: And health?]. *Politique Africaine*, 4, 156.

Baxerres, C., & Marquis, C. (Eds.). (2018). *Regulations, markets, health: Questioning current stakes of pharmaceuticals in Africa.* (Conference proceedings). HAL, Ouidah, Benin. https://hal.archives-ouvertes.fr/hal-01988227.

Benoist, J. (1996). *Soigner au pluriel. Essais sur le pluralisme médical [Providing care in the plural. Essays on medical pluralism]*. Paris, France: Karthala.

Bonah, C., & Gaudillière, J.-P. (2007). Faute, risque ou accident iatrogène. La régulation des évènements indésirables du médicament à l'aune des affaires stalinon et distilbène [Error, risk, or iatrogenic accident. The regulation of adverse drug events in light of the stalinon and distilbene cases]. *Revue Française Des Affaires Sociales*, 3–4, 123–151.

Borchers, A. T., Hagie, F., Keen, C. L., & Gershwin, M. E. (2007). The history and contemporary challenges of the US Food and Drug Administration. *Clinical Therapeutics*, 29(1), 1–16. https://doi.org/10.1016/j.clinthera.2007.01.006.

Callon, M. (Ed.). (1998). *The laws of the markets*. Oxford, UK: Wiley Blackwell.

Callon, M. (2017). *L'emprise des marchés: Comprendre leur fonctionnement pour pouvoir les changer [The sway of markets: Understanding how they work so they can be changed]*. Paris, France: La Découverte.

Canzler, W., Kaufmann, V., & Kesselring, S. (2008). *Tracing mobilities towards a cosmopolitan perspective*. Farnham, UK: Ashgate Publishing.

Cassier, M. (2013). Pharmaceutical patent law in-the-making: Opposition and legal action by States, citizens and generics laboratories in Brazil and India. In J.-P. Gaudillière, & V. Hess (Eds.), *Ways of regulating drugs in the 19th and the 20th centuries* (pp. 287–317). Hampshire, UK: Palgrave Macmillan.

Cassier, M., & Correa, M. (2003). Patents, innovation and public health: Brazilian public sector laboratories' experience in copying AIDS drugs. In J.-P. Moatti, B. Coriat, Y. Souteyrand, T. Barnett, J. Dumoulin, & Y. A. Flori (Eds.), *Economics of AIDS and access to HIV/AIDS care in developing countries. Issues and challenges* (pp. 89–107). Paris, France: ANRS.

Cassier, M., & Correa, M. (Eds.). (2019). *Health innovation and social justice in Brazil*. Cham, Switzerland: Palgrave Macmillan. https://www.palgrave.com/fr/search?query=cassier.

Chaudhuri, S. (2005). *The WTO and India's pharmaceutical industry: Patent protection, TRIPs and developing countries*. New Delhi, India: Oxford University Press.

Chauveau, S. (2008). La demande de sécurité : L'épreuve des crises sanitaires depuis les années 1980 [The demand for security: The health crises ordeal since the 1980s]. *L'Atelier du Centre de Recherches Historiques (online)* 2, 183–203. https://doi.org/10.4000/acrh.993.

Chorev, N. (2020). *Give and take: Developmental foreign aid and the pharmaceutical industry in East Africa*. Princeton, NJ: Princeton University Press.

Collin, J., & David, P.-M. (2016). *Vers une pharmaceuticalisation de la société? [Towards a pharmaceuticalization of society?]*. Quebec, Canada: Presses de l'Université du Québec.

Correa, M., Cassier, M., & Loyola, M. A. (2019). Regulating the copy drug market in Brazil: Testing generics and similar medicines (1999 to 2015). In M. Cassier, & M. Correa (Eds.), *Health innovation and social justice in Brazil* (pp. 241–276). Cham, Switzerland: Palgrave Macmillan.

Cramer, T. (2010, December). *A case of internationalization before World War II: Bayer's marketing strategies in Latin America*. Paper presented at the CERMES Colloquium, Drugs, standards and the practices of globalization, EHESS, Paris, France.

Damien, B. G., Baxerres, C., Apetoh, E., & Le Hesran, J.-Y. (2020). Between traditional remedies and pharmaceutical drugs: Prevention and treatment of "palu" in households in Benin, West Africa. *BMC Public Health, 20*, 1425.

Desclaux, A., & Egrot, M. (Eds.). (2015). *Anthropologie du médicament au Sud. La pharmaceuticalisation à ses marges [Anthropology of medicines in the South. Pharmaceuticalization at its margins]*. Paris, France: L'Harmattan.

Desclaux, A., & Lévy, J.-J. (2003). Présentation: Cultures et médicaments. Ancien objet ou nouveau courant en anthropologie médicale? [Presentation: Cultures and medicines. Ancient object or new trend in medical anthropology?] *Anthropologie et Sociétés, 27*(2), 5–21.

Fabrega, H. (1974). *Disease and social behavior: An interdisciplinary perspective*. Cambridge, MA: The MIT Press.

Fassin, D. (1996). *L'espace politique de la santé, essai de généalogie [The political space of health, genealogy essay]*. Paris, France: Presses Universitaires de France.

Faure, O. (1993). Le succès du remède au 19ème siècle et ses significations [The success of the remedy in the 19th century and its meanings]. In J.-C. Beaune, & C. Vallon (Eds.), *La philosophie du remède : Instruments et philosophie [The remedy philosophy: Instruments and philosophy]* (pp. 216–25). Seyssel, France: Champ Vallon.

Faure, O. (1996). Les officines pharmaceutiques françaises: De la réalité au mythe (fin 19ème, début 20ème). [French pharmacies: From reality to myth (late 19th, early 20th)]. *Revue d'Histoire Moderne et Contemporaine, 44*(3), 672–685.

Faure, O. (2005). Les pharmaciens et le médicament en France au 19ème siècle [Pharmacists and medicines in France in the 19th century]. In C. Bonah, & A. Rasmussen (Eds.), *Histoire et médicament aux 19ème et 20ème siècles [History and medication in the 19th and 20th centuries]* (pp. 65–85). Paris, France: Éditions Glyphe.

Garcia, V. (2020). *La construction et la régulation de l'industrie et du marché de médicaments en Colombie (1914–1971). Contribution à une histoire de la mondialisation du médicament [The construction and regulation of the drug industry and market in Colombia (1914–1971). Contribution to a history of the globalization of medicines]*. Unpublished doctoral dissertation, Ecole des Hautes Etudes en Sciences Sociales, Paris, France.

Gaudillière, J.-P. (2005). Une marchandise pas comme les autres. Historiographie du médicament et de l'industrie pharmaceutique en France au 20ème siècle [A commodity like no other. Historiography of medicines and the pharmaceutical industry in France in the 20th century]. In C. Bonah, & A. Rasmussen (Eds.), *Histoire et médicament aux 19ème et 20ème siècles [History and medication in the 19th and 20th centuries]* (pp. 115–158). Paris, France: Éditions Glyphe.

Gaudillière, J.-P., Beaudevin, C., Gradmann, C., Lovell, A. M., & Pordié, L. (Eds.). (2020). *Global health and the new world order: Historical and anthropological approaches to a changing regime of governance*. Manchester, UK: Manchester University Press.

Gaudillière. J.-P., & Hess, V. (Eds.). (2013). *Ways of regulating drugs in the 19th and the 20th centuries*. Hampshire, UK: Palgrave Macmillan.

Gbenou, A. S. (2017). *Accès aux soins et aux médicaments au Bénin: Pratiques des soins au sein des familles [Access to care and medicines in Benin: Care practices within families]*. Unpublished master's thesis, Université UPMC Paris 6, France.

Greene, J. A. (2014). *Generic: The unbranding of modern medicine*. Baltimore, MD: Johns Hopkins University Press.

Greffion, J. (2014). *Faire passer la pilule. Visiteurs médicaux et entreprises pharmaceutiques face aux médecins : Une relation socio-économique sous tensions privées et publiques (1905–2014) [Pass the pill. Medical visitors and pharmaceutical companies confronting doctors: A socio-economic relationship under private and public tensions (1905–2014)]*. Doctoral dissertation, Ecole des Hautes Etudes en Sciences Sociales/ENS, Paris, France. Retrieved from http://www.theses.fr/2014EHES0133.

Hauray, B. (2006). *L'Europe du médicament. Politique, expertise, intérêts privés [The Europe of medicines. Politics, expertise, private interests]*. Paris, France: Presses de Sciences Po.

Hayden, C. (2013). Distinctively similar: A generic problem. *UC Davis Law Journal, 47*(2), 101–132.

Horner, R., & Murphy, J. T. (2018). South–North and South–South production networks: Diverging socio-spatial practices of Indian pharmaceutical firms. *Global Networks, 18*(2), 326–351.

Jianfang, Z. (Ed.). (2013). *A detailed chronological record of project 523 and the discovery and development of qinghaosu (artemisinin)*. K. Arnold, & M. Arnold (Trans.). Houston, TX: Strategic Book Publishing and Rights Co. (Original work published 2006).

Kleinman, A. (1988). *The illness narratives. Suffering, healing, and the human condition*. New York, NY: Basic Books.

Krikorian, G. (2014). *La propriété ou la vie ? Économies morales, actions collective et politiques du médicament dans la négociation d'accords de libre-échange. Maroc, Thaïlande, Etats-Unis [Property or life? Moral savings, collective actions and drug policies in the negotiation of free trade agreements. Morocco, Thailand, United States]*. Doctoral dissertation, Ecole des Hautes Etudes en Sciences Sociales, Paris, France. Retrieved from http://www.theses.fr/2014EHES0035.

Lachenal, G. (2014). *Le médicament qui devait sauver l'Afrique: Un scandale pharmaceutique aux colonies [The drug that was supposed to save Africa: A pharmaceutical scandal in the colonies]*. Paris, France: La Découverte.

Lantenois, C., & Coriat, B. (2014). La «préqualification» OMS: Origines, déploiement et impacts sur la disponibilité des antirétroviraux dans les pays du Sud [WHO "prequalification": Origins, deployment, and impacts on antiretroviral availability in Southern countries]. *Sciences Sociales et Santé*, *32*(1), 71–99.

Lavigne Delville, P. (2010). La réforme foncière rurale au Bénin. Émergence et mise en question d'une politique instituante dans un pays sous régime d'aide [Rural land reform in Benin. Emergence and questioning of an institutional policy in a country under an aid regime]. *Revue Française de Science Politique*, 60(3), 467–491.

Leon, J. K. (2015). *The rise of global health: The evolution of effective collective action*. New York, NY: State University of New York Press.

Mackintosh, M., Banda, G., Tibandebage, P., & Wamae, W. (Eds.). (2016). *Making medicines in Africa: The political economy of industrializing for local health*. London, UK: Palgrave Macmillan.

Marks, H. M. (1997). The progress of experiment: Science and therapeutic reform in the United States, 1900–1990. *Cambridge History of Medicine*. Cambridge/New York: Cambridge University Press.

Marks, H. M. (2000). Confiance et méfiance dans le marché: Les statistiques et la recherche clinique (1945–1960) [Confidence and mistrust in the market: Statistics and clinical research (1945–1960)]. *Sciences Sociales et Santé*, *18*(4), 9–27.

Mattern, C. (2017). *Le marché informel du médicament à Madagascar : Une revanche populaire [The informal drug market in Madagascar: Vindication by the people]*. Doctoral dissertation, Université catholique de Louvain, Louvain-La-Neuve, Belgium. Retrieved from tps://dial.uclouvain.be/pr/boreal/en/object/boreal%3A191542.

Mertens, M. (2014). Chemical compounds in the Congo: Pharmaceuticals and the "crossed history" of public health in Belgian Africa (ca. 1905–1939). Doctoral dissertation, Ghent University, Belgium. Retrieved at https://biblio.ugent.be/publication/4443278/file/4443346.pdf.

Monnais, L. (2014). *Médicaments coloniaux : L'expérience vietnamienne, 1905–1940 [Colonial medicines: The Vietnamese experience, 1905–1940]*. Paris, France: Les Indes savantes.

Montalban, M. (2011). La financiarisation des big pharma. De l'insoutenable modèle blockbuster à son dépassement ? [The financialization of big pharma. Moving beyond the unsustainable blockbuster model?]. *Savoir Agir*, 2(16), 13–21.

Nichter, M. (1996). Pharmaceuticals, the commodification of health, and the health care-medicine use transition. In M. Nichter and M. Nichter (Eds.), *Anthropology and international health, Asian case studies* (pp. 265–326). Amsterdam, The Netherlands: Gordon and Breach.

Nouguez, E. (2017). *Des médicaments à tout prix: Sociologie des génériques en France [Drugs at all costs: Sociology of generics in France]*. Paris, France: Presses de Sciences Po.

Pelletan, C. (2019). *Le médicament, l'Etat et les marchés: La co-construction de l'industrie pharmaceutique et de l'Etat en Afrique du Sud [Medicines, the State, and markets: The co-construction of the pharmaceutical industry and the State in South Africa]*. Doctoral dissertation, Université de Bordeaux, France. Retrieved from http://www.theses.fr/2019BORD0099.

Peterson, K. (2014). *Speculative markets: Drug circuits and derivative life in Nigeria*. London, UK: Duke University Press Books.

Pourraz, J. (2019). *Réguler et produire les médicaments contre le paludisme au Ghana et au Bénin : Une affaire d'Etat ? Politiques pharmaceutiques, normes de qualité et marchés de médicaments [Regulating and producing malaria drugs in Ghana and Benin: A State affair?*

*Pharmaceutical policies, quality standards, and drug markets]*. Doctoral dissertation, Ecole des Hautes Etudes en Sciences Sociales, Paris, France. Retrieved at http://www.theses.fr/2019EHES0014.

Quet, M. (2018). *Impostures pharmaceutiques: Médicaments illicites et luttes pour l'accès à la santé [Pharmaceutical deceptions: Illicit drugs and struggles to access health]*. Paris, France: La Découverte.

Quet, M., Pordié, L., Bochaton, A., Chantavanich, S., Kiatying-Angsulee, N., Lamy, M., & Vungsiriphisal, P. (2018). Regulation multiple: Pharmaceutical trajectories and modes of control in the ASEAN. *Science, Technology and Society, 23*(3), 485–503. https://doi.org/10.1177/0971721818762935.

Ravelli, Q. (2015). *La stratégie de la bactérie. Une enquête au coeur de l'industrie pharmaceutique [The bacteria strategy. An investigation at the heart of the pharmaceutical industry]*. Paris, France: Seuil.

Ridde, V. (2005). *Politiques publiques de santé et équité en Afrique de l'ouest. Le cas de l'Initiative de Bamako Au Burkina Faso [Public policies for health and equity in West Africa. The case of the Bamako Initiative in Burkina Faso]*. Doctoral dissertation, Université Laval, Quebec, Canada. Retrieved from http://hdl.handle.net/20.500.11794/18117

Saillant, F., & Genest, S. (2005). *Anthropologie médicale. Ancrages locaux, défis globaux [Medical anthropology. Local roots, global challenges]*. Quebec, Canada: Presses de l'Université de Laval.

Scheper-Hughes, N. (1992). *Death without weeping: The violence of everyday life in Brazil*. Berkeley, CA: University of California Press.

Schwartz, D. (1996). *Méthodes statistiques à l'usage des médecins et des biologistes [Statistical methods for use by physicians and biologists]*. Paris, France: Flammarion.

Sunder Rajan, K. (2012). Pharmaceutical crises and questions of value: Terrains and logics of global therapeutic politics. *The South Atlantic Quarterly, 111*(2), 321–346.

Tilly, M. (2017). *Perception et mode de traitement du 'palu' dans les familles à Cotonou au Bénin [Perception of and treatment methods for 'palu' among families in Cotonou in Benin]*. Unpublished master's thesis, Université UPMC Paris 6, France.

Van der Geest, S. (1987). Self-care and the informal sale of drugs in South Cameroon. *Social Science & Medicine, 25*(3), 293–305.

Van der Geest, S. (2017). Les médicaments sur un marché camerounais. Reconsidération de la commodification et de la pharmaceuticalisation de la santé [Medicines on a Cameroonian market. Reconsidering commodification and the pharmaceuticalization of health]. *Anthropologie & Santé, 14*.

Vaughan, M. (1991). *Curing their ills: Colonial power and African illness*. Cambridge, UK: Polity Press.

Whyte, R. S., Van der Geest, S., & Hardon, A. (2002). *Social lives of medicines*, New York, NY: Cambridge University Press.

# Part I

# Varying choices for State regulation and their consequences

This first section of the book mobilizes sociohistorical and anthropological approaches. It describes the choices made by the governments of the countries studied—Benin, Ghana, Côte d'Ivoire, and Cambodia—with regard to pharmaceutical production, supply, and distribution from colonial times to the present day. Although these choices result in part from historical legacies and are constrained by the countries' economic and geopolitical contexts, they are nonetheless deliberate decisions made by the national authorities and thus have a considerable effect on how pharmaceutical markets are organized in these countries, including in the current globalized period.

# 1 Strengthening national pharmaceutical regulation through local production

*Jessica Pourraz, Claudie Haxaire, Daniel Kojo Arhinful*

## Introduction

This chapter provides a history of administrative pharmaceutical regulation from independence to the present in Ghana, Côte d'Ivoire, and Benin—three countries that are geographically close but have unique itineraries and contrasting pharmaceutical profiles, whether from an institutional perspective or in terms of their industrial or commercial structures. In order to underscore the comparison, we have added Côte d'Ivoire to the two countries specifically studied in this book. Its economic resources are close to Ghana, but at the time of independence, Côte d'Ivoire opted to enact different development policies than its anglophone neighbor (Eberhardt & Teal, 2010).

As highlighted briefly in the Introduction, the legal framework and pharmaceutical distribution, supply, and production systems vary from country to country, depending on their colonial legacies and post-independence policies for industrial, economic, and health development. The three countries' State pharmaceutical regulations also differ considerably. They fall under the national drug policy covering the spectrum of the various ways the State is involved in pharmaceuticals, such as defining the rules and overseeing their implementation. It is therefore incumbent on the States to establish a drug regulatory system through the intermediary of a national authority. The structure, operations, and legal status of this body vary depending on the countries' administrative organization and economic resources (OMS, 2006). Thus, while Benin has had a technical directorate since the 1960s, Ghana, where the pharmacy industry's infrastructure is much denser, established a semiautonomous agency with more resources in 2012. Falling between Benin and Ghana in terms of industrial pharmaceutical development, Côte d'Ivoire initiated its process to create an agency in 2015 that culminated in 2019. An analysis of these three case studies reveals how the evolution of State pharmaceutical regulatory systems is linked to which pharmaceutical policies were chosen for procurement and support of local drug production. We will examine various models of administrative pharmaceutical regulation in place in West Africa and how they were constructed over time. This will shed light on how local drug production played a role in constructing regulatory systems.

Using a sociohistoric approach, we have structured our narrative chronologically around the major global events confronting the States in equal measure. These include the debt crisis that caused the oil price shocks of the 1970s, the enforcement of structural adjustment policies in the 1980s, and the devaluation of the Financial Community of Africa (CFA) franc in 1994 in francophone countries. From the 2000s onwards, these regulatory systems evolved in response to how diverging industrial dynamics interacted with their regulatory methods. Focusing on the role of States, non-State private actors—including private pharmacists, pharmaceutical firms, and wholesalers—as well as transnational actors[1] provides a deeper analysis of how regulatory systems were created. This perspective also reflects the broader reform movements at play in the region, characterized by the process to harmonize pharmaceutical regulations at the community level and the trend to create agencies, as did Ghana and, very recently, Côte d'Ivoire.[2] More broadly, this chapter encourages an examination of how States construct pharmaceutical sovereignty as they take ownership of their drug policies. This issue allows for an analysis of public action, including pharmaceutical and industrial policies, and the role of national and transnational actors and how they interconnect at various levels.[3] By doing so, we will investigate how local production, combined with States' considerable capacity to regulate drugs, is a powerful tool in constructing pharmaceutical sovereignty.[4]

## Contrasting development policies (1960–1973)

At the time of their independence, Côte d'Ivoire and Benin were following the French Public Health Code dictating that pharmacists maintain a monopoly and, in return, perform their job duties in person and on site.[5] Meanwhile, until 1960, Ghana applied British laws under the authority of the Pharmacy and Poison Board,[6] which legislated a limited monopoly, did not require a pharmacist to operate the business, and allowed the jobs of manufacturer, wholesaler, retailer, and drug representative to be combined. Moreover, Ghanaian pharmacists were also not required to hold the majority of pharmaceutical companies' capital as was the case for manufacturers in Côte d'Ivoire from 1986 to 2015. In the francophone countries, the monopoly and its associated obligation to perform tasks in person reduced the sources of capital that could be mobilized to create industrial or commercial pharmaceutical enterprises, since they needed consolidated capital from pharmacists. In anglophone countries, combining jobs promoted faster accumulation of concentrated capital and allowed smaller companies to start up. After independence, the three countries chose contrasting development policies, whereby Ghana prioritized industrialization but Côte d'Ivoire and Benin promoted the exploitation of agricultural resources. This resulted in the establishment of pharmaceutical manufacturing in Ghana, while the two francophone countries strengthened the drug supply circuits inherited from the colonial period.

### *In Ghana: Prioritizing industrialization and the underpinnings of pharmaceutical regulation*

At the time of its independence in 1957, Ghana—which had substantial mineral and agricultural resources—was poorly industrialized. Kwame Nkrumah, who would become President of the First Republic of Ghana in 1960, turned to the economist William Arthur Lewis who recommended a free-enterprise production model and encouraged the use of foreign investors while dissuading the State from becoming a shareholder in or owner of industries (Lewis, 1953). Kwame Nkrumah committed the country to a vast industrialization program to foster economic development by substituting locally produced goods for imports. When local production began in 1957, Ghana was importing most of its medicines from Europe and the United States.[7] This demanding and specialized industrial sector required public infrastructure (water, electricity, road networks), skilled human resources, and access to capital (Simonetti, Clark, & Wamae, 2016), conditions that Ghana did not fulfill. The government created policies to overcome these technological shortcomings and to mobilize the necessary investments. Since efficient technologies were located in the former colonial empires (Swainson, 1987), Kwame Nkrumah called on investors from the United States and Europe to develop a local industrial foundation. He initiated an industrial policy in support of setting up pharmaceutical factories through administrative, financial, and fiscal facilities and market protections for locally produced medicines that penalized imports. As a result, the British firm Major & Company began producing medicines in Ghana in 1957, followed by Ghana Laboratories Ltd. Pioneer Companies Relief Incorporation in 1958; the English companies J. L. Morrison & Sons and Kingsway Chemists; Sterling Products Ltd. (United States); Dumex Limited (Denmark); Pharco Laboratory (India); and the Netherlands African Manufacturing Company-NAMCO, a joint venture between a Dutch company and a Ghanaian wholesaler (Boateng, 2009). The public company Ghana Industrial Holding Corporation (GIHOC) Pharmaceuticals Ltd., formed through a partnership with Hungary, began operations in 1967. A few private local initiatives arose on the sidelines (Gaizer, 2015), such as the still active Ayrton, created in 1965 by a Ghanaian pharmacist trained in England. The law in force in Ghana did not prohibit production units from holding shares in companies performing other functions in the sector,[8] making it easier to set up a company there. These companies were even more economically viable because they could combine manufacturing activities with wholesaling, as was the case for NAMCO, or with acting as an agent-importer, in the case of Major & Company (Baxerres, 2018).

Under Kwame Nkrumah, local pharmaceutical production was better able to meet public health priorities by providing medicines as well as the need for industrial and economic development. Local production went hand in hand with the development of a regulatory framework focused on enacting new legislation primarily on medicines approval and regulating the practice of the pharmacy as a profession. In 1961, the first Ghanaian legislation regulating the pharmacy profession, pharmaceuticals, and narcotics was passed: the Pharmacy and Drugs Act.

This act also provided for the creation of a new authority, the Pharmacy Board, responsible for regulating the pharmacy profession and issuing authorizations to practice and licenses to distribute medicines in the private sector, inspecting manufacturers and granting their authorizations, registering products, and controlling the import and distribution of narcotics.[9]

### *Côte d'Ivoire and Benin: Prioritizing strengthened supply chains inherited from the colonial period*

The two francophone countries focused on maintaining and strengthening the supply systems inherited from the colonial era through central procurement offices located in France that, from their point of view, guaranteed the safety and quality of imported medicines. No plans were made to build any drug production facilities. In Côte d'Ivoire, the public sector continued to be supplied by the Central Pharmacy (Pharmacie Centrale), which replaced the colonial Pharmapro in 1958, while the two private "wholesaler-distributors"[10] established before independence supplied the few distributors that worked in the country at the time[11]: Laborex, a subsidiary of the West Africa Trading Company (SCOA; Société Commerciale d'Afrique de l'Ouest), an importer since 1949, and the Pharmaceutical Group of Côte d'Ivoire (GOMPCI; Groupement Pharmaceutique de Côte d'Ivoire).[12] During the first 10 years following independence, Ivorian pharmacists, primarily trained in France, opened private pharmacies or held positions in pharmaceutical companies or Ministry of Health directorates.

At this time, Dahomey, which would become the People's Republic of Benin in 1975, was experiencing political instability that hampered investment. From independence in 1960 to Mathieu Kérékou's assumption of power in 1972, the industrial sector remained underdeveloped and the pharmaceutical industry was inexistent. As will be discussed in the next chapter, the public sector was still supplied by Pharmapro, backed since 1964 by the Benin National Office of Pharmacies (ONP, Office National des Pharmacies du Bénin) that oversees drug distribution to a few private pharmacies and health facilities.

From a legislative standpoint, the French Public Health Code required some modifications in terms of regulating the profession and the conditions for importing and registering medicines. The National Order of Pharmacists of Côte d'Ivoire was established in 1960,[13] and its Beninese counterpart was set up in 1973.[14] In addition to protection from the Order, pharmacists in Côte d'Ivoire are also protected by trade unions, and in this liberal economy are even able to establish *mutuelles* (insurance cooperatives), buy shares in pharmaceutical companies, and then set themselves up as financial holding companies,[15] whose importance will be explained later. In Benin, these groups would establish themselves much later (see Chapter 2). The 1960 decree defining the powers of the Ivorian Ministry of Public Health[16] created the Directorate of Pharmaceutical Services (DSP, Direction des Services Pharmaceutiques); Benin's General Directorate of Pharmacies (DGP, Direction Générale des Pharmacies) was established that same year. Both issue installation licenses and inspect pharmaceutical establishments.

In addition to private pharmacies, these directorates oversee the Chemistry and Fraud Laboratory and the Central Pharmacy in Côte d'Ivoire; and Pharmapro and the ONP in Benin.

In 1965,[17] Côte d'Ivoire reaffirmed the criteria governing drug registration, which did not occur in Benin until between 1973 and 1976 through the enactment of an initial series of ordinances[18] that decreed that only State-approved structures are authorized to import drugs and are required to report to the DGP.[19] The two countries recognized the need to control imported pharmaceuticals through a sales authorization in Côte d'Ivoire and a visa in Benin, issued by the respective pharmaceutical regulatory authority (DSP in Côte d'Ivoire and DGP in Benin) after checking the manufacturing conditions. In Côte d'Ivoire, the Law of 1965 established a registration fee paid to the Treasury for pharmaceuticals, whose rate and payment conditions are fixed by decree, as is also the case in Benin. This law also provided for the creation of a registration commission (or technical commission in Benin) whose composition and function were also defined by decree. However, registration fees paid to the Treasury are not transferred to the Beninese DGP and are only partially transferred to the Ivorian DSP, thus limiting their resources. At that time, drug registration was fairly lax, essentially consisting of paying registration fees to the Public Treasury and providing a technical dossier.

## A turning point in the 1980s: The global debt crisis and structural adjustment programs

The oil crisis of the 1970s slowed industrial activity and foreign investments in the pharmaceutical sector in Ghana until the late 1980s (Mackintosh, Banda, Tibandebage, & Wamae, 2016). The crisis also raised countries' costs of imported medicines. In Côte d'Ivoire and Benin, this affected public pharmaceutical supply structures and pushed the countries to consider producing medicines locally, a move that challenged the global trend to deindustrialize. At the international level, the essential medicines policy, initiated by World Health Organization (WHO) in 1977, encouraged the use of generics and establishing production units in the Global South.

### *The flight of multinationals from Ghana and the advent of Indian initiatives*

Throughout the 1970s and early 1980s, the Ghanaian economy experienced a severe crisis that forced many health professionals to leave the country (Senah, 1997). Jerry John Rawlings, who assumed power through a military coup d'état in 1981, was compelled to adopt structural adjustment programs imposed by the Bretton Woods financial institutions until 1992 (Whitfield & Jones, 2007). The launch of an economic recovery program in 1983, combined with trade liberalization, brought an end to the protectionist measures implemented under Kwame Nkrumah. Opening the market to competition, however, highlighted the lack of competitiveness of pharmaceutical companies based in Ghana. Starting in the late 1980s, the global crisis, coupled with economic reforms, led pharmaceutical multinationals to decrease, if not cease, activities with their subsidiaries (Boateng, 2009). During this period, only two Indian-owned companies were established: Letap Pharmaceuticals Limited in 1983 and M&G Pharmaceuticals Ltd. in 1989. Development of the pharmaceutical industry in India, starting in the 1970s (Chaudhuri, 2005), triggered changes in the structure and circulation of global drug markets, especially from Asia to Africa. Indian companies began to play a major role in technology transfer to the African continent.

### *Reorganizing public procurement and the start of an industrial policy in francophone countries*

In Côte d'Ivoire, local actors developed initiatives in response to the international events. In his pursuit for long-term economic sovereignty, the first president, Felix Houphouët-Boigny, sought to develop local pharmaceutical production.[20] This required training for pharmacists. Although planned for several years, the School of Pharmacy was not opened until 1977.[21] The school offered international-level training reserved for Ivorian citizens, adapted to the needs of local populations.[22]

However, Ivorian pharmacists envisaged pharmaceutical sovereignty from a financial perspective. A type of association based on capital drawn from professionals emerged in Côte d'Ivoire that would play a major role there. These were holding companies that gave pharmacists considerable influence on the

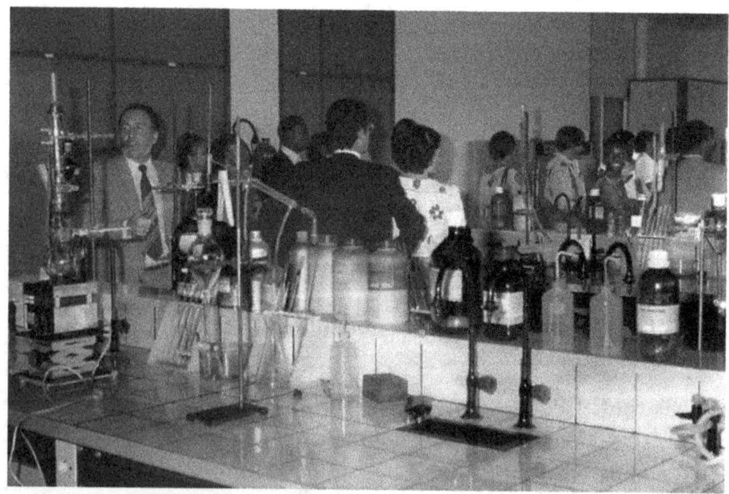

*Figure 1.1* Visit to the practical work chemistry room of the Abidjan Faculty of Pharmacy during the 5th Abidjan Medical Days, March 1981, where training has begun for pharmacists who will fill positions in control laboratories.

Source: © Pr.hon.Dean André Rambaud, March 1981

companies in which they were shareholders. Private pharmacists primarily owned shares in the two wholesaler-distributors (Laborex and GOMPCI). In 1975, some of these pharmacist shareholders united in the Eurapharma holding company, so they could pressure the French central procurement office, Continental Pharmaceutique, based in Rouen, the office that Laborex depended on.[23]

In 1980, the consequences of the global crisis, structural adjustment programs, and the withdrawal of French development aid programs led Felix Houphouët-Boigny to enlist actors from the pharmaceutical sector to consider setting up a drug production facility in Côte d'Ivoire. With no support from wholesaler-distributors or French industrials, it took 6 years to carry out the project. Côte d'Ivoire benefited from the problems of Rhône-Poulenc, which planned to outsource its production abroad in units acting as manufacturers and working under a license (Barral, 2008). The first Ivorian law on the pharmaceutical industry was enacted in 1986, requiring Ivorian pharmacists to hold senior-level manufacturing and control positions, as well as stipulating that they be the majority shareholders of the company's capital. Ivorian private pharmacists could then join forces to mobilize the necessary capital and, like the wholesaler-distributors, invest in the first production company, Cipharm, opened in May 1988, operating under the Rhône-Poulenc license.[24] From the time of its creation until the International Monetary Fund (IMF) put an end to it, this firm enjoyed a reserved market.[25] A second private production company, Galefomy, specializing in dermatological preparations, was established in 1989 in Bouaké, the country's second largest city. It was financed by a private pharmacist[26] who had accumulated capital through his shares in the wholesaler-distributors' capital fund, just as Western pharmacies of the nineteenth century once did (Ruffat, 1996). He was able to get around the rules requiring a pharmacist to run the company and forbidding pharmaceutical functions from being combined through a one-time agreement with the president of the Order of Pharmacists, who wanted to promote the establishment of production facilities.

This process resulted in strengthening the institutions that oversee regulation in Côte d'Ivoire. Following the 1983 Etats Généraux de la Santé, a citizens' forum to gather health information, the Ministry of Health was reorganized to favor the relative autonomy of its subsidiary structures. The Central Pharmacy became the Côte d'Ivoire Pharmacy of Public Health (PSPCI, Pharmacie de la Santé Publique de Côte d'Ivoire), established as a Public Institution of an Industrial and Commercial Nature (EPIC in French).[27] In 1984, the Laboratory of Chemistry and Fraud became a central autonomous directorate of the Ministry of Health. Later, a National Pharmacovigilance Commission was created.[28] The first national list of essential medicines was created in 1989.

Benin was also facing a dire economic situation, and in 1980, the ONP and Pharmapro went bankrupt, causing severe drug shortages. In response, the Beninese State, which had minimal financial resources of its own, entered a phase to privatize the pharmaceutical supply and distribution systems. The private sector, thus far repressed by the Marxist government, found a place in the pharmaceutical landscape (Baxerres, 2013). In 1982, President Mathieu Kérékou used the family-owned capital of a Beninese biologist living in France who created the private firm Pharmaquick to produce medicines locally and reduce the cost of imports. The industrialist's arrival crystalized numerous tensions among Beninese private pharmacists, who accused him of violating the monopoly rules since he was not a pharmacist. In 1987, IMF programs imposed economic measures on Benin aimed at decreasing public expenses and thus endorsed State withdrawal from the health sector (Baxerres, 2013). Benin was subject to two structural adjustment programs, first from 1989 to 1991 and then from 1991 to 1994. The Central Purchasing Office of Essential Medicines and Medical Consumables, or CAME was created in 1989 to replace the ONP and Pharmapro, prompted by the World Bank and other development partners (see Chapter 2).

## Privatization of the pharmaceutical sector in the 1990s

Serious drug shortages continued in the 1990s in the three countries, generated in part by the phenomenon of deindustrialization described earlier in Ghana and by the devaluation of the CFA franc in 1994 in Benin and Côte d'Ivoire. No longer able to pay the bills for imported drugs, these two francophone countries used less expensive generic medicines. This was all the more necessary because the cost recovery policy promoted by the Bamako Initiative required that populations cover a portion of medicine prices. In Ghana, this meant the implementation of the "cash and carry" policy starting in 1992 (Arhinful, 2003). From then on, privatization of the pharmaceutical sector then underway seemed to solve the availability problems surrounding pharmaceuticals.

### *Recovering industrial investment through local private capital and strengthening drug regulation in Ghana*

Since the mid-1990s, industrial investment has picked up in Africa, in large part due to local investors (Mackintosh et al., 2016). In Ghana, the flight of multinationals allowed private Ghanaian entrepreneurs, some who were pharmacists, to buy back production facilities created after independence and to start manufacturing drugs, thus contributing to the "indigenization" of the pharmaceutical sector.[29] The capital mobilized by this new generation of Ghanaian industrialists came from their business activities in medicine importation, promotion, and distribution (see Chapter 3). The Ghanaian State continued to play a determining role in supporting local industry by promoting the creation of markets reserved for local manufacturers using a list of 14 medicines prohibited for import and reserved for local production[30] and a 15% discount on prices for public tenders. Fiscal advantages were also granted to local producers, such as tax exemptions on imported raw materials, machines, and equipment needed to manufacture finished products[31] and simplified registration. Thus, the interventionist policy implemented by the Ghanaian State offers the market conditions that local industries need in order to develop and is a form of "educational protectionism"

(Guennif & Mfuka, 2003, p. 85). It does not, however, solve the problem facing local companies that want access to capital and technology.

Besides the need to regulate, support, and guide increased local production, Ghana's national regulatory authority was confronted with increasingly more generic medicines coming from Asia during the 1990s that needed quality and origin inspections before registration. It became necessary to separate the regulation of products from the regulation of professional practice and to create an independent authority solely for regulating products, whether imported or produced locally. The Pharmacy Board disappeared and was replaced by the newly created Pharmacy Council and the Food and Drugs Board (FDB). In 1994, Pharmacy Act 489 created the Pharmacy Council to control the pharmacy practice and the registration of pharmacists and licensed chemical sellers. The FDB, created in 1997 following the enactment in 1992 of the Food and Drugs Law, managed the control of drug manufacturing, import, export, distribution, use, and advertisement. Overseen by the Ministry of Health, the FDB enjoys relative autonomy and independence in its decision-making. Comprising two divisions at its beginnings—with one dedicated to medicines, cosmetics, medical devices, and household chemical substances and the other dedicated to foods—the governing board was composed of 14 individuals, including 5 pharmacists. Operationally the FDB seeks the support of external actors to implement some activities: USAID for quality surveillance, and the United States Pharmacopeia (USP) and WHO for laboratory equipment and training. The industrial policy was combined with strengthening the regulatory authorities' capacities and competencies since the FDB was gradually acquiring a pool of pharmacist-inspectors who, on average, conducted about 20 inspections of manufacturing plants each year in Ghana. Over time, the expertise acquired during these inspections gradually gave FDB officials the necessary expertise to conduct inspections abroad. Pharmaceutical companies exporting their medicines to Ghana had to pay a fee when registering their medicines to cover the costs associated with conducting inspections at their production sites.[32] Ghanaian inspectors carried out about 30 inspections abroad per year, mainly in Asia where most of the generic medicines came from (FDA-Ghana, 2011–2015). They also received training within multinationals, such as Cipla in India, the US Food and Drug Administration (FDA), and the Medicines and Healthcare products Regulatory Agency in the United Kingdom.

### *The indigenization of the industry and distribution in francophone countries*

In Côte d'Ivoire, the early 1990s witnessed the deployment of Ivorian pharmacists' competencies and capital throughout the pharmaceutical sector. The cooperative of private pharmacists, Copharm, promoted financial assistance within the profession,[33] based on the model of cooperatives described by Sueur (2017) in France. Two new pharmaceutical companies were created, with an even more uncertain future than Cipharm: Dermopharm[34] in 1992 and Pharmivoire in 1991. Pharmivoire, created by two university pharmacists who got loans from Proparco, a subsidiary of the French Development Agency (AFD), which supports the private sector by granting loans. It would become Pharmivoire Nouvelle in 1999, following a recapitalization by Copharm (Aouely, Bih, & Kacou, 2017).

At the same time, the process to indigenize wholesaler-distributors' capital continued when 161 Ivorian private pharmacists,[35] who were shareholders of the Ivorian branch of Laborex, or Laborex-CI, repurchased the majority of the capital of this company (55%) in 1990. They did this by exchanging their Laborex shares for shares in Pharmafinance, the holding company provided for by Ivorian law that they had just created and that they used to take control of this former Ivorian subsidiary from the SCOA group, namely, Laborex-CI. Thus, in 1991, Pharmafinance created Pharmaholding, which became Ubipharm, and, in 2000, acquired a purchasing platform, Planet pharma, approved by the French Agency for the Safety of Health Products. Today, Ubipharm is the leading drug distributor in francophone African countries, "a 100% African success story" (Coulegnon, 2013). Owners of private pharmacies also sat on wholesaler-distributors' boards of directors. Therefore, Ivorian pharmacists continued to seek economic sovereignty with share buyouts in order to claim majority ownership in two new wholesaler-distributors: Copharmed in 1996 and DPCI in 1999.[36]

Confronted with drug shortages caused by the devaluation of the CFA franc, the local firms Cipharm and Pharmivoire Nouvelle were able to provide some essential medicines and infusion solutions. They were joined by the Pharmaceutical Laboratory of Côte d'Ivoire (LPCI, Laboratoire Pharmaceutique de Côte d'Ivoire), created in 1997 by Ivorian university pharmacists to prepare herbal medicines, but whose activity was limited to repackaging, and by Lic Pharma, created in 2002 with Chinese capital.[37] Lic Pharma has a unique financial arrangement relative to the 1986 law on pharmaceutical companies, which requires that pharmacists hold the majority of a company's capital. This resulted in a bilateral agreement between the government of the new president Henri Konan Bédié and the Chinese State in 1995, resulting in a series of projects funded by the Chinese Exim Bank in 1996 (Caubin, 2010). Loans to the Ivorian government were lent on to private operators to fund productive projects through joint ventures, including Lic Pharma. In Benin, the devaluation of the CFA franc and the procurement crisis helped strengthen the role of the CAME, which purchases and distributes generic medicines, as well as the private company Pharmaquick, which produces them locally. The second structural adjustment program from 1991 to 1994 strengthened the country's commitment to a phase of economic liberalism (Gbetoenonmon, 2013). The procurement system was gradually expanding with the establishment of two new private wholesaler-distributors (see Chapter 2).

Just as in Ghana, sourcing generics from Asia and creating new local industries in Côte d'Ivoire required strengthening Beninese and Ivorian regulations on importation and registration. As a result, the technical directorates of the Ministries of Health were restructured. In Côte d'Ivoire in 1994, President Bédié reorganized the Directorate of Pharmaceutical Services, which became the Directorate of Pharmacy, Medicine, and Laboratories (DPML, Direction de la Pharmacie et du Médicament et des Laboratoires) in 1997. In Benin, the Directorate of Pharmacies and Laboratories' prerogatives were broadened to become the Directorate of Pharmacies and Diagnostic Investigations (DPED, Direction des Pharmacies et des Explorations Diagnostiques). Between 1994 and 1995 in Benin, the WHO essential medicines program supported strengthening registration procedures for medicines for human use.[38] These procedures were revised in 1997 with Decree no. 97-632 of December 31 to increase pre-regulation screening and make the registration process more transparent and rigorous.[39] This went hand-in-hand with creating or strengthening quality control systems. In Benin, an analytical laboratory was created in 1999. In Côte d'Ivoire, the national laboratory, created in 1991,[40] was upgraded to a Public Establishment of an Administrative Nature (an EPA in French) and became the National Laboratory of Public Health (LNSP).

Despite these institutional reforms, the skills developed by Beninese and Ivorian technical directorates particularly for inspection remained very limited in comparison to those of the FDB in Ghana, where a dense industrial infrastructure platform encouraged the FDB to build up production site inspection capacities early on. This last factor is key to highlighting how local production processes are entangled with pharmaceutical regulation.

## The 2000s: Differing local industrial dynamics

### *Continuing Ghana's industrial policy*

Throughout the 2000s in Ghana, continuation of the industrial policy led to the creation of drug manufacturing pharmaceutical companies by Ghanaian pharmacists—such as Kinapharma, Danadams, and Ernest Chemists—bringing the total number of companies to 36. Most started out as import wholesalers for international companies. Once seen as intermediaries, these wholesaler-retailers became manufacturers by accumulating capital (Baxerres, 2018; Braudel, 1985). They received Indian and/or Chinese technical assistance: for example, Danadams was created through a Sino-Ghanaian partnership. In the same period, new Indian Ghanaian companies[41]—such as Eskay Therapeutics Ltd. in 1998, Pharmanova Limited in 2005, and Unichem Industries in 2010—opened in Ghana, taking advantage of an environment that made it easier for them to produce generic versions of drugs still under patents.[42]

### *How the Ivorian political crisis affected the industrialization process*

In Côte d'Ivoire, the military-political crisis that began in 2000 saw Laurent Gbagbo's accession to the presidency and ignited 10 years of turbulence and deregulation resulting in clashes, after which Alassane Ouattara came to power.

The wholesaler-distributors Ubipharm and Eurapharma managed to hold on during the crisis, as did the local pharmaceutical companies Cipharm[43] and Pharmivoire Nouvelle. Despite the 1986 law in force, in 2007 the Gbagbo government authorized the establishment of the Olea company using Italian capital and belonging to non-pharmacist Milanese businessmen. The new initiatives fall

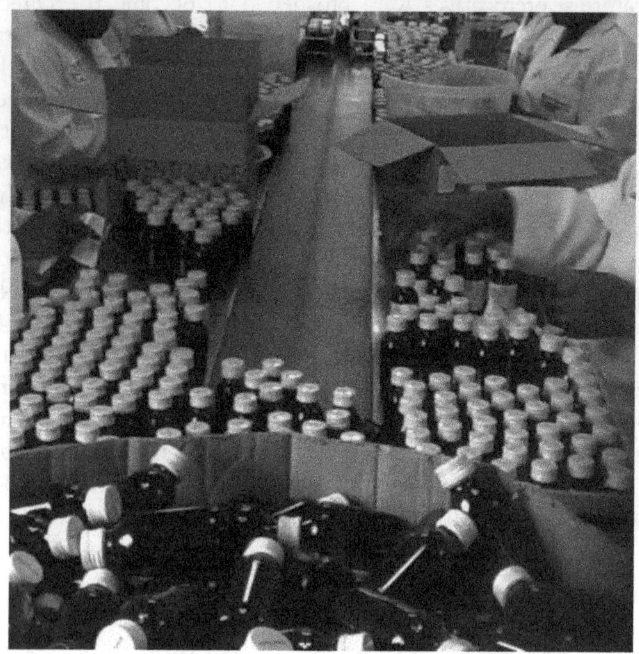

*Figure 1.2* Packaging area of a pharmaceutical company in Ghana.

Source: © IRD/Jessica Pourraz, Accra, January 2017

under a form of capitalism that bypasses the rules on monopolies and the origin of capital. Other companies tried to start up with no lasting success, including a subsidiary of the Canadian firm Rougier. However, in those troubled times, wholesaler-distributors no longer risked investing in local production as they did when Cipharm was created.

Starting in 2011, the government of Alassane Ouattara set out to promote the development of local pharmaceutical companies to ensure better access to medicines, seeing more investment opportunities in a booming market (Coulibaly, 2018). Conditions for setting up manufacturers were facilitated by the creation of free zones.[44] A new law, promulgated in 2015,[45] finally allowed non-pharmacists to inject capital into the pharmaceutical industry (Amari & Pabst, 2016). Two Moroccan pharmaceutical companies and Asian generic manufacturers, including the Indian firm Pharmanova, were approved and began building factories at the end of 2018. The Tunisian company SAIPH broke ground for its production facility in June 2017,[46] joining the 10 already-established Ivorian companies in 2015 (DPML, 2015).

### *Failed industrial projects in Benin*

In Benin, none of the technological, financial, or economic conditions encouraged local pharmaceutical production. While drug imports were tax-exempt, imported raw materials were not. Energy, such as electricity, was also very expensive. Local manufacturers were disadvantaged compared to foreign firms that exported medicines in Benin (West & Banda, 2016), which explains why requests to create firms never materialized, other than one from Pharmaquick in 1982. Of the 11 requests submitted to the Directorate of Pharmacies, Medicine, and Diagnostic Investigations (DPMED) between 2001 and 2009,[47] primarily from Beninese, Cameroonian, North African, and Chinese developers, only 5 companies received authorization to establish in Benin, primarily for the production of solutes, generics, and medical consumables, but none of these projects ever came to fruition.[48] With no industrial policy supporting local medicine production over imports and because of the way its supply chains operated, Benin became an enclave reserved for medicine imports.

The industrial dynamics described earlier appear to be linked to the regulatory models adopted by the countries and the resources available to them, as we shall see next.

## Different administrative regulatory modes: Technical directorate versus agency

### *Limits placed on regulation by the Ivorian and Beninese technical directorates*

In the course of the 2000s, technical directorates in Côte d'Ivoire and Benin underwent several institutional reforms to raise their level of expertise. In Côte d'Ivoire, the Gbagbo government reformed operations in the Pharmacy of Public Health (PSP, Pharmacie de la Santé Publique) in 2002[49] and reorganized the DPML in 2006 to make it responsible for applying the government's health policy for pharmaceutical matters. The role of the National Laboratory of Public Health (LNSP, Laboratoire National de Santé Publique) was strengthened through Order no. 198/MSHP of 2009, which made quality control mandatory for all imported medicines. Despite these reforms, these institutions were not satisfactory. In 2008, the National Program for the Development of Pharmaceutical Activity (PNDAP, Programme National de Développement de l'Activité Pharmaceutique)[50] was created. Directly attached to the Directorate General of Health Services (DGS), it was charged with implementing the National Pharmaceutical Plan. However, it seemed its mission partially overlapped with the DPML until its role was better defined. In Benin, functions pertaining to diagnostic explorations were reassigned to the DPM in 2010, which has now become the DPMED.[51] The National Quality Control Laboratory (LNCQ, Laboratoire Nationale de Contrôle de Qualité) was created in 2005 with French support from the Chirac and Pierre Fabre Foundations, which provided equipment to improve the quality control of imported medicines.

Although the DPML and the DPMED were made up of sub-directorates that carved up the pharmaceutical sector along different lines, and despite Côte d'Ivoire having better staffed human resources than Benin, these technical directorates shared similar dysfunctions. First, in terms of human resources, the DPML in Côte d'Ivoire has about 30 pharmacists, but most of them do not work full-time and/or have not been trained in regulatory matters.[52] It employs young contract pharmacists who are waiting to open their own pharmacies. The Beninese DPMED suffers from an even greater lack of staff. In December 2016, they numbered six pharmacists (DPMED, 2016): two were civil servants and four were young contractors who were graduates with no specialized training, just as in Côte d'Ivoire. The precariousness of contract employees adds to staff instability and prevents having a body of specialized experts in pharmaceutical regulation.

Moreover, the skills developed by the Beninese[53] and Ivorian technical directorates in inspection remained quite limited given the industry's small scale. There are still no legally recognized and sworn pharmacist-inspectors in Benin or Côte d'Ivoire, thus rendering their recommendations and decisions ineffective and without legal value. This legal vacuum means that none of the national regulatory authorities of UEMOA member States[54] conduct inspections abroad. For its part, Côte d'Ivoire does not conduct inspections but rather makes site visits, organized by the companies themselves when requested by the Ivorian directorate. The experts' impartiality might be challenged, knowing that the pharmaceutical companies cover all mission expenses and offer luxury services to the visitors.[55] More specifically in Benin, the DPMED's lack of resources means employees cannot ensure medicines undergo quality control, conduct inspections abroad, or evaluate Marketing Authorization (MA) applications. For these functions, Benin relies on the expertise of international regulatory authorities and importers based in France and Europe, delegating the bulk of the evaluation and quality control work to them for imported drugs. In the eyes of DPMED regulators, these intermediaries offer sufficiently reliable and robust quality assurance systems. This last point, especially evident in the case of Benin, clearly shows how processes that mutually reinforce local production and pharmaceutical regulation are entangled. Côte d'Ivoire, which has strengthened the capacities of its National Laboratory, performs these controls and evaluations itself. However, since products come from central procurement offices located in France, such as Planet pharma, a subsidiary of Ubipharm, the country takes advantage of the guarantees offered by established supply chains.

In closing, the DPMED's organization complicates the effective performance of its duties since it has five units that focus on all regulatory functions.[56] The Pharmaceutical Legislation, Regulation, and Governance Unit, for example, covers five of the regulatory functions on its own (OMS, 2003; 2006),[57] each of which must be assigned to a single unit. The lack of financial resources adds to these shortcomings. Both countries have a backlog of MA applications and follow-up monitoring.[58] The fees charged for MAs by the two directorates are low, and their lack of resources prevents them from developing sufficiently solid expertise that would justify raising their fees.

In summary, the technical directorates of Benin and Côte d'Ivoire have little functional autonomy compared to the Ministry of Health and suffer from inefficient internal organization and inadequate financial resources and technical staff, hampering their analytical capacities and offering minimal scientific expertise to the State. We will now use the case of Ghana and more recently Côte d'Ivoire, to see whether an agency can serve as a model to address the dysfunctions noted in the technical directorates.

### *An agency model: The Food and Drug Authority in Ghana*

In October 2012, the Ghanaian parliament approved the *Public Health Act*, which created the Food and Drugs Authority (FDA), a legal entity separate from the State, responsible for providing and enforcing norms and standards for the sale of medicines (Republic of Ghana, 2012). One year after its creation, the organization that transitioned to the FDA was restructured and five specialized divisions were created, including the drug registration and inspectorate division[59] (WHO, 2014), which oversees the departments that support local industry and law enforcement. This reform also prompted the hiring of 10 additional pharmacist-inspectors, primarily from the industrial sector, who were assigned to the new Drug Enforcement Department. The quality control laboratory is under the direct responsibility of the FDA chief executive officer and is located within the FDA's institutional headquarters in Accra, which has housed the entire staff since 2013 in a brand-new three-story building.[60] The FDA has nearly 500 employees, including about 50 pharmacists (FDA-Ghana, 2014). That same year, the FDA department supporting local industry developed a road map to guide local companies in the process to meet the standards of good manufacturing practices (GMP) by 2020, ensuring the drug's quality at each step of its production.[61] The road map also provides for the creation of a regional center in Ghana for bioequivalence studies so that Ghanaian companies can conduct these studies locally at a lower cost. These studies are required for WHO prequalification certification, in addition to GMP standards, to guarantee a generic's similarity with the reference medicine (Lantenois & Coriat, 2014). The FDA has a dual goal: to guarantee the quality of medicines distributed on the private market and to support Ghanaian companies in their quest to obtain WHO prequalification, a precondition for access to markets subsidized by transnational actors, such as the Global Fund.

Although it remains under the Ministry of Health, the FDA's new status grants it greater autonomy than that of a conventional public service administration. Nevertheless, its fiscal plans are still subject to approval by the Ministry of Finance and Economic Planning, since it receives an annual operating budget, allocated by the State and approved by the parliament, defined according to planned activities. Until 2012, approximately 75% of the operating budget came from the government (WHO, 2014). Drug registration fees are another source of considerable funding. The FDA keeps half of the amounts received and pays the other half to the State.[62] The Public Health Act authorizes the FDA to hire the staff needed to perform its functions, but like all public health institutions, it must obtain a financial authorization for each new hire (FDA-Ghana, 2012), causing delays. The government would ultimately like the FDA to pay its staff with its

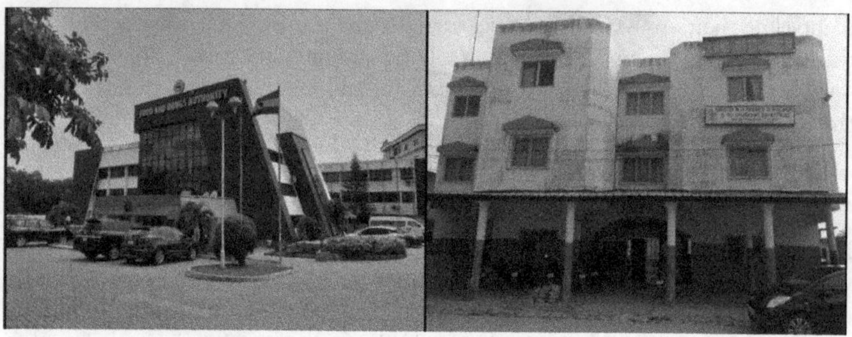

*Figure 1.3* FDA-Ghana and DPMED-Benin headquarters in 2020.

Source: © IRD/Emelia Agblevor and Stéphanie Mahamé

own funds, which will give it greater autonomy and independence (Benamouzig & Besançon, 2005).

Hence, the FDA in Ghana has gradually come into being through an endogenous process since the 1990s with occasional financial and technical support from external partners (USAID, WHO, USP), with the primary goal of ensuring the quality of drugs distributed on the domestic market.

## Creation of the Ivorian Pharmaceutical Regulatory Agency (AIRP, Agence Ivoirienne de Régulation Pharmaceutique)

In Côte d'Ivoire, plans to create an agency, driven by Ivorian specialists in the pharmaceutical sector, materialized much faster on the recommendations of the Economic Community of West African States (ECOWAS) and international experts,[63] and with technical and financial support from the AFD. In 2015, the Ivorian government set out to reorganize the existing regulatory institutions to create an agency through the Debt Reduction-Development Contract (C2D)[64] and the Project to Support the Revitalization of Côte d'Ivoire's Health Sector (PARSSI, Projet d'Appui à la redynamisation du Secteur de la Santé en Côte d'Ivoire) funded and managed by the AFD (Allemand, 2017). First, the Pharmacy of Public Health changed its status to become an N-PSPCI, a nonprofit organization, thus granting it the autonomous management that it had lacked. The National Laboratory of Public Health's capacities were bolstered through staff training and the provision of equipment and reference samples. The DPML's legal powers were also strengthened, and the various sub-directorates' responsibilities were redefined. This process prepared for reconfiguring the existing institutions by redefining their functions, organizing them into the three specializations covered by the Ivorian agency (Ouattara, 2018). At the same time, various legal provisions point to the Ivorian system's similarities to the Ghanaian model. For example, the Order of Pharmacists of Côte d'Ivoire was reorganized in 2015 and now categorizes producers, wholesaler-distributors, and promotion agencies together.

Launched in 2015, the process to create the Ivorian Pharmaceutical Regulatory Agency culminated in 2017 with a vote on Act no. 2017-541 of August 3 and its implementation decree in February 2019. Responsible for the management of the pharmaceutical sector, it conducts surveillance and enforces penalties for violators,[65] which entails establishing a body of inspectors made up of sworn pharmacists (Ouattara, 2018). According to these promoters, this agency should be able to guarantee industrial investments by cleaning up the market, especially by eliminating informal circuits (Ouattara, 2018). While it is difficult to assess the effects of such recent changes, an analysis of the creation process for the AIRP in Côte d'Ivoire highlights the role played by local medicine production in constructing regulatory systems. The local protagonists supporting the AIRP defended the plan to create the agency as a way to install a regulatory system that is robust enough to meet the development goals of the national pharmaceutical industry.

## Conclusion

Where medicines are made and how they are procured—direct imports, via a central procurement office and/or local production—affect the instruments deployed by States to guarantee the quality of the products distributed to their populations. Control systems, applied through factory inspections and drug registration, are key factors, requiring learning and investment. In Ghana, the presence of local drug production developed since independence and the importation of generics directly from Asia helped build robust national regulation. The phenomenon of cooperation (Hauray, 2006) between the regulatory authority and the local companies also plays an important role by creating a space for mutual learning between manufacturers and regulators. Comparing this to the situations of Benin and Côte d'Ivoire highlights the importance of strengthening institutional regulatory capacities to attract direct foreign investment and to structure the industrial landscape. More than the legal form of the national regulatory authority, the training and number of pharmacists dedicated to regulatory issues promote the emergence of regulatory systems and industry growth.

In order to eliminate the heterogeneity of regulation between West African States, a regulatory harmonization process was launched at the regional level to homogenize laws and transform technical directorates into autonomous agencies.[66] Desired by the region's countries themselves, this process is seen as a public health tool with a goal to promote access to quality medicines. It is accompanied by the creation of a common market aimed at increasing trade in the region. Far from being complete or free of any challenges, this homogenization does help develop and support local drug production, making it instrumental in establishing pharmaceutical sovereignty for countries in the West African region.

## Notes

1. These include multilateral United Nations agencies, such as WHO and the United Nations Industrial Development Organization (UNIDO), and the United States (USAID), French (Expertise France), German (GIZ), and British (DFID) bilateral aid agencies.

2. At the beginning of 2020, the DPMED (Direction des Pharmacies, du Médicament et des Explorations Diagnostiques) in Benin became the Beninese Agency for Pharmaceutical Regulation (ABRP-Agence Béninoise de Règlementation Pharmaceutique). In view of these very recent developments, we have not been able to study this transformation process to report on it in this book.
3. Sovereignty is a legal concept governed by public law: "Sovereignty is the quality for a State not to be bound except by its own will, within the limits of the superior principle of law and according to the collective objectives that it is called upon to achieve" (Louis Le Fur, 1896, p. 443).
4. See the Introduction of the book for more information on the data collection methodology.
5. Reaffirmed in Côte d'Ivoire by Act no. 65-250 of August 4, 1965. See Chapter 3 for Benin.
6. January 1960, Public Records and Archives Administration Department (PRAAD), Ministry of Industry, GH/PRADD/RG.7/1/39, Accra, Ghana.
7. January 1960, Public Records and Archives Administration Department (PRAAD), Ministry of Industry, GH/PRADD/RG.7/1/39, Accra, Ghana.
8. Information confirmed by former officials from the Pharmacy Council and the FDB of Ghana during the Globalmed symposium in Ouidah in 2018.
9. Interview with a former FDB executive in Accra on April 1, 2015.
10. This profession will be discussed in Chapter 3.
11. There were 42 private pharmacists in 1970.
12. Created by Jean Mazuet, the first French pharmacist posted in Côte d'Ivoire in 1936, and later developed in other francophone African countries (Mazuet, 1987).
13. By Act no. 60-272 of September 2, 1960, followed by a code of ethics, established through Act no. 62-249 of July 31, 1962. For the industry, owner-pharmacists who are manufacturing are in one section (B) as opposed to pharmacists who are distributing (C), which clearly separates the two functions, unlike in Ghana. Pharmacists who are salaried employees in industry management fall under section D, distinct from that of owners.
14. Ordinance no. 73-38 of April 21, 1973.
15. These are companies whose shareholders could have an influence on the company's decisions.
16. Decree no. 61-34 of January 14, 1961, on the reorganization of the Ministry of Public Health, later changed to Decree no. 69-48 of January 20, 1969.
17. Act no. 65-250 of August 4, 1965.
18. For example, Ordinance no. 75-7 of January 27, 1975, on governing medicines in Dahomey.
19. Ordinance no. 73-68 of September 27, 1973, defining the conditions for the importation of pharmaceuticals and wound care products in Dahomey.
20. Interview with the first faculty dean, André Rambaud, (November 2018) and his presentation in June 2018 during the 40-year commemoration of the Research and Training Unit (UFR, Unité de Formation et de Recherche) for pharmaceutical sciences at the Houphouët-Boigny University in Cocody (Abidjan).
21. By President Felix Houphouët-Boigny, Professor Michel Attiso, and pharmacist Jean Baptiste Mokey.
22. By 2015, it had trained over 2000 graduates (DPML, National Pharmaceutical Policy, 2015, p. 18).
23. These actors are also present in Benin, which will be discussed in the next chapter.
24. The capital was distributed as follows: Rhône-Poulenc 26%, Roussel-Hoechst 13%, Sanofi 13%, Ivorian pharmacists 28%, GOMPCI 10%, and Laborex 10%. CIPHARM manufactured the specialties of three pharmaceutical companies: Nivaquine®, aspirin, and Flavoquine®.

25. Interview with Assane Coulibaly, head pharmacist and Deputy Director of Cipharm until December 2014: medicines produced by Cipharm are not imported.
26. Interview with Dr. Mamadou Yacine Fofana in February 2018.
27. By Decree no. 84-764 of June 6, 1984.
28. By Order no. 249 MSP DSPH of November 18, 1988.
29. "Indigenization" describes the origin of capital and indicates that it comes from local private individuals. It differs from nationalization, which means that capital belongs to the State.
30. This includes paracetamol, ampicillin, chloramphenicol, tetracycline, aspirin, and diazepam.
31. Compared to 10% import taxes on finished products.
32. In 2009, this fee was USD 700 for a local firm and USD 20,000 for a foreign firm (source: FDA).
33. In 1993, the Order of Pharmacists of Côte d'Ivoire entrusted a colleague trained in management with the task of "creating a cooperative, COPHARM, to mobilize savings, provide financial assistance between pharmacists, and carry out joint projects" (interview with Elisabeth Kakou conducted by Sabine Cessou for *Afrique Méditerranée Business*, April–May 2017, p. 32–35).
34. Dermopharm presents itself as a family business created by an Ivorian private pharmacist, who died in 2016.
35. Interview with the Director General of Ubipharm, Gérard Mangoua, for *Forbes Afrique* (Coulegnon, 2013).
36. Through the creation of a holding company with Ivorian capital in 1996, Copharmed, to control their shares in Eurapharma (repurchased by the CFAO Group in 1996). However, unlike Laborex-CI, Copharmed remains a partner of the Eurapharma group.
37. According to our sources, the capital is now entirely Chinese, coming from a construction company, and is not a branch of a Chinese pharmaceutical company. The Chinese staff is also not from the pharmaceutical industry; instead, they are chemical and agribusiness technicians supervised by Ivorian pharmacists.
38. WHO Archives, E19-445-3BEN, WHO Action Programme on Essential Drugs-Benin, 1989, Jacket No. 3.
39. The decree grants the Technical Commission for Medicines, in charge of issuing the Marketing Authorization (MA), the power to consult experts in order to deepen document assessment and analysis.
40. By Decree No. 91-654 of October 9, 1991.
41. These three companies are owned or were set up by Indians who had Ghanaian nationality.
42. Ghana is one of the countries that is not bound to the World Trade Organization (WTO) agreements on Trade-Related Aspects of Intellectual Property Rights (TRIPS).
43. Because of the crisis, when international firms withdrew capital from Cipharm, their stocks were purchased by the current Director (Ibrahim Diawara), who had still kept some of their licenses.
44. The Decree of December 6, 2012 created a Public Establishment of an Administrative nature, facilitating the "one-stop shop" approach that could give the pharmaceutical industry advantages: the CEPICI, Center for the Promotion of Investments in Côte d'Ivoire.
45. Act no. 2015-533 of July 20, 2015 on the practice of pharmacy.
46. See the daily newspaper *Ivoire Matin*, November 26, 2018.
47. Source: DPMED Pharmaceutical Establishments Unit, August 2016.
48. These were the International Pharmaceutical Solutes Company (*Société Internationale de Solutés Pharmaceutiques*), a Beninese NGO project; the Benin-Pharma BTL SA company for generics production; Biovegemed SA from a technology transfer from the French Pharmaceutical Group Michel Iderne to develop local medicine

products based on plant extracts; a Chinese company producing medicines and mineral water, Texmed-Bénin SARL; and another Beninese enterprise to manufacture and package medical consumables.

49. It gave the PSP the opportunity to manufacture and package some medicines commonly used in hospitals: Act no. 202-334 of June 13, 2002.
50. It was created by Order no. 308/MSHP/CAB of December 11, 2008.
51. According to Order no. 4482/MS/DC/SGM/CTJ/DPMED/SA of August 12, 2010 on the attributions, organization, and functioning of the Directorate of Pharmacy, Medicine, and Diagnostic Investigations (DPMED).
52. The majority of deputy directors are professors at the School of Pharmacy.
53. Its employees have only conducted one inspection of the Pharmaquick production site, on March 15–17, 2010. To our knowledge, it is the only inspection carried out, for which documents were archived in the Pharmaquick files at the DPMED in Cotonou (Source: observation within the DPMED Pharmaceutical Establishments Unit between 2014 and 2016).
54. Created in 1994, the West Africa Economic and Monetary Union is composed of eight francophone member States, with the goal of creating a harmonized and integrated economic zone. Source: http://www.uemoa.int/fr/presentation-de-luemoa, accessed March 3, 2019.
55. Interview in August 2017 with a staff member from the regional pharmaceutical sector.
56. A Pharmaceutical Legislation, Regulation, and Governance Unit; a Pharmaceutical Establishments Unit; a Diagnostic Investigations Unit; a National Medical Imaging and Radiation Protection Unit; and a Medicinal Plants Unit.
57. Drug regulation, evaluation, inspection, quality control, and monitoring of medicines on the market, and pharmacovigilance.
58. Sources: Interview with Professor Anglade Malan in Abidjan, 2015; observations conducted at the DPMED in Cotonou.
59. At the time it was created, it had four departments: drug evaluation and registration, drug enforcement, herbal medicine, and tobacco.
60. The FDA has its headquarters in Accra, nine regional offices, set up between 2003 and 2011 across the country, along with control offices at the country's official entry and exit points for goods (the Port of Tema and Kotoka International Airport).
61. UNIDO, the United Nations Industrial Development Organization, has supported this initiative on a regional scale since 2015.
62. In 2013, the cost of registering an imported drug was USD 3600 and USD 270 for locally produced drugs.
63. Sources: minutes from the seminar to share results of the experts' work (Professor Amor Toumi, Professor of Pharmacy, Tunisia; and legal experts Bernard Hody of Belgium and Victoire Ayeoura of Côte d'Ivoire) and discussions with the various involved regulatory bodies, April 27, 2015 in Abidjan.
64. The 1st C2D—Debt Reduction-Development Contract—managed by AFD for Côte d'Ivoire, was signed on December 1, 2012 in Abidjan for an amount of 630 million euros, or CFA 413.25 billion. The second C2D (2014–2020) was signed on December 3, 2014 in Paris for an amount of CFA 738 billion. The C2D enables countries to reconvert French debt through grants to fund development (C2D.gouv.CI, accessed November 25, 2018).
65. Penalties may range from suspension to permanent withdrawal of the authorization to practice, cancellation of the MA, or destruction of products. They may also be financial (up to one billion CFA francs) or criminal (ranging from 2 months to 10 years in prison).
66. http://www.nepad.org/programme/african-medicines-regulatory-harmonisation-amrh, accessed July 1, 2019.

## Reference list

Allemand, C. (2017). *La mise en place des agences du médicament dans la région UEMOA, transfert, hybridation et convergence d'un modèle d'action publique [The establishment of drug agencies in the UEMOA region, transfer, hybridization, and convergence of a public action model]*. Unpublished master's thesis, University of Political Science, Lyon, France.

Amari, A. S., & Pabst, J.-Y. (2016). 2015, les évolutions législatives du secteur pharmaceutique ivoirien: Un progrès attendu depuis plus d'un demi-siècle [2015, legislative developments in the Ivorian pharmaceutical sector: Awaited progress for over a half century]. *Revue Générale de Droit médical, 22*, 203–214.

Aouely, P., Bih, N., & Kacou, E. (2017). La production locale de médicaments face aux enjeux d'accessibilité: L'exemple de Pharmivoire Nouvelle [Local drug production in the face of accessibility issues: The example of Pharmivoire Nouvelle].[Blog post]. *Secteur Privé & Développement, La revue de Proparco, SP&D 28*, 30–33. Retrieved from https://blog.secteur-prive-developpement.fr/2018/04/23/english-local-production-of-medicine-and-accessibility-challenges-the-example-of-pharmivoire-nouvelle/.

Arhinful, D. K. (2003). *The solidarity of self-interest. Social and cultural feasibility of rural health insurance in Ghana*. Doctoral dissertation, African Studies Centre, Leiden University, The Netherlands. Retrieved from https://openaccess.leidenuniv.nl/handle/1887/12919.

Barral, E. (2008). *Rhône-Poulenc: des molécules au capital [Rhône-Poulenc: Molecules in the capital]*. Paris, France: Ateliers Fol'Fer.

Baxerres, C. (2013). *Du médicament informel au médicament libéralisé : Une anthropologie du médicament pharmaceutique au Bénin [From informal to liberalized drugs: An anthropology of pharmaceutical drugs in Benin]*. Paris, France: Les Éditions des Archives Contemporaines.

Baxerres, C. (2018). D'intermédiaire informel, devenir détaillant, grossiste puis producteur pharmaceutique : Les trajectoires « vertueuses » des hommes d'affaires du médicament au Ghana [From informal intermediary to becoming a retailer, wholesaler, and then pharmaceutical producer: The "virtuous" trajectories of drug businessmen in Ghana]. In C. Baxerres, & C. Marquis (Eds.), *Regulations, markets, health: Questioning current stakes of pharmaceuticals in Africa* (pp. 30–40). (Conference proceedings). HAL, Ouidah, Benin. https://hal.archives-ouvertes.fr/hal-01988227.

Benamouzig, D., & Besançon, J. (2005). Administrer un monde incertain: Les nouvelles bureaucraties techniques: Le cas des agences sanitaires en France [Managing an uncertain world: The new technical bureaucracies: The case of health agencies in France]. *Sociologie du Travail, 47*(3), 301–322.

Boateng, K. P. (2009). *A study to determine the factors affecting the compliance of local pharmaceutical manufacturers to international best practices in the pharmaceutical industry*. A case study of Danadams Pharmaceutical Industry Limited. Unpublished master's thesis, Paris Graduate School of Management, France.

Braudel, F. (1985). *La dynamique du capitalisme [The dynamics of capitalism]*. Paris, France: Arthaud.

Caubin, A. (2010). *La coopération économique chinoise en Afrique de l'Ouest: Exemple de la Côte d'Ivoire [Chinese economic cooperation in West Africa: The example of Côte d'Ivoire]*. Doctoral dissertation, University of Toulouse, France. Retrieved from https://docplayer.fr/5270977-La-cooperation-economique-chinoise-en-afrique-de-l-ouest-l-exemple-de-la-cote-d-ivoire.html.

Chaudhuri, S. (2005). *The WTO and India's pharmaceutical industry: Patent protection, TRIPs and developing countries*. New Delhi, India: Oxford University Press.

Coulegnon, T. (2013, November). UBIPHARM, n°1 de la distribution de médicaments en Afrique francophone [UBIPHARM, no. 1 in drug distribution in francophone Africa]. *Forbes Afrique*, 34–35.

Coulibaly, A. (2018). *West Africa inside the African market. Presentation at the International Business and Investment Forum.* Bonn, Germany. https://www.unido.org/sites/default/files/files/2018-03/Assane%20Coulibaly_%20UNIDO_West%20Africa_Inside%20the%20African%20Pharma%20Market_01032018%20Bonn.pdf.

DPMED. (2016). *Liste du personnel de la Direction de la Pharmacie, du Médicament et des Explorations Diagnostiques [List of staff from the Directorate of Pharmacy, Medicine, and Diagnostic Investigations].* Cotonou, Benin.

DPML. (2015). Politique Pharmaceutique Nationale 2015 [National Pharmaceutical Policy 2015]. *Ministère de la Santé et de la Lutte contre le Sida [Ministry of Health and AIDS Control].* Yamoussoukro, Côte d'Ivoire.

Eberhardt, M., & Teal, F. (2010). Le Ghana et la Côte d'Ivoire: Une inversion des rôles [Ghana and Côte d'Ivoire: A role reversal]. *Revue internationale de politique de développement, 1*, 37–54.

FDA-Ghana. (2011). *Annual report FDB.* Accra, Ghana: Ministry of Health, FDB.

FDA-Ghana. (2012). *FDA 2012 annual report.* Accra, Ghana: Ministry of Health, FDA.

FDA-Ghana. (2013). *FDA 2013 annual report.* Accra, Ghana: Ministry of Health, FDA.

FDA-Ghana. (2014). *FDA 2014 annual report.* Accra, Ghana: Ministry of Health, FDA.

FDA-Ghana. (2015). *FDA 2015 annual report.* Accra, Ghana: Ministry of Health, FDA.

Gaizer, S. (2015). *Local pharmaceutical industry in Ghana.* Accra, Ghana: Chairman of Industrial Pharmacist Association.

Gbetoenonmon, A. (2013). *Le Bénin en Afrique de l'Ouest: visions, défis et contraintes économiques [Benin in West Africa: Visions, challenges, and economic constraints].* Cotonou, Benin: Friedrich Ebert Stiftung. https://library.fes.de/pdf-files/bueros/benin/10691.pdf.

Guennif, S., & Mfuka, C. (2003). La lutte contre le sida en Thaïlande: De la logique de santé publique à la logique industrielle [The fight against AIDS in Thailand: From public health logic to industrial logic]. *Sciences Sociales et Santé, 21*(1), 75–98.

Hauray, B. (2006). *L'Europe du médicament. Politique, expertise, intérêts privés [The Europe of drugs. Politics, expertise, private interests].* Paris, France: Presse Sciences Po.

Lantenois, C., & Coriat, B. (2014). La « préqualification » OMS: Origines, déploiement et impacts sur la disponibilité des antirétroviraux dans les pays du Sud [WHO "prequalification": Origins, deployment, and impacts on antiretroviral availability in Southern countries]. *Sciences Sociales et Santé, 32*(1), 71–99.

Le Fur, L. (1896). *État fédéral et confédération d'États [Federal State and confederation of States].* Paris, France: Marchal et Billard.

Lewis, W. A. (1953). *Report on industrialisation and the Gold Coast.* Accra: Gold Coast Government.

Mackintosh, M., Banda, G., Tibandebage, P., & Wamae, W. (Eds.). (2016). *Making medicines in Africa: The political economy of industrializing for local health.* London, UK: Palgrave Macmillan.

Mazuet, J. (1987). Portrait. Jean Mazuet: souvenirs d'Afrique [Portrait. Jean Mazuet: Memories of Africa]. *Afrique pharmacie, Bulletin de liaison de l'association pharmaceutique interafricaine*, 4, 7.

Ministry of Industry. (1960). *Public Records and Archives Administration Department (PRAAD), Ministry of Industry*, Archives, GH/PRADD/RG.7/1/39, Accra, Ghana.

OMS. (2003). Une réglementation pharmaceutique efficace: Assurer l'innocuité, l'efficacité et la qualité des médicaments [Effective pharmaceutical regulation: Ensuring the safety, efficacy, and quality of drugs]. Geneva, Switzerland: World Health Organization. https://apps.who.int/iris/handle/10665/68502.

OMS. (AFRO). (2006). La réglementation pharmaceutique dans les pays francophones de la région africaine [Pharmaceutical regulation in francophone countries in the African region]. *Lettre d'information pharmaceutique*, 3(1), 1–4.

Ouattara, M. (2018, June). *La loi n° 2017-541 du 03 aout 2017: Quel apport pour la régulation du secteur pharmaceutique en Côte d'Ivoire [Law no. 2017-541 of August 3, 2017: What it has contributed to the regulation of the pharmaceutical sector in Côte d'Ivoire]*. Paper presented at the Nineteenth International Pharmaceutical Forum, Ouagadougou, Burkina Faso.

Republic of Ghana. (2012). *Public Health Act 851*. Accra, Ghana: Assembly Press.

Ruffat, M. (1996). *175 ans d'industrie pharmaceutique française. Histoire de Synthélabo [175 years of French pharmaceutical industry. History of Synthélabo]*. Paris, France: La Découverte.

Senah, K. A. (1997). *Money be man. The popularity of medicines in a rural Ghanaian community*. Amsterdam, The Netherlands: Het Spinhuis.

Simonetti, R., Clark, N., & Wamae, W. (2016). Pharmaceuticals in Kenya: The evolution of technological capabilities. In M. Mackintosh, G. Banda, P. Tibandebage, & W. Wamae (Eds.), *Making medicines in Africa: The political economy of industrializing for local health* (pp. 25–44). London, UK: Palgrave Macmillan.

Sueur, N. (2017). *La Pharmacie Centrale de France. Une coopérative pharmaceutique au XIXe siècle [The Central Pharmacy of France. A pharmaceutical cooperative in the XIXth century]*. Tours, France: Presses universitaires Francois Rabelais.

Swainson, N. (1987). Indigenous capitalism in postcolonial Kenya. In P. M. Lubeck (Ed.), *The African bourgeoisie: Capitalist development in Nigeria, Kenya and the Ivory Coast* (pp. 137–163). Boulder, CO: Lynne Rienner Publishers.

West, A., & Banda, G. (2016). Finance and incentives to support the development of national pharmaceutical industries. In M. Mackintosh, G. Banda, P. Tibandebage, & W. Wamae (Eds.), *Making medicines in Africa: The political economy of industrializing for local health* (pp. 279–297). London, UK: Palgrave Macmillan.

Whitfield, L., & Jones, E. (2007). *Ghana: The political dimensions of aid dependance*. GEG Working Paper 2007/32. Global Economic Governance Programme. https://www.geg.ox.ac.uk/publication/geg-wp-200732-ghana-political-dimensions-aid-dependence.

WHO. (2014). *Report of the preliminary assessment of the National Medicines Regulatory Authority of Ghana*. Geneva, Switzerland: World Health Organization.

# 2 Strengths and weaknesses of State-controlled wholesale distribution

## Benin's CAME and wholesaler-distributors

*Stéphanie Mahamé, Roch Appolinaire Houngnihin, Adolphe Codjo Kpatchavi*

### Introduction: Colonial-era system of wholesale pharmaceutical distribution

In the pharmaceutical world, wholesale drug distribution has been described as subordinate to suppliers (manufacturers) and customers (pharmacies), which share the bulk of the sector's profits between them (Lomba, 2014). In Benin, however, where manufacturing is minimal, the pharmaceutical system is centered around importation and wholesale distribution by a very small number of actors: a mere five, as we will see. This wholesale distribution is based on the pharmacist's monopoly, which will be discussed in the next chapter. The monopoly is strictly controlled by the State and mobilizes significant capital, which affects the position of these actors and crystallizes economic and political challenges—challenges that have at times led to crises and redefined power relations. The current configuration of this wholesale distribution system, the result of a series of choices by political actors combined with various economic and ideological factors, will be discussed in this chapter.

In Benin, as in most former colonies, pharmaceutical drugs were introduced during the colonial era (Baxerres, 2013; Fassin, 1987). The National Supply Pharmacy (Pharmapro) was created at that time to supply the public health system of dispensaries and military garrisons; similar structures existed throughout France's other African colonies. In addition to this colonial system, religious missionaries distributed medicines to rural populations, while trading posts or warehouses run by European commercial enterprises supplied the country's three main coastal cities of Cotonou, Porto-Novo, and Ouidah.

After gaining independence on August 1, 1960, the new Beninese State chose to retain the system it had inherited. Pharmapro continued as a department in the Ministry of Health, bolstered by the creation in 1964 of the National Pharmacy Office (ONP, Office National de la Pharmacie). Both were funded through government budget allocations but had slightly different functions: Pharmapro continued to supply medicines to public health facilities, while the ONP was responsible for importing and distributing medicines through public pharmaceutical warehouses and for mobile sales using trucks, to compensate for the lack of pharmacies in rural areas.

Private-sector pharmacies were provisioned by the Groupement des Pharmaciens du Dahomey et du Niger (Dahomey and Niger Pharmacist Group), which later became the Groupement des Pharmaciens Bénin-Niger (GPBN, Benin-Niger Pharmacist Group). This entity, the country's first private wholesale structure, was set up by the French pharmacist Jean Mazuet[1] (Baxerres, 2013).

In 1972, as in many African countries during the Cold War, political power in Benin shifted to a regime that advocated a Marxist-Leninist ideology. Private initiatives were severely curtailed as the prerogatives of the two public entities increased. Private pharmacies were forced to source their supplies through the ONP, which had been granted an exclusive monopoly by the government to import pharmaceutical products. However, the ONP and Pharmapro faced a host of problems in the 1980s, similar to most francophone African countries (Van der Geest, 1987). Budget allocations became hard to mobilize from the financially strapped government, and debts mounted. The situation was further complicated by management issues such as poorly run warehouses, an excessive number of workers, and cash flow problems; suppliers required orders to be prepaid. Benin experienced disruptions in the supply of medicines on a regular basis. In the face of these difficulties, the import monopoly that had been granted to the ONP was reviewed, initially to give pharmacists the opportunity to provision themselves,[2] but was later completely abandoned. With an increasing number of Beninese pharmacists[3] setting up private pharmacies, the private sector was reorganized in 1980 with the birth of the very first private wholesaler-distributor, the Cooperative of Private Pharmacists in Benin (COPOB, Coopérative des Pharmaciens d'Officine du Bénin), which 2 years later became the Private Pharmacist Purchasing Association of Benin (GAPOB, Groupement d'Achat des Pharmaciens d'Officine du Bénin). Its shareholders were almost exclusively Beninese pharmacists. This was followed by a second private wholesaler in 1985, the Benin Pharmacy Company (Sophabé, Société des pharmacies du Bénin) (Baxerres, 2013).

The ONP and Pharmapro closed their doors for good in 1989 as part of the country's first structural adjustment program (SAP) and were replaced by a new entity, the Central Purchasing Office for Essential Medicines and Medical Consumables (CAME, Centrale d'Achat de Médicaments Essentiels et consommables médicaux). The private sector was joined by two new wholesaler-distributors: the Beninese Union of Pharmacists (UBPHAR, Union Béninoise des Pharmaciens) in 1990 and Promopharma, a subsidiary of the international group Eurapharma, in 1991.[4] This occurred at the time of the Conference of Active Forces of the Nation (*Conférence des forces vives de la Nation*), which marked Benin's transition to democracy and a degree of State disengagement, particularly in the education and health sectors (Boidin & Savina, 1996).

This chapter describes the wholesale distribution system that was subsequently established. The creation and functioning of the CAME, a private and later associative entity with a public service mission, is examined, as is the formation of a private distribution system and the economic conflicts that drive it. We demonstrate that, apart from the dysfunctions and tensions inherent in the financial interests at stake, this public and private wholesale distribution system has undeniable advantages in terms of efficiency and fulfilling public health needs. However, it also crystallizes the public-sector political issues of State sovereignty vis-à-vis transnational actors and the private-sector ideological issues within the pharmacy profession in a postcolonial context. The Conclusion will address the current circumstances, in which this system is being challenged by Beninese political actors.[5]

## CAME: Caught between public service and the quest for autonomy

### *History of a recommended but contested institution*

Created by Decree no. 89-307 of July 28, 1989, the CAME began operating in October 1991 as part of the World Bank Health Services Development Project (Brown, Cueto, & Fee, 2006; Cling & Roubaud, 2008). The first stage of the project was an audit of the ONP and Pharmapro, which led to these entities being liquidated. Various health actors were then invited to discuss setting up a structure to replace them. In addition to the World Bank, the government, and health professionals (professional physician, pharmacist, and academic societies), the discussions included other transnational actors, such as UNICEF and the German and Swiss foreign development agencies, which are heavily involved in health through various projects. The discussions favored creating an entity that could supply the country with medicines to replace Pharmapro and the ONP, but one without their weaknesses, especially their dependence on budget allocations from the State. The very first director of the CAME explains it this way:

> You know, the ONP was a State office [...] whose director changed as ministers came and went. It was a structure subordinate to the Ministry of Health that operated under a budget allocation, so we wanted to change all that by putting a number of principles in place. First of all, we wanted this Central Purchasing Office to be autonomous: we wanted the director to be hired rather than appointed by a ministerial body, and to have a performance contract with its board of directors. And we wanted to set up a management committee that would be completely free to make decisions, with government control through a steering committee, where the Ministry of Health, the Ministry of Finance, and... a few other ministries are represented, along with donors. And this must be able to guarantee a certain autonomy for the organization. That's how we started. And an organization that must be quite light. Compare it to the ONP, which used to employ more than 500 people, whereas the Central Purchasing Office started with 11 people.
>
> (Interview, Cotonou, January 15, 2016)

The World Bank advocated for an autonomous institution, while the State wanted to keep the public supply of medicines under its control.

As the discussions dragged on, the State adopted a decree establishing the CAME in the form of a project executed by the Ministry of Health, with the condition that it become autonomous after 2 years. The CAME was thus created in a dual context, one health-related and one economic. Its health mandate echoes the 1987 Bamako Initiative of 2 years earlier (Ridde, 2004; Tizo & Flori, 1997), the recommendations of which were implemented in Benin in 1988, and the introduction of essential medicines into the public sector.[6] By allowing the sale of medicines in public health facilities, the Bamako Initiative resolved one of the key questions regarding how a public procurement agency operates: financial autonomy. In economic terms, as mentioned earlier, the procurement agency was created in the context of the SAPs Benin committed to from 1989 to 1991 and from 1991 to 1994. The goal of these SAPs, promoted by the World Bank and the International Monetary Fund (IMF), was to limit government spending by reducing public employment and gradually privatizing national companies (Baxerres, 2013). These economic and public health policies are described as having opened the door to changing the roles of both the State and the private sector in supplying medicines and structuring the pharmaceutical system. Whereas the State model passed down from colonial days was based on significant involvement of public authorities, the Bamako Initiative and SAPs introduced government disengagement, in particular moving supply and distribution activities to private actors, and a reconsideration of public social benefits (Boidin & Savina, 1996). Nevertheless, the State was increasing its investment in regulation and control, as highlighted in the previous chapter.

Although the CAME began operating in 1991, our research shows it took until 1996 to revise the legislation making the CAME an autonomous entity. During the discussions, the Minister objected to the use of the term "association," even though the CAME operates as such. The articles of association therefore state that "a Central Purchasing Office for Essential Medicines and Medical Consumables is established in the Republic of Benin, governed by private law and subject to the government's obligation of control" (Article 1, 1996 articles of association). The State thus stressed its intention to maintain a right to exert control over the group. According to a former director, "It was very difficult, because the health authorities we had at that time wanted to take it over. I met ministers who told me 'I will never give this entity independent status'" (interview, Cotonou, January 15, 2016). Autonomous management, which had been strongly affirmed from the outset, was supposed to make the CAME an apolitical system with purely technical management to avoid political blockages, power struggles, and corruption. Part of the World Bank's technocratic vision was having the board of directors hire the CAME director, which the articles of association stated must be a pharmacist with at least 12 years' experience in managing a pharmaceutical establishment. In practice, however, this vision only exacerbated power conflicts. "I was called a ministry within a ministry. (…). The CAME was irritating… it was an autonomous body and people didn't like that, they didn't like that," says a former director. The other actors in the system (physician and pharmacist unions, transnational actors) argued against the State, supporting an autonomous organization. A former chairman of the CAME management committee[7] gave his perspective on how association status was eventually obtained:

> We were fighting to have the CAME's status revised, in an appropriate way, hoping to make it an entity… managed by the 1901 law. So, the pharmacists' union… and then other bodies were working towards that. There was a workshop, a seminar… a delegation from the seminar went to see the minister, all that… In short, there were all of those pressures, including from technical and financial partners who were also pushing for independent status to ensure better stability, a stable entity, so that it wouldn't be a ploy and we wouldn't know whether it was still in government hands or if it was autonomous.
>
> (Interview, Cotonou, March 23, 2015)

The transition to association status was finally made when the Global Fund to Fight AIDS, Malaria and Tuberculosis became involved. Another former director explains:

> There was the Global Fund, supporting priority diseases—malaria, tuberculosis, and AIDS—and they wanted to go through the CAME. But they said, in order to go through the CAME, it must have a clear legal identity. So we started working on it again for a third time, and this time the donors hired a lawyer, or two specialists, to help the government establish a truly unambiguous and clear status, and we arrived at the current statutes that make the CAME a nonprofit association. So, it was clearly defined, and it was from that point that we began to enter into contracts with partners.
>
> (Interview, Cotonou, March 17, 2016)

In 2010, the CAME adopted new articles of association stipulating "a nonprofit-making association called Centrale d'Achat des Médicaments Essentiels et

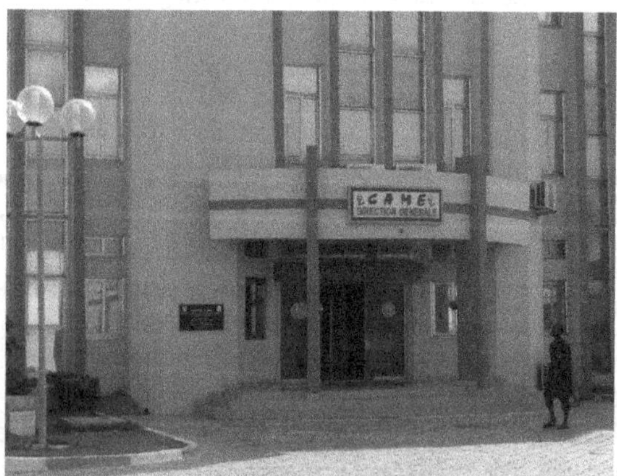


*Figure 2.1* New headquarters of the powerful CAME open in October 2014.

Source: © IRD/Stéphanie Mahamé, Cotonou, avril 2016

Consommables Médicaux is created in the Republic of Benin, with the acronym CAME" (Article 1, 2010 articles of association).

### *Procurement challenges*

Article 1 of the agreement between the CAME and the Beninese government[8] expressly establishes: "under the terms of this Agreement, the Government entrusts the CAME, which accepts, with performing the following mission of general utility: to regularly supply quality essential medicines, laboratory reagents, and medical consumables and equipment to the following clients: public and private nonprofit health facilities, private pharmaceutical establishments,[9] and private hospitals with monopoly products[10] at a price that is accessible to the population...." The organization's core business is, therefore, supplying and distributing essential medicines (see Figure 2.1).

To obtain supplies, the CAME issues a call for applications every 2 years to preselect suppliers for the products it needs. Selection is based on criteria related to company structure and operations (legal and financial documents) and their products (quality assurance, international inspections). After selection, the "list of pre-qualified suppliers" is set, and only the selected companies receive the calls for tenders. This is not WHO prequalification,[11] but CAME selection is based on the WHO model for both products and companies, albeit with less stringent requirements. The CAME also has significant concerns about product prices, volumes to be provided, and suppliers' terms of payment. In accordance with the WHO definition of essential medicines (OMS, 2002), the most important selection criterion is the "quality-price" ratio: suppliers who offer the best product at a reasonable price are chosen.

This "quality-price" factor means the CAME is constantly balancing public health requirements with economic issues. The pharmaceutical form offered by the supplier is also taken into account because the market of prescribers and patients must be satisfied in addition to public health priorities.

### *Distributing essential generic drugs and inputs from vertical health programs*

The CAME is commonly perceived as the entity responsible for provisioning public health centers. When it was created in 1989, transnational actors specified that it would supply public health centers as well as private nonprofit centers. This has been enshrined in its articles of association, with a particular focus on mission and humanitarian health centers, which play an important role in providing access to health care for the country's most disadvantaged populations (Baxerres, 2013). But as the CAME has evolved, a series of negotiations have resulted in the current configuration, i.e., provisioning private pharmacies and private for-profit health centers in addition to the original clients. Private pharmacies have officially been able to obtain supplies from the CAME since 1994, when the CFA franc was devalued. Medicines sold in pharmacies had doubled in price, becoming inaccessible for the vast majority of the population, while the CAME, with the help of French and Danish aid agencies, had managed to hold its prices steady. The government asked the agency to make certain products available to pharmacies. Small health centers and large private clinics have played a major role in urban health services since the 1980s (Boidin & Savina, 1996). The consultation fees in small centers are quite low, with most of the income coming from the sale of medicines (Baxerres, 2013). These centers are supposed to use their medicines on-site for the care they provide, not sell them. According to the head storekeeper of the CAME in Cotonou,[12] some of these centers recast themselves as NGOs to gain access to the CAME's medicines and circumvent this limitation. Others used personal contacts to go through authorized centers in order to access these drugs, and the vast majority simply obtained their supplies from the informal market (Baxerres, 2013). The CAME became aware of this situation in the early 2010s; the director then pushed the management committee to accredit these private health centers so that they would have direct access and the CAME would have the right to monitor and control their pharmaceutical activities.[13] A former director recalls:

> Ordinarily, private health centers do not have access to the CAME. But I find this to be an injustice, because there is no such thing as a private patient. All the patients are Beninese, so [the centers] juggle, they go through approved health facilities to obtain supplies, [...] and yes, they are given approval. Because in any case, if you refuse, they'll go through another entity to get supplies. I know of cooperative clinics that used to buy for private centers. But I say, this is a joke. It's better that... the private center just comes to us.
>
> (Interview, Cotonou, January 15, 2016)

Although the legislation governing the CAME had not yet been amended to account for this category of actor, in practice, the management committee grants private centers an accreditation allowing them to be customers.

The CAME is also in charge of storing and distributing products for vertical health programs.[14] Because the AIDS epidemic erupted in the early 1980s, in the midst of an economic crisis and the IMF- and the World Bank-advocated disengagement of African governments, treatments did not become available on the continent until the late 1990s (Desclaux & Egrot, 2015). As observed in most countries in the global South, the fight to control the AIDS epidemic has had a major impact on how the public supply of medicines and more broadly pharmaceutical policy in these countries are structured (Chabrol, 2012; Desclaux & Egrot 2015; Loyola, 2009). In Benin, the CAME's current configuration and performance are partly linked to this fight. Transnational actors provided the initial stocks of medicines to launch CAME activities but only began actively participating in distributing medicines in Benin in the 2000s with antiretrovirals (ARVs), when the National AIDS Control Program (French acronym: PNLS) began storing ARVs at the CAME. According to our sources, these first products were funded by the United Nations Development Programme (UNDP). Reagents and products to treat opportunistic infections were added in 2002. UNICEF and Médecins Sans Frontières also entrusted the CAME with storing their ARVs, to be distributed by the PNLS. The stakes for the CAME were high; the volume of medicines it managed was unparalleled, which helped to cast its activities in a new light.

By integrating the AIDS system, in 2008 the Global Fund created a management unit within the CAME that absorbed the previous initiatives and centralized the supply and management of ARVs and products to treat opportunistic infections. In 2010, after discussions between the government, the CAME, and transnational actors, the Global Fund management unit was expanded to include other actors and programs to become the Specific Program Management Unit (French acronym: UGPS). This is a department within the CAME, headed by a responsible pharmacist and a health logistics specialist who manages the stocks. The CAME thus took on another mandate, added to the 2010 articles of association, to "acquire, store, manage, and distribute medicines and medical equipment provided by the Beninese government or external partners for national health programs" (Article 1, Government/CAME Agreement, 2010).

Although the arrival of transnational actors significantly transformed the CAME's structure, the value of the drugs distributed by the UGPS appears marginal compared to the CAME's total sales. The following table 2.1 compares the CAME's sales figures to the value of medicines distributed by the UGPS.

In 2018, the CAME had sales of nearly CFA 13 billion (about EUR 20 million) and distributed more than CFA 4 billion worth of medicines (about EUR 6 million) on behalf of transnational actors, for a total of about 17 billion products distributed (about EUR 26 million). But these figures represent only a portion of Benin's pharmaceutical market, which is dominated by private actors.[15]

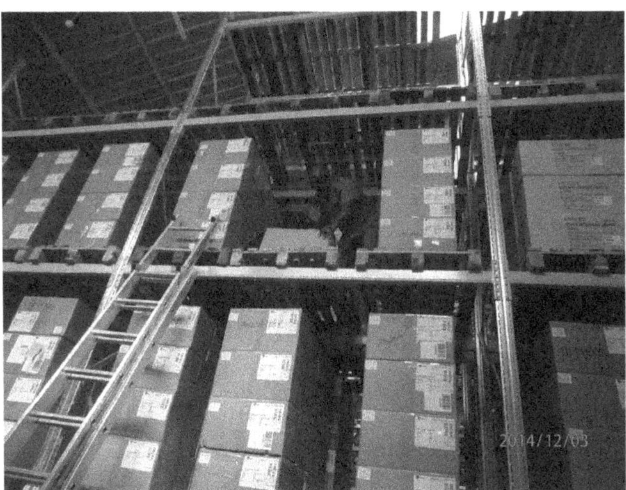

*Figure 2.2* UGPS warehouse at CAME's headquarters.

Source: © IRD/Stéphanie Mahamé, Cotonou, March 2014

*Table 2.1* UGPS's medicines within the CAME sales

| *Year* | *CAME sales figures (CFA franc)* | *Value of UGPS products*[a] *(CFA franc)* |
|---|---|---|
| 2018 | 12,794,044,095 | 4,316,393,857 |
| 2017 | 12,582,299,098 | 3,716,213,396 |
| 2016 | 11,354,224,129 | 3,818,190,875 |

Source: UGPS Accounting Department, CAME, July 2019.

[a] These are not products sold to generate revenue, but the market value of the products that are distributed free of charge on behalf of transnational actors, including the Global Fund, USAID, UNICEF, and the UNFPA. Note: 100 CFA francs = 0.15 €; 1,000,000,000 CFA francs = 1,524,000 €.

## Private wholesale distribution: Supply under pressure

### *Conflicting paths for wholesaler-distributors*

In Benin, private wholesale companies are often formed in a contentious environment, as illustrated in this interview excerpt:

> You see, it's always personal, people who got angry with someone, to create that. Nothing has ever been created in Benin, in the pharmaceutical sector, for the good of Beninese consumers.
>
> (Interview with the general manager of one of the wholesale distribution companies located in Benin, Cotonou, July 15, 2015)

In the 1980s, a time when the ONP had difficulties supplying pharmacists and the State asked private pharmacists to organize among themselves to obtain their own supplies, two competing concepts took hold among these pharmacists. The GPBN functioned and supplied them, but was perceived as a "French" entity since, as mentioned earlier, it was created and initially managed by the French pharmacist Jean Mazuet. Some pharmacists felt the GPBN should take over and become an umbrella organization responsible for supplying all Beninese pharmacies with pharmaceutical products. Another group of pharmacists advocated establishing a "purely Beninese" type of wholesale entity. In 1980, this latter group created the COPOB, which later became the GAPOB. By refusing to support the GPBN, this group of pharmacists ascribed to an ideology that denounced Western hegemony. Misunderstandings have been part of the private wholesale drug distribution network in Benin since its inception and are associated with ideological issues that are still prevalent today. As Didier Fassin asserts, the social sciences have under-researched medicines as ideological investments, defining ideology as "a set of discourses that legitimize or contest an order of things" (Fassin, 2007, p. 94). Despite the desire for a purely Beninese company, the COPOB was created with the support of a French organization, the Central Procurement Office (Office Central d'Achat, OCA SARL). The first group of pharmacists eventually created the Benin Pharmacy Company (Sophabé, Société des Pharmacies du Bénin) in

1985 after significant opposition and with the technical and financial support of the GPBN, which had ceased its activities. According to a wholesale company director, a group of pharmacists opposed to the creation of Sophabé lobbied the Minister of Health at the time, who initially wrote in a letter that he would "maintain my ministry's refusal to Sophabé indefinitely."[16]

On March 18, 2014, 29 years after Sophabé was established (but before this organization became Medipharm), the Beninese daily *Fraternité* published a story on a wholesaler-distributor who wanted to set up business in Benin: "For six years, the Ubipharm case has been the subject of disagreement between the Minister of Health and the National Order of Pharmacists of Benin. The leaders of Ubipharm-Benin applied to the Minister of Health on March 23, 2009 for a license to open and operate a wholesale company (...). However, to date, no action has been taken on Ubipharm-Benin's request, either by the National Order of Pharmacists of Benin or by the Minister of Health."[17] One month later, on April 18, 2014, the newspaper *Le Matinal* wrote on its website: "Ubipharm affair: Professional health care organizations gave a press conference yesterday, Thursday, April 17, 2014, at the headquarters of the National Order of Pharmacists of Benin in Cotonou. They denounced the government's illegal decision to authorize the multinational Ubipharm-Benin SA (...) to operate. They called for the general mobilization of all the professional health care organizations in Benin and the Beninese people to dissuade flagrant violations of the law by the Head of State aimed at destabilizing national organizations." The spokesperson for one of Benin's two pharmacists' unions used this same article to accuse the National Order of being motivated by "conflicts of interest, abuse of power, insider trading, abuse of corporate assets, and influence peddling."

The nationalist and anti-hegemonic ideology on display since the very beginnings of the private wholesale distribution system resurfaced as soon as Ubipharm took steps to become established.

Didier Fassin discusses protests against biomedicine as a "Western" concept in the context of AIDS in South Africa; in this case, the protests were in fact against Western companies initially and continue against multinationals today, to the benefit of national companies. Wholesalers who claim to be "local" describe themselves as "dominated," stating they "reveal the domination they experience in order to free themselves from it, by denouncing it as a plot and by countering it with a nationalist project" (Fassin, 2007, p. 94). In this vein, we collected comments like this one, from the director of a wholesale company:

> Multinational companies are there to divide the profession because they know that if it is not divided, they will not be able to get established and sell in the market. And the president of the republic is behind it. (...) Look at UBPHAR, Médipharm, and GAPOB: all of the shareholders are Beninese. We are unique! This is the only country where locals perform most of the distribution. They can buy the others, but they won't get me. They can't buy me!!
>
> (Interview on October 7, 2015)

There is more than just ideology involved here, however. The economic stakes are a major factor in the tensions and conflicts sending tremors through Benin's wholesale distribution sector. In the course of their history, GAPOB and Sophabé have had other conflicts with private pharmacists over their access to a greater number of shares, which led the pharmacist-owners of the three largest pharmacies in Cotonou to withdraw from these organizations. At the end of the 1980s, these pharmacists joined forces to create Mareli Distribution, a wholesale company, but this had difficulty taking off. At the time it was created, the public Beninese pharmaceutical sector was bankrupt, so suppliers would not offer them deferred payment terms to allow them time to develop their business. They received a proposal for technical support from Eurapharma, the multinational mentioned earlier, which also acts as a central procurement agency and has its own logistics, which they accepted. Mareli Distribution became Promopharma, a subsidiary of Eurapharma, in 1991.[18] In 2011, while Ubipharm was trying to obtain its license to open and operate in Benin, the Order of Pharmacists was suing Promopharma's managing director and commercial director, a French pharmacist and a Congolese pharmacist, respectively, on the grounds that as foreigners they could not legally practice in Benin. Beninese legislation does in fact state that to establish in Benin, a wholesale company must "be managed by a pharmacist of Beninese nationality hired exclusively for this activity; this pharmacist may be of another nationality provided that there are reciprocity clauses between their country and Benin; this person is called the responsible pharmacist."[19] To comply with this clause, Eurapharma was careful to appoint a Beninese responsible pharmacist, but this individual was neither the managing director nor the commercial director. According to the commercial director at the time of our interviews, the Order of Pharmacists of Benin wanted to use the trial to "send a strong signal, they wanted to land a blow. It was intimidation against Ubipharm to show them that those who have been here for a long time are being attacked, so don't think you will be spared." That trial resulted in the complaint being withdrawn in 2015 following the election of the Order's officers, all of whom were new.[20]

The arrival of other private pharmacists on the market as well as internal conflicts (around money, power, and ideology) in various wholesale companies led some pharmacists to leave and create the UBPHAR in 1995, which is wholly owned by Beninese pharmacists. As the pharmaceutical market continued to grow, new pharmacists and those unable to access larger shares in existing wholesale companies were drawn to Ubipharm by their operating model. It is similar to Eurapharma's in that it acts as a single procurement group, but the Ubipharm model also gives them an opportunity to access shares in the "parent" or holding company, in addition to shares in the local wholesale company.

Under the combined effects of these ideological and economic challenges, the wholesale pharmaceutical distribution sector in Benin was divided into two types of actors: the three "locals" that are wholly owned by Beninese pharmacists who primarily run their private pharmacies, and the two multinational wholesalers, subsidiaries of large pharmaceutical groups based in Rouen, France, which provide wholesale distribution through a central procurement office and local wholesalers in various countries. Whether local or international, wholesale companies are subject to significant constraints by Beninese lawmakers that they try to either respect or circumvent in order to increase their share of the pharmaceutical market and grow their business.

### *Wholesale distribution practices: Legal obligations and circumvention strategies*

Under Article 1 of Decree no. 2000-450 of September 11, 2000 and Article 7 of Inter-ministerial Decree no. 006 of February 18, 2002, wholesaler-distributors are responsible "for the import, wholesale purchase, and distribution of medicines to private pharmacies and public health facilities and to all other pharmaceutical establishments" (Article 1 of Decree no. 2000-450). "They are not allowed to transfer medicines directly to private health facilities, state or private companies, or pharmaceutical warehouses in rural areas" (Article 7 of Inter-ministerial Decree no. 006).

In practice, wholesaler-distributors' main clients are the pharmacies that are found throughout the country. All wholesalers supply all pharmacies, although there are differences in volumes depending on their approach, business strategies, and personal affinities. Some wholesalers supply public hospitals and private clinics as well as pharmacies.

Wholesalers deliver products once a day on average to pharmacies in Cotonou and in the large nearby cities (Abomey-Calavi, Porto-Novo, and Ouidah). Pharmacies in other cities or towns receive some supplies once or twice a week or every 10 days from some of the wholesalers, using delivery vans; the rest arrive through shipments via taxis or passenger buses. GAPOB has a branch in the city

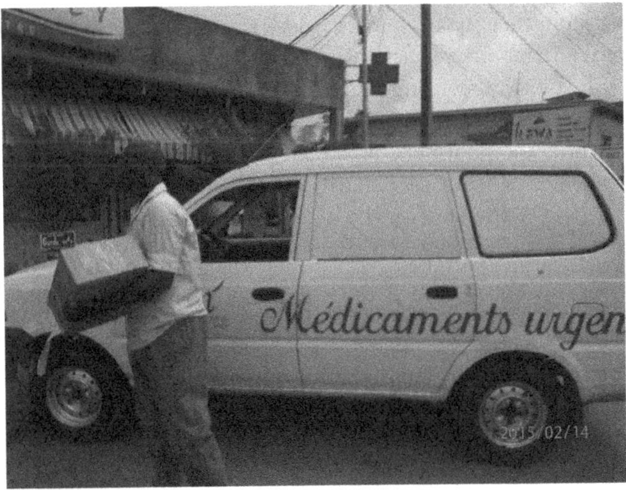


*Figure 2.3* Daily delivery of medication by a wholesaler-distributor to a pharmacy.

Source: © IRD/Stéphanie Mahamé, Cotonou, February 2015

of Bohicon and another in Parakou. UBPHAR also has a branch in Parakou, which gives these two wholesalers better coverage of the country than their competitors. Each wholesaler has its own strategy for covering its territory. UBPHAR and GAPOB have positioned themselves through their branches in the interior, while Promopharma is focusing on the country's largest pharmacies to earn its sales revenue. "I would say that most of Promopharma's sales are made to six pharmacies. Everything else is incidental… it's a different business strategy. That is, you can try to reach everyone, but you risk biting off more than you can chew. Or you can decide to only target the best and only work with them" (interview with the sales manager of one of the wholesale distribution companies, Cotonou, October 21, 2015). Our sources tell us that Ubiparm, which started operating while we were collecting data, has set up an Internet platform that provides access to complete product availability information and the ability to place orders online for pharmacies anywhere in Benin, anytime. It ships daily to pharmacies located in the interior of the country and makes deliveries to those in Cotonou and its surroundings. Pharmacists are given 15 days for payment, although some pay cash on delivery.

Faced with Beninese legislation that prohibits them from competing on price by setting their profit margins (a topic addressed in Chapter 3), wholesalers have developed strategies to increase their market share. One of the main sales strategies is to be the preferred wholesaler for as many pharmacies as possible. Pharmacists generally choose a main wholesaler to order from on a daily basis. They contact a second wholesaler, then a third, and so on down the list, only when the products they need are out of stock with their preferred supplier. This preferred wholesaler is not selected after years of doing business with the pharmacy; instead, it is generally chosen when the pharmacy first opens.

Given the significant financial resources required to set up a private pharmacy, banks often ask pharmacists for a wholesaler's backing as a guarantee. This backing entails providing a pharmacist with the initial stock of medicines, which the pharmacist will pay for according to a schedule negotiated between the two parties. Some wholesalers even lend the necessary money to pharmacists without interest. In return, the pharmacy is obligated to purchase its supplies primarily from this wholesaler and only secondarily from others until the loan for its initial stock is fully repaid to the bank or the wholesaler in question. The sales manager of a wholesale structure expressed it this way:

> We are in the business world; let's be honest, there are no perks. We don't set you up for your pretty face. We set you up because we want you as a client. So, you set up shop, you start buying from your main wholesaler. When you can't find a product with them, you move on to the next one, if they don't have it you move on to the third, and so on and so forth.
>
> (Interview, Cotonou, October 21, 2015)

Every 3 years the Ministry of Health publishes the national pharmaceutical map, at which point wholesalers approach the new pharmacists who have been authorized to open a business and propose their business conditions; these pharmacists then compare their options and make a choice. In this system, a wholesaler who has a branch in Bohicon and another in Parakou has a major advantage with the pharmacies located in those areas, who often choose them as their primary wholesaler for the ease of supply. This explains the domination of GAPOB and UBPHAR in specific areas of the country, which may be viewed as wholesalers dividing up the territory. The process of setting up a new pharmacy is therefore a key driver in how wholesale distribution is structured in Benin.

Wholesalers' sales strategies can also be seen in the support they offer to pharmacies, which may include visiting their premises and offering advice on store layout and product availability. Some wholesalers visit the Faculty of Pharmacy during scientific meetings to introduce themselves to young pharmacy students.

Another sales strategy used by some "local" wholesalers is to act as the distribution agents for certain firms in Benin. As such, they have the exclusive right to supply their own products, which they then use to supply both other wholesalers and pharmacies. Although the law requires wholesalers to stock "an assortment of pharmaceutical products representing at least nine-tenths of those authorized in Benin," it does not address the possibility of being the distribution agent for a trademark or product. This legal vacuum is exploited by wholesalers to increase their sales. These are important changes that are beginning to modify the practices of Beninese wholesalers, gradually approximating those of more liberal systems such as in Ghana (Baxerres, 2013); these are discussed in Chapters 3 and 6.

Another sales strategy we identified is for wholesalers to monitor the availability of certain commonly used drugs and ensure that they are in stock, bringing them in by the more expensive air route if necessary, when these products are out of stock with competitors. Wholesalers also use parapharmacy products, the prices of which are not fixed, to stimulate economic competition with their competitors. As the director of one of the wholesalers put it, "parapharmacy is not registered [with the government] so everyone does what they want" (interview, Cotonou, July 15, 2015). Competition is a daily factor in order-delivery speed, discounts, gifts, flexible payment terms, corporate calls,[21] and so forth. Some wholesalers offer trips to their best customers at the end of the year. These are professional or leisure trips, generally to Europe or the United States, paid for by the discounts offered to these high-volume customers throughout the year. One popular destination is the Pharmagora exhibition held every year in Paris, which brings pharmacists together from all over the world.

The financial challenges surrounding the private pharmaceutical market share are, in our opinion, the source of the conflicts disrupting this private wholesale pharmaceutical distribution sector in Benin. These conflicts are particularly evident when new actors arrive or when new pharmacies are authorized to open. They also result in fairly strong power and alliance relationships with the Order of Pharmacists and the Ministry of Health, the two regulatory authorities for pharmaceutical distribution.

## Conclusion: A buzzing pharmaceutical system

Benin's public and private wholesale distribution system has undeniable advantages in terms of efficiency and compliance with public health needs. The CAME has gradually established itself as an essential actor in Beninese pharmaceutical distribution, both public and private. Despite the challenges of conducting business in the context of a low-income country (mainly stock shortages), it was demonstrating a clear level of performance at the time of our study. In 1991, the CAME started with an EU-funded stock of medicines worth a mere CFA 450,000 (EUR 686); by 2017 sales revenue topped CFA 16 billion (nearly EUR 25 million)—2.5 billion (about EUR 19 million) from their own sales and 3.7 billion (about EUR 6 million) from government vaccine procurement—not to mention distributing products on behalf of transnational actors worth CFA 3.7 billion. The CAME's revenue has risen consistently over time, as its technical and human capacities have improved and its legal autonomy has grown. Sales revenue increased from CFA 5 billion (EUR 7.6 million) in 2007 to CFA 7 billion in 2010 (EUR 10.7 million), 10.5 billion in 2013 (EUR 16 million), and 12 billion from 2015 (EUR 18.3 million).[22] Moreover, since its supply system had been open from the outset to generic manufacturers, primarily in India, the association has been able to adequately fulfill its mission of providing essential medicines per the "price-quality" ratio mentioned earlier. Through the UGPS, it also provides an efficient logistics platform for distributing medicines funded by transnational actors. Wholesaler-distributor operations, strictly regulated, provided good levels of product availability and traceability at the time of our study. This will be discussed further in the next chapter and compared to the private wholesale sector in Ghana. Nevertheless, supply sources remained limited and focused exclusively on France (Baxerres, 2013), and the prices of drugs sold in private pharmacies were relatively high. However, as we have seen, this sector of activity, both public and private, is steeped in political, ideological, and economic challenges.

The tensions in Benin's wholesale distribution system since 2014 and Ubipharm's arrival in the country have led to a power struggle between the Ministry of Health and the Order of Pharmacists and, in turn, to upheavals and "a reconfiguration of the social space, a redefinition of fields of expertise and the lines that separate them, and a new relationship between professionals, society, and the State" (Aïach & Fassin, 1994, p. 1). This situation has been greatly exacerbated since the new president was elected in 2016. From his first months in office, President Talon's "disruptive" administration showed a desire to completely differentiate itself from all previous practices in the pharmaceutical sector and others.[23] Eradicating the informal market for medicines has been at the top of the president's agenda for this sector.

Several campaigns to clean up the pharmaceutical system have been undertaken since the 1990s, including by various health ministers, but none had had the scale and media coverage of Operation Pangea IX, launched on February 24, 2017. In his February 27 press conference, the Minister of the Interior declared "the operation was meticulously prepared and will be implemented on an ongoing basis throughout the country."[24] A man transporting pharmaceutical products was arrested as part of this operation, which led to the arrest, trial, and conviction of the directors of five of Benin's wholesalers as well as an elected deputy from the opposition party who also represented a pharmaceutical company. On March 13, 2018, the directors were all sentenced to 48 months in prison and two fines: one for CFA 10 million (EUR 15,300) to be paid by each individual, and the other for CFA 100 million (EUR 153,000) in damages to be paid jointly to the State. On appeal, the penalty was reduced to 48 months' imprisonment, including 18 before being eligible for parole, and a fine of CFA 100 million.[25]

At the close of the Council of Ministers meeting on March 14, 2018, the day after the wholesalers' conviction, the government suspended the National Order of Pharmacists for 6 months. On June 20, 2018, the government dropped another bombshell, issuing a decree withdrawing its approval from the CAME.[26] Another decree was signed on the same day concerning the entire pharmaceutical sector: Decree no. 2018-252 of June 20, 2018 establishing the Steering Committee to reform the pharmacy, medicines, and diagnostics sector in Benin. Known as the "Pharmed Committee," its mission is to "propose a new legal and institutional framework for pharmacy, medicines, and diagnostics operations and to assist the Ministry of Health in managing the period following the suspension of the Order of Pharmacists of Benin." Two years later and quite recently, in June 2020, the CAME was dissolved and replaced by the Beninese Society for Health Product Supply (SoBAPS, Société Béninoise pour l'Approvisionnement en Produits de Santé), a public limited company (SA) with the Beninese State as sole shareholder.

This situation echoes events in Burkina Faso, where the Central Purchasing Office for Essential Medicines and Generics (CAMEG), modeled entirely on the Beninese CAME, was disrupted for several months (approximately May 2016 to April 2017) by what the Burkinabe press described as a "political, economic, legal, and judicial battle."[27] That crisis began when a new government tried to replace the executive director and the chairman of the CAMEG board of directors through its Minister of Health.

How are we to understand such dramatic events and new strong measures by a government? As a reminder of State presence, particularly in the face of transnational actors? As a State that has become strong and capable? As one trying to regain control? The controversies surrounding the CAME's autonomy (not unlike Burkina Faso's CAMEG, perhaps) seem to argue in this direction, since the CAME is a major actor in Benin—where pharmaceutical production is low and the financial stakes center on importing and distributing medicines—facing off against the Ministry of Health. President Patrice Talon's speech at the International Conference on Access to Quality Medicines and Other Medical Products in Francophone Africa in Geneva on May 22, 2018 also suggests this position:

> The fight must become sincere, from every point of view. The major laboratories must stop developing production lines exclusively dedicated to poor countries [silence]. Such discrimination is immoral! It violates ethics, borders

> on being illegal, and weakens our fight against counterfeit drugs. Is it possible to have drugs made for the poor that are not recommended for the rich within the same country? Around the world, why are some drugs made for poor countries and not developed countries? (...). Developed countries don't really want to combat counterfeit medicines. What we are doing in Cotonou makes us sadly realize that we are alone in this fight. In Benin, there are deputies who are in prison because they are barons of counterfeit drug trafficking. There are expatriates who are in prison because they are involved in counterfeit drug trafficking.[28]

Recent events in Benin's pharmaceutical sector illuminate both the sector's strategic importance in the country and its structural weaknesses. These weaknesses were highlighted in the previous chapter and are evidenced by the current government's uncertainty about how to proceed.[29] The question we might ask after conducting a thorough inventory of the pharmaceutical system is: "Does the government in power intend to radically reform this domain?" If so, in what direction: away from the colonial French system and laws? Toward economic liberalization, or increasing investment in local production? Whatever the direction, our research shows that it will need to include significantly strengthening the technical, material, and qualified human resources capacities and skills of the national pharmaceutical regulatory authority.

## Notes

1. Jean Mazuet is a French pharmacist some call the "father of African pharmacy." In the 1950s and 1960s, he set up "wholesale" drug distribution companies managed by pharmacists in several francophone African countries: Benin, Burkina Faso, Cameroon, Côte d'Ivoire, Niger, and Senegal (Mazuet, 1987). He is also discussed in Chapter 1 on Côte d'Ivoire.
2. Pharmacists could import medicines directly but had to pay the ONP 2% of the purchase price (Baxerres, 2013).
3. There were no pharmacy schools in Benin at that time. Most pharmacists were trained in France, Russia, or Senegal.
4. The Eurapharma group, discussed in the previous chapter, belongs to the multinational CFAO, itself a subsidiary of the Pinault-Printemps-Redoute group. Its head office is based in Paris. It specializes in the distribution of medicines, initially to the French Overseas Departments and Territories and later to former French colonies in Africa. There are now 23 Eurapharma offices in Africa, including 7 in non-francophone countries (Angola, Kenya, and Uganda, and since 2008 Ghana, Nigeria, Tanzania, and Zambia) that were added beginning in the early 2000s as the group expands its presence beyond the French-speaking world. Sources: www.eurapharma.com and www.cfaogroup.com, accessed May 2019.
5. See the Introduction of the book for more information on the data collection methodology.
6. The concept of "essential medicines" emerged in the early 1970s. It emphasizes the need for low-income countries to prioritize the purchase of a limited number of essential and low-cost medicines for the health of their populations. Essential medicines should have four constituent properties: therapeutic efficacy, safety, meeting the health needs of populations, and cost-effectiveness. In the late 1970s, the

World Health Organization (WHO) established a list of "essential medicines," and international agencies, national governments, and nongovernmental organizations (NGOs) adopted this new policy beginning in the 1980s (Whyte, Van der Geest, & Hardon, 2002). The first national list of essential medicines dates to 1987–1988.

7. Composed of 13 members elected by each stakeholder category present at the general meeting, the management committee is the CAME's executive body. It meets once a quarter. A representative of the CAME staff participates in management committee meetings as an observer, and its director and his or her deputy also participate, but in an advisory capacity. Management committee members' terms are unpaid and last three years, renewable once. They are only reimbursed for the expenses they incur in the performance of their mission, on a flat-rate basis.
8. The agreement was signed in 1997 and updated in 2010.
9. These are private wholesaler-distributors and pharmacies.
10. Monopoly products are those for which the CAME has an import monopoly. These include all narcotic drugs and essential medicines still under patent.
11. WHO prequalification is a certification procedure set up by WHO in the early 2000s to ensure the quality of medicines to treat HIV, tuberculosis, and malaria. It was later extended to the certification of medicines to treat other diseases, raw materials, and quality control laboratories (Pourraz, 2019).
12. The CAME has three branches throughout the country: one in Cotonou to supply the south of the country, one in Natitingou to supply the north-west, and the third in Parakou for the north-east.
13. We were unable to obtain the precise date on which the CAME began issuing these accreditations.
14. These are health programs launched by transnational actors. The largest two in Benin are the Global Fund and USAID.
15. A previous study using 2007 figures reported that the financial volume of the private sector was more than four times that of the public sector: about CFA 21 billion (EUR 32 million) versus CFA 4.6 billion (about EUR 7 million) (Baxerres, 2013). Benin's pharmaceutical market appears to have increased considerably since 2007, but we were unable to obtain figures to determine the respective trends in the public and private sectors.
16. The letter was shown to us and read during an interview with one of that organization's managers. Interview conducted in Cotonou on July 15, 2015.
17. The Ubipharm company was discussed in Chapter 1. A spin-off of the Eurapharma group, this company has become one of the leaders in distributing medicines in French-speaking African countries through its local branch in Côte d'Ivoire.
18. It is a subsidiary of Eurapharma, just like Laborex Côte d'Ivoire, which Ivorian pharmacists rebelled against (see Chapter 1). The Ivoirian pharmacists created Pharmaholding, the future Ubipharm, which that same year acquired a procurement platform (Planet pharma) that was very similar to Eurapharma's (Continental pharmaceutique). The Eurapharma group's policy is to set up wholesaler-distributors in various countries in partnership with local companies.
19. See Article 2 of Decree no. 2000-450 of September 11, 2000, Implementing Act no. 97-020 of June 11, 1997, establishing the conditions for private practice in the medical and paramedical professions and relating to the opening of wholesale distribution companies in the Republic of Benin.
20. In comparison to Ghana, where a public entity—the Pharmacy Council—is responsible for regulating pharmacy practice, it is interesting to note that in Benin (as in France), the Order of Pharmacists is responsible for this regulation. This puts pharmacists in the positions of both jury and defendant, as our Ghanaian contacts pointed out to us. In the United Kingdom, a similar public entity has only existed since 2010—the General Pharmaceutical Council, which in that year succeeded the Royal Pharmaceutical Society of Great Britain (Mahalatchimy, 2017).

21. This is an arrangement whereby the wholesaler distributes mobile phones to its customers so that they can place orders at its own expense. This is a service offered by GSM operators that allows a limited number of numbers to be called at no additional charge for a fixed prepaid rate.
22. UGPS Accounting Department, CAME, July 2019.
23. Other examples include the reappropriation of public space, the appointment of deans and heads of institutions in public universities, and the practice of biomedicine in the private sector.
24. Source: *Les Pharaons* daily newspaper, https://www.lespharaons.com/le-benin-interdit-la-vente-des-medicaments-contrefaits/, accessed March 2019.
25. See the March 14, 2018 edition of the Beninese daily newspaper *La Nation*.
26. See Decree no. 2018-253 of June 20, 2018, withdrawing the approval granted to the Central Procurement Agency for Essential Medicines and Medical Consumables, according to which "the Minister of Health is authorized to terminate the partnership agreement between the Central Procurement Agency for Essential Medicines and Medical Consumables and the government, signed on September 29, 2010."
27. See the *Burkinabe news*, website Lefaso.net of April 9, 2017, http://lefaso.net/spip.php?article76583, accessed March 2019.
28. One of the imprisoned wholesaler-distributor directors is a French national.
29. Following the withdrawal of accreditation from the CAME on June 20, 2018, a subsequent press release on June 28, 2018 announced that the organization would continue until further notice. https://lanouvelletribune.info/2018/06/benin-retrait-dagrement-a-la-came-le-ministre-hounkpatin-clarifie-son-homologue-de-la-justice-menace/, accessed April 2019. Also, in 2019, a presidential announcement called on the CAME to source only from internationally certified suppliers and WHO; this decision was later reversed. The very recent creation of SoBAPS and the dissolution of the CAME nevertheless shows the government's current direction in this regard.

## Reference list

Aïach, P., & Fassin, D. (1994). *Les métiers de la santé. Enjeux de pouvoir et quête de légitimité [Health careers. Power issues and the quest for legitimacy]*. Paris, France: Anthropos.

Baxerres, C. (2013). *Du médicament informel au médicament libéralisé : Une anthropologie du médicament pharmaceutique au Bénin [From informal to liberalized drugs: An anthropology of pharmaceutical drugs in Benin]*. Paris, France: Les Éditions des Archives Contemporaines.

Boidin, B., & Savina, M.-D. (1996). Privatisation des services sociaux et redéfinition du rôle de l'État : Les prestations éducatives et sanitaires au Bénin [Privatization of social services and redefinition of the role of the State: Educational and health services in Benin]. *Tiers Monde*, *37*, 853–874.

Brown, T. M., Cueto, M., & Fee, E. (2006). The World Health Organization and the transition from "international" to "global" public health. *American Journal of Public Health*, 96(1), 62–72.

Chabrol, F. (2012). *Prendre soin de sa population. Le sida au Botswana entre politiques globales du médicament et pratiques locales de citoyenneté [Taking care of its people. AIDS in Botswana between global drug policies and local citizenship practices]*. Doctoral dissertation, Ecole des Hautes Etudes en Sciences Sociales, Paris, France. Retrieved from https://tel.archives-ouvertes.fr/tel-00766707v1.

Cling, J., & Roubaud, F. (2008). Introduction. In J.-P. Cling (Ed.), *La Banque mondiale [The World Bank]* (pp. 3–6). Paris: La Découverte.

Desclaux, A., & Egrot, M. (Eds.). (2015). *Anthropologie du médicament au Sud. La pharmaceuticalisation à ses marges [Anthropology of medicines in the South. Pharmaceuticalization at its margins]*. Paris, France: L'Harmattan.

Fassin, D. (1987). La santé, un enjeu politique au quotidien [Health, a daily political issue]. In E. Le Roy (Ed.), *Politique africaine n 28: Politiques de santé [African politics no. 28: Health policies]* (pp. 1–8). Paris, France: Karthala.

Fassin, D. (2007). Entre désir de nation et théorie du complot. Les idéologies du médicament en Afrique du Sud [Between national hopes and conspiracy theories. Drug ideologies in South Africa]. *Sciences Sociales et Santé, 25*(4), 93–114.

Lomba, C. (2014). Les grossistes de médicaments : Juste-à-temps et normes sanitaires [Drug wholesalers: Just-in-time systems and health standards]. In P. Fournier, C. Lomba, & S. Muller (Eds.), *Les travailleurs du médicament. L'industrie pharmaceutique sous observation [Drug workers. The pharmaceutical industry under observation]* (pp. 251–273). Toulouse, France: ERES.

Loyola, M. A. (2009). Sida, santé publique et politique du médicament au Brésil : Autonomie ou dépendance? [AIDS, public health, and drug policy in Brazil: Autonomy or dependence?]. *Sciences Sociales et Santé, 27*(3), 47–75.

Mahalatchimy, A. (2017). Le monopole pharmaceutique en Grande Bretagne [The pharmaceutical monopoly in Great Britain]. In A. Leca, C. Maurain, I. Moine-Dupuis, & G. Rousset (Eds.), *Le monopole pharmaceutique et son avenir [The pharmaceutical monopoly and its future]* (pp. 109–127). Bordeaux, France: LEH Édition.

Mazuet, J. (1987). Portrait. Jean Mazuet: Souvenirs d'Afrique [Portrait. Jean Mazuet: Memories of Africa]. *Afrique pharmacie, Bulletin de liaison de l'association pharmaceutique interafricaine, 4*, 7.

OMS. (2002). La sélection des médicaments essentiels [The selection of essential medicines]. Perspectives politiques de l'OMS sur les médicaments [WHO policy perspectives on medicines]. 4. https://apps.who.int/iris/bitstream/handle/10665/67376/WHO_EDM_2002.2_fre.pdf?sequence=1.

Pourraz, J. (2019). *Réguler et produire les médicaments contre le paludisme au Ghana et au Bénin : Une affaire d'Etat ? Politiques pharmaceutiques, normes de qualité et marchés de médicaments [Regulating and manufacturing antimalarial drugs in Ghana and Benin: A State affair? Pharmaqceutical policies, quality standards, and drug markets]*. PhD thesis. http://www.theses.fr/2019EHES0014/document.

Ridde, V. (2004). Kingdon à Bamako: Conceptualiser l'implantation d'une politique publique de santé en Afrique [Kingdon in Bamako: Conceptualizing the implementation of a public health policy in Africa]. *Politique et Sociétés, 23*(2–3), 183–202.

Tizio, S., & Flori, Y. (1997). L'initiative de Bamako: Santé pour tous ou maladie pour chacun? [The Bamako Initiative: Health for all or disease all around?]. *Tiers Monde*, 38(152), 837–858.

Van der Geest, S. (1987). Self-care and the informal sale of drugs in South Cameroon. *Social Science & Medicine, 25*(3), 293–305.

Whyte, R. S., Van der Geest, S., & Hardon, A. (2002). *Social lives of medicines*, New York, NY: Cambridge University Press.

# 3 Distribution and access to medicines

## Role of the pharmacist monopoly

*Carine Baxerres, Adolphe Codjo Kpatchavi, Daniel Kojo Arhinful*

### Introduction

The States of the world, whether in the "North" or the "South," use a variety of mechanisms to regulate pharmaceutical distribution, chosen at different points in history for various reasons. These mechanisms are built around the issue of the pharmacist's monopoly, granted by the State, and the scope of this monopoly, which varies by country.

France is the emblematic example of a country where this monopoly is most broadly applied (Fouassier, 2017).[1] The monopoly of French pharmacists is an ancient institution that gradually formed between the 11th and 18th centuries (Leca, Maurain, Moine-Dupuis, & Rousset, 2017) and was established by the "Germinal law" under Napoleon Bonaparte on 21 Germinal year XI (1803), even before the advent of industrial drug production. This monopoly was granted to pharmacists in exchange for their incorporation as a true profession, one requiring competence guaranteed by a diploma (Guerriaud, 2017). The French pharmacy sector was built up over the 20th century through the consolidation of the pharmacist profession (Van den Brink, 2017). Development was very different in the United Kingdom, where this sector was formed by the market using the free trade model. Stuart Anderson (2005) notes that, through the Pharmacy Act of 1868, "the emphasis on 'trade' as opposed to dispensing activities was maintained" (p. 79). The English retail distribution model is now described as "based on opening private pharmacies' capital and an economic approach to the profession. (…). Opening the capital of private pharmacies should increase competitiveness and promote lower prices, since economic interests are at the forefront" (Debarge, 2011, p. 202).

This monopoly can be applied to various aspects of pharmacy practice. It may be a professional monopoly, i.e., access to the profession in which only pharmacists can manufacture and/or distribute medicines. It may be a retail sales monopoly, i.e., a dispensing monopoly in which retail drugs may only be sold in pharmacies. Finally, it may be a monopoly of ownership in which only pharmacists can own an establishment in which pharmacy-related activity is practiced, be this the manufacture and/or wholesale and/or retail distribution of a drug (Leca et al., 2017). In France, only pharmacists may prepare medicines for human use, regardless of context—industrial, compounding, hospital, or dispensary—and engage in wholesale or retail sales of medicines. In return for this monopoly, pharmacists have an obligation to perform their public health missions. "One of the most important considerations is personal and exclusive practice: 'pharmacists who have a private pharmacy must personally practice their profession. (…). The same is true for managing pharmacists (along with their delegates and deputies) involved in bulk drug manufacturing or distribution'" (Guerriaud, 2017, pp. 24–25). Such personal practice is especially required for a private pharmacy, where the pharmacy owner cannot be engaged in any other activity. In addition, private pharmacists must provide the necessary information and advice for the proper use of the medicinal product. This point is another strong argument for justifying the monopoly in France, one repeated in the pharmacist's code of ethics. In France, one often hears that "medicines are unlike any other product, and as such require compliance with precautions for use or contraindications. (…). Whenever they feel it is necessary, pharmacists should encourage their patients to consult a qualified practitioner. (…). Thus, private pharmacists must yet again put the interests of public health before their own economic interests" (Guerriaud, 2017, p. 25).

But historians remind us that the French government granting this monopoly is part of a broader movement through which the State has, since the French Revolution, maintained a privileged and protective relationship with the legal, medical, and pharmaceutical professions, known as the liberal professions.[2] According to Jean-Paul Gaudillière, "in this system of professions, the status of medicines was initially intended to defend the monopoly in drug preparation and sales granted to degreed pharmacists on the basis of their scientific skills" (Gaudillière, 2005, p. 133). Thus, restricting actions to pharmacists alone also guarantees them an economic monopoly, "by defending access to the profession and exclusive sales" (Guerriaud, 2017, p. 12). Pharmacists are not only health professionals; they also have "commercial status or practice their profession within a commercial enterprise." They nearly always perform "commercial acts remunerated by a mark-up that is also commercial in nature" (Fouassier, 2017, p. 52).

The current debates on the pharmaceutical monopoly in Europe are especially polarizing. Proponents and opponents of the monopoly regularly inveigh against each other, one side propounding the demands of public health and the other the primacy of economic freedom and competition between economic actors. It is frequently noted, particularly in France, that this monopoly maximizes the ability to fulfill public health requirements. It is "a remarkable tool in the service of safeguarding health security" (Guerriaud, 2017, p. 11). This is something that British and American pharmacy experts generally disagree on. In this chapter, we examine this monopoly and the consequences of the different ways it is applied to retail and wholesale distribution in Benin and Ghana as a result of the institutional and legal legacies of their former colonial powers.[3]

## Legislative differences in pharmaceutical distribution

### *Pharmacies, pharmaceutical warehouses, and over-the-counter medicine sellers*

In Benin, as in France, the pharmacist's monopoly prevails. It was established by Order no. 73-38 of April 21, 1973, establishing and organizing the Ordre national des pharmaciens or National Order of Pharmacists.[4] Private pharmacy is defined as "a health facility opened and managed by an owner-pharmacist," dedicated to dispensing prescriptions and preparing medicines and pharmaceutical products. Retail medicines in Benin can only be legally distributed in these private pharmacies.[5] As in French law, a licensed pharmacist must be registered with the Order of Pharmacists and may only own one pharmacy. In 2015, there were 243 private pharmacies in operation in the country,[6] which are authorized to sell all drugs registered in Benin.[7]

In Ghana, two types of licenses are granted for the retail sale of pharmaceuticals. One is the general license for pharmacies managed by a qualified pharmacist who is registered with the Pharmacy Council, but who may be an employee and not necessarily the owner.[8] The other is the limited license granted to "over-the-counter (OTC) medicine shops," commonly known as "chemical shops," which are managed by non-pharmacists with a minimum academic level (Middle School Leaving Certificate[9]) who must attend mandatory post-registration training sessions on a regular basis.[10] Shops are inspected by Pharmacy Council agents and must comply with certain conditions, such as space and ventilation, before obtaining authorization.[11] Unlike pharmacies, the OTC medicine sales license is granted for an individual who operates a single store.

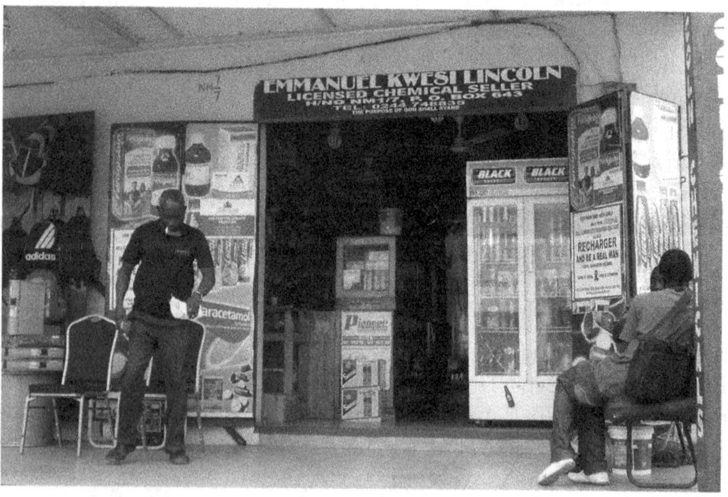


*Figure 3.1* OTC medicine shop in Accra.

Source: © IRD/Carine Baxerres, mai 2015

There were 2175 pharmacies and 10,424 OTC medicine shops in Ghana in 2015.[12] Ghanaian pharmacies are allowed to sell all Food and Drugs Authority (FDA) categories of pharmaceuticals, i.e., prescription-only medicines (also known as Class A drugs), those pharmacists can recommend based on their scientific expertise (pharmacy-only medicines, called Class B drugs), and OTC medicines (Class C drugs).[13] The only drugs permitted to be sold in OTC medicine shops are those designated as Class C by the authorities, including some public health program products such as antimalarials or contraceptives. Antibiotics are not officially to be sold in these stores, with the exception of cotrimoxazole.

In Benin, although the status of OTC medicines is not recognized, since 1975 there have been private pharmaceutical warehouses in rural areas, the owners of which do not have a degree in pharmacy; they must have an education at least equivalent to the Certificate of Primary Studies and receive "appropriate training" when they first open (Article 1, Decree no. 2000-410 of August 17, 2000). These shops are authorized to sell essential medicines from a limited list[14] and were established to expand pharmacy services in the country. However, they are subject to strict legislation that, in our opinion, impedes their development.[15] In keeping with the pharmacist's monopoly, these facilities are under a pharmacist's supervision and shut down if a pharmacy opens within a 10-km radius. Warehouse owners must obtain their supplies from a private pharmacist. Products must be sold at the retail price even though they are purchased at a pre-established margin from the pharmacists, who sell them to the warehouse at a price marked up from the wholesale prices they paid. This category is therefore both underdeveloped and shrinking in Benin: there were 279 such facilities in 2006, 250 in 2007, 179 in 2013, and only 165 in 2018.[16]

Pharmacies are not equitably distributed throughout either Ghana or Benin, but instead are concentrated in urban areas. In Benin, 97 of the 243 pharmacies operating in 2015 were in the economic capital (Cotonou), 29 were in the adjacent cities to the west (Godomey and Abomey-Calavi), and 33 were in the administrative capital (Porto-Novo) located 42 km northeast of Cotonou, meaning all were located in cities and the southern part of the country. In Ghana, 1323 of the country's 2175 pharmacies operating in 2015 were located in the Greater Accra area. In Accra itself, our field surveys showed that pharmacies were mainly found in the city's most exclusive districts (Agblevor, 2016). The semirural area where we worked in this country, Breman Asikuma in the Central Region, had no pharmacies at all. The semirural area where we conducted our surveys in Benin, in the Mono department, had one pharmacy at that time, in the city of Comé.

Retail distribution in these two countries thus differs significantly. What about wholesale distribution?

### *Wholesaler-distributors versus private wholesalers*

The legislation governing private wholesaler operations in Benin and Ghana is radically different. In Benin, wholesalers are considered full public service actors and legislation significantly limits their activity, whereas in Ghana, they have much greater leeway in how they conduct business.

In France, pharmaceutical wholesaler practices were codified and the profession of "wholesaler-distributor" was recognized by legislation in 1962 with the introduction of social security. The expansion of social security to include the costs of treatment required stronger regulation by the State, which sought to more effectively control product costs (Chauveau, 2005).[17] Drug prices and distributor profit margins also began to be established at that time (Lanore, 2008; Le Guisquet & Lorenzi, 2001). Prior to that, when the first pharmaceutical distribution companies appeared at the end of the 19th century, they freely advertised their services and engaged in unbridled competition (Chauveau, 2005; Faure, 2005; Sueur, 2018). In Benin, although the country had only recently gained independence when the French legislation on wholesaler-distributors was introduced and the country had no universal system for covering health expenses,[18] very similar regulation was adopted specific to pharmaceutical distribution. The first wholesalers set up their businesses in Benin in the 1980s before there was any specific legislation for that industry (see Chapter 2); provisions were later ratified by Decree no. 2000-450 of September 11, 2000, implementing Act no. 97-020 of June 11, 1997. These provisions stipulate that "wholesale distribution companies" are a "pharmaceutical and wholesale establishment for medicines and wound-care products opened and managed by a pharmacist (…) of Beninese nationality engaged exclusively in this activity." The company must be "owned by a pharmacist or a company whose general management is provided by a pharmacist. The chairperson and the majority of the members of the board of directors must be pharmacists." As in French legislation (Lomba, 2014), these companies have binding public service obligations. They must "carry an assortment of pharmaceuticals representing at least nine-tenths (9/10) of those authorized in Benin," which they import. Each must also "carry stock, at all times and at a minimum, covering three months of typical customer use." In addition, "the sales prices charged for medicines registered in the Republic of Benin by a wholesaler-distributor company to retail pharmacists or public health facilities are fixed by decree adopted by the Council of Ministers." Therefore, as public health actors, these companies are not in competition with each other through their products or their prices.[19] They cannot legally invest in promoting medicines, nor can they engage in retail sales. Because of these binding obligations, at the time of our research study, five players shared the private pharmaceutical market.

Completely different legislation governs private wholesalers operating in Ghana. These laws provide the actors who invest capital in this domain with significant room for maneuvering. Again, as noted previously regarding pharmacies, these individuals may or may not be pharmacists. Those who are not are required to employ a registered pharmacist (see Act no. 489 and Act no. 857). They do not sell all the medicines authorized in the country; some only distribute a single product or drugs manufactured by a single pharmaceutical company. These factors explain why there are so many: 576 were operating in the country at the end of 2013, only a small portion of whom (38 companies) had multiple branches in

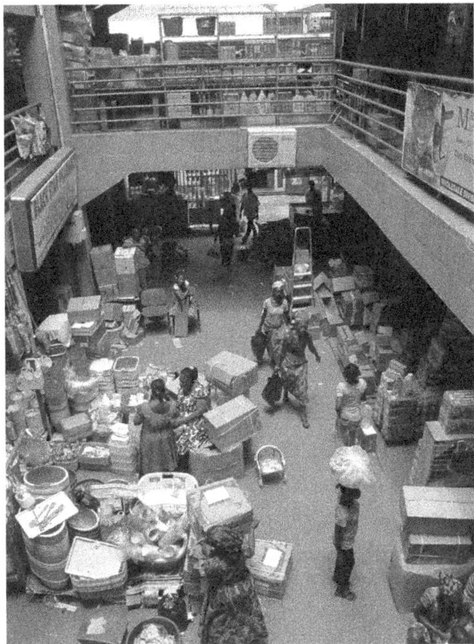

*Figure 3.2* Inside one of the seven private buildings of the Okaishie market where the wholesale distribution of medicines takes place.

Source: © IRD/Carine Baxerres, août 2014

different parts of the country.[20] Most of these companies (377) were both wholesalers and retailers, and 199 were wholesalers only. A significant proportion of them imported drugs after registering with Ghana's FDA.[21] Many were located in the so-called drug lane section of the Okaishie market in Accra (see Figure 3.2 above).

Unlike their Beninese counterparts, private wholesalers in Ghana promote the medicines they distribute, especially when they import the products as well. Depending on their company's capital and number of employees, owners either hire "sales reps" or "medical reps" or handle promotion themselves (see the section in Chapter 9 on this subject). Another major difference in pharmaceutical distribution between the two countries is that drug prices and wholesaler and retailer distributor profit margins are freely set by the market in Ghana, whereas they are set by public authorities in Benin, as we noted earlier.[22] In Ghana, therefore, private wholesalers compete on the basis of both price and products.

The legislative elements described earlier show that, for both wholesale and retail distribution, the pharmacist's monopoly is very strong in Benin but quite limited in Ghana, similar to what Aurélie Mahalatchimy (2017) notes for the United Kingdom. What consequences can we demonstrate when the pharmacist's monopoly is applied so differently?

## Consequences for pharmacy practice

Rather than presenting an exhaustive review of all current pharmacy practices in Benin and Ghana, in this section, we will examine only those aspects that best illustrate the consequences of how the pharmacist monopoly is applied in the two countries. We could have described some of the informal practices in pharmacies and pharmaceutical depots in Benin, such as the sale of drugs without a prescription, but these have been discussed elsewhere for Benin (Anago, Djralah, Kpatchavi, & Baxerres, 2016) and other countries (Kamat & Nichter, 1998; Van Der Geest, 1987).

### *A large informal drug market in Benin*[23]

The below figure (see Figure 3.3) summarizes the information presented earlier, clearly highlighting one of the major consequences of these legislative differences (in bold). Ghana's population and size are more than double that of Benin, but that does not explain the disproportionate number of legal retail pharmaceutical distribution structures in the two countries. While Ghana had 2175 private pharmacies in 2015, Benin had a mere 243. More than 10,000 (10,324) OTC medicine shops were operating that year in Ghana, compared to 179 pharmaceutical depots in 2013 in Benin. Admittedly, private pharmacies in Ghana, like wholesalers operating in that country, do not distribute most authorized medicines, so the profile of these structures differs between the two countries. Nevertheless, it is clear that the gap left by official distribution structures in Benin is filled by a large informal market for medicines.[24]

**Benin**
(population 9.9 million; area 112,622 km²)

- Pharmacist's monopoly strongly enforced
- **243** private pharmacies
- **179** pharmaceutical depots in rural areas
- 5 private wholesaler-distributors
- Wholesalers must offer 9/10 of the products authorized in the country. They cannot promote drugs
- Drug prices are set by the authorities

**Ghana**
(population 24 million; area 239,460 km²)

- Pharmacist's monopoly very limited
- **2175** private pharmacies
- **10,324** OTCMS
- 199 private wholesalers
- 377 private wholesalers who are also retailers
- Wholesalers can distribute a single company's products if they wish. They promote medicines
- Drug prices are not regulated

*Figure 3.3* Summary of formal pharmaceutical distribution data in Benin and Ghana.

Source: Pharmacy Council Ghana 2015, DPMED Benin 2013 (2015 population figures)

We did observe informal itinerant sellers in the Accra city center, who generally sold medicines they had just purchased from private wholesalers in the surrounding area.[25] In rural areas around Breman Asikuma, we met some street vendors, several of whom were in fact associated with a local OTC medicine seller and, as such, peddled medicines to the most remote villages and hamlets.[26] During an observation of an OTC medicine shop in a rural area, one of these vendors, who had come to obtain supplies, explained: "I have been in the drug business for about 10 years now. I started with one man whom I peddled with, but now that man owns a chemical shop. But me, I haven't been able to establish my own" (field diary, June 10, 2015). Several OTC medicine shop owners we interviewed in rural areas had been street vendors in the 1980s, 1990s, and even 2000s. We also observed informal itinerant vendors on public transport, particularly inter-municipal or interregional buses.[27] The foregoing is not to deny the presence of an informal drug market in Ghana but to emphasize that that market has nothing in common with the one we have been studying since the mid-2000s in Benin. From the most remote villages of Ghana to the densely populated working-class neighborhoods and even shantytowns, OTC medicine shops with a Pharmacy Council authorization can be found absolutely everywhere in the country.

The informal market in Benin was highly developed at the time we conducted our research. A previous study we conducted in Cotonou with retailers as well as with the wholesalers in the sprawling Dantokpá market (Baxerres, 2013) focused on describing the gradual emergence of this informal market in the early 1950s, how it functioned, and the role it played for the city's residents, primarily as a distribution outlet. Some 4–6 years later, not much had changed. The quantitative survey we conducted among nearly 600 households on access to health care in Cotonou revealed that when pharmaceutical drugs are needed, 26% of respondents said they had used informal (generally female) vendors even though they preferentially obtain supplies from official pharmacies (65%).[28] As we had observed previously, such vendors were omnipresent in the city, in a variety of forms: in shops and stalls, as roving street vendors, set up along roadsides, and selling from homes or in neighborhood markets (Baxerres, 2013) as well as near construction sites (Kpatchavi, 2012).

The reality of the informal market was significantly different in rural and semirural areas of the Mono department where we worked. Informal sellers were qualitatively more present, since formal distribution actors were much less represented than in urban areas. For example, in Lobogo, where we conducted a quantitative study of 580 households, people reported that they obtained their medications in almost equal proportions from the health center pharmacy (39%) as from informal vendors (35%). Only 23% of purchases were made from private pharmacies and warehouses. In addition, these saleswomen in rural settings appear to have quite a bit more influence on what their customers purchase than vendors in urban areas do. They advised their clients on what medicines to buy 30% of the time; in contrast, in Cotonou, this was true for less than 6% of purchases (Baxerres, 2013). This can be seen in an excerpt from an interview with a middle-class mother: "I said that my child had started a fever. She asked me what fever, how long ago it started, and I told her three days. She asked what I had been doing at home for three days. I told her I was giving para [paracetamol] and other medicines, that's why I waited to see if there would be any improvement, but since there wasn't any, that's why I brought him. So she sold him the drugs (…), she said she was going to sell him the deworming and I said I already have some. (…). She sold me a lot… she sold me a lot of medicine that looks like para… she sold me a lot of medicines, including the malaria drug with the drawing of mosquitoes" (interview, January 4, 2015).

Apart from self-imposed rules and standards and the trade licenses that those who work in these locations pay to market management companies, these legions of informal sellers are not regulated by any institutional entity. Their activity is completely unregulated. According to Joseph Nyoagbe, then head of the Pharmacy Council of Ghana, the massive development of the informal drug

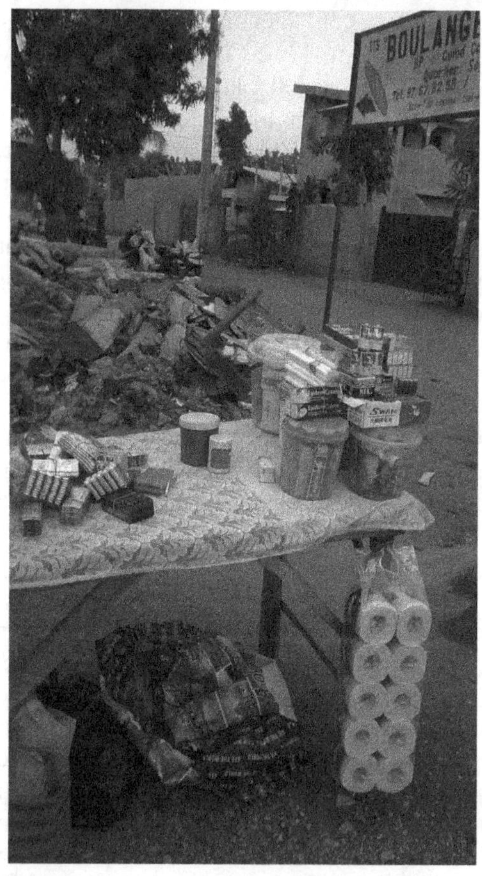

*Figure 3.4* Stall of an informal saleswoman in semirural Benin.

Source: © IRD/Anani Agossou, février 2015

market in French-speaking West African countries can be explained by the fact that there is no system of private pharmaceutical distribution below the level of pharmacies in these countries[29] (interview conducted during a previous study in July 2007 in Accra). We will see in the next two sections that although Ghanaian pharmaceutical regulatory authorities exercise real control over pharmacy practices, informal practices in both retail and wholesale activities continue to flourish in that country as well.

### *Informal practices among Ghanaian retailers*

Although all the OTC medicine shops operating in the locations we surveyed in Ghana are licensed by the Pharmacy Council, several of their practices fall outside the scope of the legislation presented earlier (Act no. 489 and Act no. 857).

First, the people who receive the license and participate in the continuing education are not necessarily the ones who actually work in the stores on a daily basis, something Pharmacy Council agents are not fooled by: "If you are doing the training (…) how would you be very sure that this man who is participating is actually sitting in the facility? (…). The majority of those people who have their names on the licenses are not there" (Pharmacy Council Head of Education and Training, Accra, June 3, 2016). In fact, many of these are family businesses involving multiple family members: husband, wife, children, including middle and high school students who work after school, and sometimes even more distant family members (such as an uncle, cousin, or nephew). Stores that are not family businesses generally see a succession of employees one after another, who may or may not work alongside the owner.[30] These employees are rarely "Medicine Counter Assistants,"[31] although this is more often the case in urban areas. More commonly they are referred to simply as "shop attendants." Another phenomenon occurs when the official owner dies or transfers their license, yet the license remains in their name and continues to be renewed for several years. Finally, some OTC medicine shop owners open multiple stores, using the identity of other people to obtain the authorization, which is not allowed.

We observed several OTC medicine shops, both rural and urban, engage in other unauthorized activities, delivering health-care services in addition to medicine distribution (offering injections, infusions, diagnostic microscope tests, occasionally even "hospitalization"), in a room either directly adjacent to the store or located nearby. Some open a drug sales business after retiring as a health worker (nurse, midwife), but this is not always the case. Surprisingly, although Ghanaian health authorities appear to have cracked down on the illegal practice of medicine—evidenced by the fact that our field studies show far fewer informal health structures or health workers even in semirural areas than in the less-regulated 1990s (Senah, 1997)—Pharmacy Council agents do not seem focused on curtailing the health-care practices of these OTC medicine shops (Arhinful, Sams, Kpatinvoh, & Baxerres, 2018). Also outside the legal framework of their activities, some OTC medicine shops act as wholesale supply outlets for their counterparts in the neighborhood and sometimes even for nearby public health facilities (health centers and community-based health planning and services [CHPS] compounds),[32] particularly in rural or semirural areas where access to formal wholesalers is more difficult.

The biggest criticism leveled at OTC medicine shops is that they sell drugs from therapeutic classes well outside their legal purview. Antibiotics are undoubtedly of greatest concern, given the current more-than-critical issue of resistance. But other prescription drugs (Classes A and B) are also involved (to end pregnancy or treat anxiety, hypertension, diabetes, asthma, etc.).[33] In short, OTC medicine shops follow the law of supply and demand to sell what their customers want, think they need, and can afford.

Despite these criticisms, this system does have strong points. OTC medicine shops must account for their practices to Pharmacy Council inspectors, who are more numerous and more efficient than their Beninese counterparts.[34] An OTC medicine seller explained: "The Pharmacy Council does check on us. They don't give you the date that they are coming. It is impromptu. If they see an inappropriate item, they will take it. (…). Sometimes they could lock the shop and take the key to their office for a few days" (field diary, semirural area, July 24, 2015).[35] Ghanaian FDA inspectors are also supposed to inspect these businesses. In addition, OTC medicine shops distribute drugs purchased from authorized wholesalers. Finally, and we will come back to this in Chapter 10, OTC medicine shops play a key role in Ghana as first-line care providers—just as Beninese informal sellers do in rural areas—because of their very high geographical accessibility, their long business hours, and the close social proximity of their vendors (Agblevor, Missodey, Arhinful, & Baxerres, 2016).

### *Informal practices among Ghanaian wholesalers*

However, in our opinion, the informal practices found among wholesalers in Ghana pose the greater risk to public health. These practices question the validity of the very weak application of the pharmacist monopoly in that country.

As we have seen, unlike Benin, a businessman or woman can open a wholesale company in Ghana and import medicines without being a pharmacist but must employ a pharmacist. Of the 25 wholesaler owners we interviewed, 9 were pharmacists. The other 16 either had no specific training (generally the case for the older owners) or had studied marketing, accounting, business, or administration; one had completed 3 years of science studies (chemistry, geology, botany). Quite often, when the owner is not a pharmacist, the "superintendent pharmacist," i.e., the person through whom the facility obtained its authorization to open, is not actually present or is only occasionally present at the wholesale facility. These individuals usually work in teaching positions, government departments, or for other pharmaceutical establishments. They often agreed, for a fee, to provide their license to obtain authorizations from the Pharmacy Council but are not regularly present in the stores, merely stopping by from time to time.

A wholesale company employee explained these business practices this way: "The pharmacists [in the two branches they have] don't come that often, maybe once in a week or even at times once every month" (interview, Accra, September 19, 2015). An employee of another company stated: "Everyday he [the pharmacist] comes here, but he is working somewhere else as well, but every day he comes here" (interview, Accra, August 21, 2014). Again, another study participant told us: "We have a pharmacist. He doesn't come… he doesn't come here at all… we just pay him his money. He just comes for his money" (interview, Accra, November 30, 2015). This is especially true of small companies that would have real difficulty paying the salary of a full-time pharmacist.

The most influential companies on the market, which cannot afford to violate the law, do employ pharmacists who are permanently on site. But the fact that they are employees, and therefore subordinate to the owner, changes or at least influences the dynamic. Our observations showed that their activities are often limited to taking inventories of current or missing stock, or products that must be acquired at advantageous costs. As expressed by the then Pharmacy Council Head of Education and Training: "Sometimes I ask myself, if we are to actually enforce the laws on regulation, then the poor pharmacist will be finished, because there will be so many issues that the pharmacist cannot explain (…) you regulate the pharmacist…. Will the pharmacist be able to check the others? How? The pharmacist doesn't own the pharmacy. He is an employee" (interview, Accra, June 1, 2016).

What are the implications of this significant investment by non-pharmacists in the practice of wholesale pharmacy? First of all, wholesalers spend considerable time in the pharmacy sector in Ghana, through their sales representatives, maintaining their business relationships, promoting their products, and keeping abreast of market developments. This will be discussed in Chapter 9. In empirical observations, such activities, related to trade rather than pharmacy practice or health care, take a considerable amount of time. The extent of these commercial activities may be largely due to the fact that products are not sold at the same price everywhere and that wholesalers do not all sell the same products. Our field studies and interviews with wholesalers in Accra highlighted two types of significant informal dealings in addition to these relational (and not informal) activities.

First, their customers include three types of informal actors alongside those actually authorized to obtain supplies from wholesalers (pharmacies, OTC medicine shops, public and private health centers, other wholesalers). These include the few informal retailers mentioned earlier who resell drugs in Accra's city center. Second, informal wholesale vendors from French-speaking countries in the West African region (Benin, Burkina Faso, Côte d'Ivoire, Mali, Togo, etc.), as discussed earlier regarding Benin, represent an important clientele for wholesale companies in Ghana, especially those in the Okaishie market in Accra, both quantitatively (in terms of the number of vendors) and qualitatively (they buy a lot and pay cash). A feature of the Okaishie market is that it is able to accommodate this type of clientele. Finally, the third category of informal wholesale customers is the intermediaries or "independent sales reps" (for representatives), as they were called by an employee of a wholesale company (interview on June 4,

2016, Accra). These are individuals who do not have a formal authorization but who are involved in the pharmacy business by buying products from wholesalers, then reselling them to retailers or even private individuals who need them. They offer their clients extremely flexible services (delivering at very late hours, providing the desired products quickly, finding drugs that are out of stock or hard to access, etc.), which allows them to build up a clientele that prefers using them rather than wholesalers, despite the relatively higher cost. They also provide a service to wholesalers who, through them, can increase their customer base and thus their sales. They help promote products from importers, usually small companies who do not have sales representatives, and sometimes also work for larger wholesalers. These intermediaries take advantage of occasional drug shortages, seen as inevitable in the market, to sell products they had purchased earlier at a higher price during shortages, thus earning higher profits. Anyone can buy medicines from Ghana's numerous authorized wholesalers, especially in Okaishie.[36] Our observations also showed that, in practice, all customers, both formal and informal, can purchase medicines from any therapeutic category they want to from wholesalers. This was easily demonstrated by looking at how wholesale companies create invoices and how client files are compiled in the software: "A man came to buy 20 boxes of Tanzol [an anthelmintic]; for the customer's name, the young woman in charge of writing the invoice wrote 'cash'. She then explained to me that when customers do not come from a pharmacy or chemical shop and are only buying for themselves, they [the staff of the wholesale company] write 'cash'" (field diary, Accra, August 8, 2014).[37]

A second important observed informality is that despite existing inspection and control mechanisms and capacities of Ghana's FDA and Pharmacy Council (see Chapter 1), the fact that informal actors like "independent sales reps" can so easily engage in pharmaceutical distribution suggests that unauthorized products may also enter the system. This has been discussed several times in our research.[38] The work of regulatory authorities is further burdened by the presence of almost 600 formal wholesale companies involved in distributing pharmaceuticals within the country. In comparison, the pharmacist's monopoly and the specific status of "wholesaler-distributors" ensures greater product traceability in Benin's wholesale distribution operations, as noted previously (see Chapter 2).

According to many of our sources, various informalities described earlier are explained by the fact that businessmen and sometimes women run the companies, and therefore "put profit before practices" (interview with the pharmacist owner of a wholesale company, Accra, November 30, 2015) or that "it really is business, money, that determines everything here" (field journal, discussion with a pharmacist employed by a wholesale company, Accra, December 2, 2015). The head of the Pharmacy Council at the time said this about the wholesale companies based in Okaishie: "The philosophy of most of them who are running the business is profit, not practice. They are just trading. So anybody who walks in, they are just pushing commodities onto people. The necessary [things] that they have to do, they will not do… profit, profit, profit…" (interview, Accra, June 1, 2016).

## Conclusion: Is the pharmacist's monopoly evolving?

In France, the pharmacist's monopoly and its various applications are challenged on a regular basis (Fouassier, 2017). Several official reports have been published on the subject in recent years.[39] The mass retail company E.Leclerc has been developing awareness campaigns for its customers since the mid-1980s and is trying to pressure public authorities into allowing it to distribute medicines.[40] Until very recently, the French health authorities, with support from the Order of Pharmacists, which is quite active in these issues (Brutus, Fleuret, & Guienne, 2017), have favored maintaining the monopoly as it exists. Instead, new health-care functions are being proposed for private pharmacists to clearly identify them as being on the public health side of the sector rather than the commercial side: patient support and treatment follow-up, integrating pharmacists into first-line care, and dispensing certain prescription-only drugs.[41] In Europe, in accordance with the principle of subsidiarity, the pharmaceutical monopoly falls within the competence of individual States, which must nevertheless comply with competition law and the principle of free movement of goods for supply. States can therefore no longer prohibit the online or mail order sales of medicinal products not subject to compulsory medical prescription, which is why this has been allowed in France since 2012.[42] The European Commission is generally opposed to monopolies in principle, although it recognizes pharmacists as true health professionals (Debarge, 2017). Accordingly, a trend toward partial liberalization of retail drug distribution seems to have been underway in Europe since the 2000s (Denmark in 2001, Norway in 2003, Portugal in 2005, Italy in 2006, and Sweden in 2009) (Leca et al., 2017).

Changes are also evolving in Benin and Ghana. In Benin, we have seen a kind of "conquest of rural areas" by pharmacists, at least in the south of the country. There has been a greater trend of pharmacists opening pharmacies in villages than in the past.

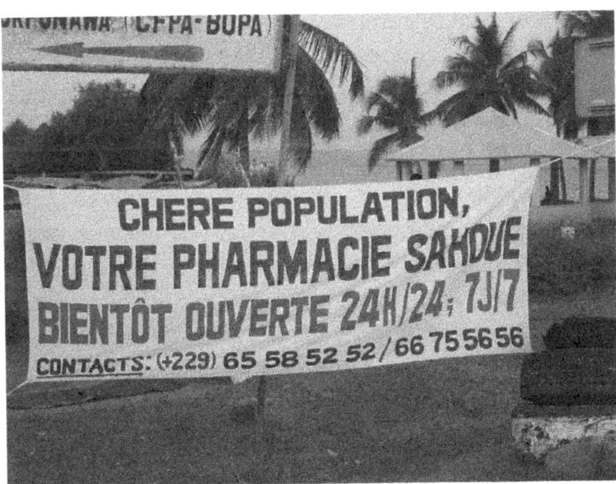


*Figure 3.5* Banner announcing the upcoming opening of a pharmacy in a Benin village.

Source: © IRD/Carine Baxerres, avril 2014

Others set up pharmaceutical warehouses in rural areas and managed them remotely with the help of employees (pharmacy assistants who may or may not have been trained in private pharmacy schools).[43] This was particularly true for four pharmaceutical warehouses in our study area, two of which opened during our research. In Ghana, the coming years may also see a change in the very large number of wholesale companies. The legislation governing their activities is similar in some respects to that in effect in the United States and the United Kingdom (a company can be both a wholesaler and a retailer, there is no obligation to distribute all approved medicines, and activities are not reserved for pharmacists) (Baxerres, 2013; Mahalatchimy, 2017). As in Ghana, these UK and US economic actors are not subject to the binding public service requirements to which wholesaler-distributors in Benin and France are held. The difference is that the US and UK actors have experienced a concentration in the sector that has not yet occurred in Ghana. At the end of 2010, there were only three main actors in "wholesale" distribution, accounting for nearly 90% of deliveries, in both the United Kingdom and the United States (Baxerres, 2013). A similar shift in concentration could begin in Ghana, although we did not observe anything like that; as noted earlier, only a few companies have multiple branches. The one exception was an interview with the pharmacist owner of a wholesale company, who proposed a franchising model that he wanted to set up in the coming years to distribute his products.

Pragmatic changes formulated by the economic actors and regulators seem to be well underway in both Ghana and Benin to address some of the dysfunctions highlighted in this chapter. The results of the Globalmed program were presented to the Ministry of Health of Benin on February 21, 2017; when we suggested there should be a discussion of opening up the pharmacist's monopoly for retail distribution,[44] the Directorate of Pharmacy, Medicine, and Diagnostic Investigations (DPMED) Director General solemnly replied that as French speakers with the pharmaceutical values that accompany a pharmacist's francophone training, it was impossible for them to conceive of businesses such as the OTC medicine shops of Ghana.[45] However, he went on to say that the health authorities should as a matter of necessity ensure that the number of pharmaceutical depots were increased throughout Benin. The problems in Benin's pharmaceutical sector at the time of this writing do not allow us to study the prospects of that statement at this time. Nevertheless, it could be seen as a very sensible way of effectively opening up the retail pharmacist monopoly without appearing to actually alter it. For the Head of the Ghana Pharmacy Council at the time of our research, many of the informalities in pharmacy practice described earlier would be greatly reduced if pharmacists were actually at the head of wholesale companies: "Those who had money were mostly non-pharmacists. It is now that with some level of consciousness we are arousing the conscience of pharmacists, that they should either have the majority shares or set up their own altogether. So gradually it is shifting. (...). What we want to clamp down on is that all steps should be supervised by the pharmacist (...). Now if we are able to reverse this trend, so pharmacists stay longer and are supervising the activities, then it is presumed that access or unlawful access or unauthorized access to these types of people and of medicines will be minimized" (interview with Joseph Nyoagbe, Accra, June 1, 2016).

Hybrid approaches like this, which would adapt how distribution functions in both countries, are necessary. They offer new ways to strike a balance between profession and capital, and between public health and commerce, gradually distancing themselves from colonial legacies. Above all, these approaches depend on the countries' regulatory capacities, which in Benin need to be significantly strengthened. These solutions to reconcile the disparate laws of various West African countries are also needed to implement the current initiatives to harmonize pharmaceutical regulation in this region.

## Notes

1. Olivier Debarge (2011) classifies the States of the European Union into three categories of retail pharmaceutical distribution legislation: the deregulated model, which includes the United Kingdom; the strictly regulated model, which includes France; and the mixed model.
2. The liberal professions involve intellectual work, performed without any subordination between the person who conducts it and the person on whose behalf it is conducted, in accordance with codes of conduct, the remuneration of which is not intended to be commercial or speculative in nature. These professionals include notaries, architects, lawyers, doctors, and certified accountants. The liberal professions are exercised in a personal capacity, under the responsibility of the workers themselves, who are considered self-employed professionals.
3. See the Introduction of the book for more information on the data collection methodology.
4. Prior to 1973, Law no. 54-418 of 1954 made this monopoly applicable to all French colonies; see Book V of the French Public Health Code applied to the colonies.
5. Since the Bamako Initiative and beginning in 1988 in Benin, the government has been introducing the sale of medicines in public and private nonprofit health centers. Only "essential generic medicines" are eligible, mainly sold under their international nonproprietary name or INN (Decree no. 88-444 of November 18, 1988). In Ghana, medicines are also officially sold in public and private health centers.
6. List of Benin's private pharmacies, updated on September 7, 2015; Directorate of Pharmacy, Medicines, and Diagnostic Investigations (DPMED); Ministry of Health, Republic of Benin.
7. According to Ordinance no. 75-7 of January 27, 1975 on medicines in the then Dahomey, now Benin, medicines are classified by degree of harm into two main categories: nonhazardous products and poisonous substances. The latter are further classified as A (toxic), B (narcotic and psychotropic drugs), or C (dangerous). Although there is no legislation requiring pharmacies to stock all authorized drugs and there are some differences by geographic areas (neighborhood type, urban, semi-rural, rural), overall pharmacies distribute the same drugs at the same prices (sources: oral communication, DPMED, June 2016).
8. See the Ghana Pharmacy Act, 1994 (Act 489).
9. Now Junior High School Certificate.
10. See the Ghana Pharmacy Act of 1994 (Act 489), recently updated by the "Health and Professions Regulatory Bodies Act" (Act 857).
11. See the OTC medicine seller authorization conditions: http://www.pcghana.org/wp-content/uploads/2017/09/GUIDELINES-ON-APPLICATION-FOR-OTCMS-LICENCE-1.pdf, accessed April 2019.

12. Personal communication with Joseph Nyoagbe, Registrar of the Ghana Pharmacy Council, September 2015, Globalmed annual meeting: "Pharmacy practice development in Ghana: Tracing the evolution through education, practice and regulation."
13. See the list of medicines in each of these three categories: https://fdaghana.gov.gh/wp-content/uploads/2017/06/NEW-DRUG-CLASSIFICATION-LIST.pdf, accessed March 2019.
14. This is the national list of essential medicines established by the Ministry of Health for use in municipal health centers. This list provides for different drugs by health pyramid level (sources: DPMED oral communication, June 2016).
15. See Decree no. 2000-410 of August 17, 2000, implementing Act no. 97-020 of June 17, 1997, establishing the conditions for private medical and paramedical practice and for opening pharmaceutical warehouses in the Republic of Benin.
16. Source: DPMED.
17. It should be noted that, as stated in the introduction of the chapter, the pharmacy sector in the United Kingdom was created by the market using the free trade model, whereas a public health insurance system, the National Health Bill, had been established as early as 1911.
18. Currently, it is said that only 8.4% of individuals are covered, mainly civil servants or employees of large companies. Universal health coverage initiatives are not yet effective despite having been launched in 2011 (Deville, Fecher, & Poncelet, 2018).
19. Nevertheless, we saw in the previous chapter that competition between them manifests in other ways.
20. See the lists as of December 31, 2013, provided by the Pharmacy Council. Most of these 38 companies had two or three branches. The largest retailers had between four and nine branches. All the branches must be licensed by the Pharmacy Council and have a superintendent pharmacist.
21. A list provided by the FDA in 2016 shows 121 such importing companies. But this number may not be reliable, as field studies indicate it is low. FDA agents themselves noted there could be omissions due to malfunctions when extracting certain information from their database (Siamed – FDA database, developed by WHO) (sources: oral communication, August 2016).
22. The price of drugs reimbursed by Ghana's National Health Insurance, on the other hand, is set by that body (Arhinful, 2003).
23. As previously mentioned, after our field studies were conducted, the informal drug market saw unprecedented repression beginning in February 2017 under the first government of the President of the Republic of Benin, Patrice Talon, elected in April 2016. According to our information, informal sales and purchasing practices still exist, but we are not in a position to describe them.
24. By informal market, we mean drug sales and purchases that occur outside the legal and administrative frameworks imposed by the State and by a country's biomedical health system (Baxerres, 2013).
25. The vast majority of these vendors sold a few boxes of anthelmintics (albendazole and mebendazole), often marketed under different trade names; some sold laxatives or antifungal vaginal creams, and some also sold painkillers, antipyretics, or anti-inflammatories. More rarely, some vendors offered a much wider variety of drugs packaged in transparent containers to promote the contents.
26. Because cocoa farming is an important source of income in this region, camps are set up temporarily for several months during the cocoa tree maintenance and harvesting season. Other crops rely on camps during harvesting season (yam, cassava, plantain bananas).
27. These primarily involved manufactured herbal medicines (see Chapter 8).
28. The informal retail medicine trade along the West African coast is mainly performed by women, unlike countries in the Sahel region, for example.

29. Or that such distribution is too constrained, according to our analyses, as in the case of pharmaceutical warehouses.
30. During our research we saw examples of recently hired employees who did not know who the store owner was for several months, since the owner merely managed the business by telephone through the employee who had been working there the longest.
31. The schools that train Medicine Counter Assistants are private, numerous, and varied, particularly with regard to the content of their training, which generally lasts 6 months. With a few exceptions, many of these schools are criticized for the qualifications of their young graduates. A Pharmacy Council agent referred to them as a "gray area." We see this as comparable to the situation in Benin regarding schools that train pharmacy assistants and medical representatives (see Chapter 9).
32. This occurred when these health facilities and regional warehouses were out of stock and the purchasing process was faster through OTC medicine shops.
33. OTC medicine shop owners do not perceive the sale of antibiotics in their stores as a public health problem. At the time of our research, they had apparently not yet been made aware of the issue of antimicrobial resistance. More generally, their view on this subject is "if you decide to sell only over-the-counter drugs, then you end up selling nothing" (field diary, Accra, October 27, 2014).
34. In 2016, 83 people were employed full-time at the Pharmacy Council. Some had worked in its regional offices (two to four people per office). Ghana has 16 regions and at the time of our study, one final region was scheduled to have a Pharmacy Council office (interview with the Head of the Pharmacy Council, June 1, 2016). There are no pharmacist inspectors among DPMED staff in Benin (see Chapter 1).
35. The owner of this OTC medicine shop had to pay a substantial fine in order to reopen his business. We were told of several inspections and store closures. Of course, we also observed methods of circumventing inspections (closing the store following a telephone call warning of the inspectors' visit) or concealing products not supposed to be sold in stores.
36. In our view, this situation is facilitated by a legislative provision (described earlier) that allows companies to open in Ghana that are both wholesalers and retailers, which further simplifies the ability of an individual who does not have a pharmaceutical retailer's authorization to purchase medicines in that country. According to the Director of the Pharmacy Council, this provision has been obsolete in major cities since 1998 (confirmed with wholesalers). But since this expiration is not retroactive, many companies were still operating in this manner at the time of our research (377 at the end of 2013). However, the practice of selling to unauthorized buyers has also been observed among non-retail wholesalers.
37. Later in our observations, the staff of wholesalers in our ethnographic studies were instructed to stop registering customers under the name "cash" in the client software. Other practices were then used, such as giving a fictitious first name and combining it with the term "chemical," or using an employee's first name. During our observations at wholesaler premises, when a new customer was created in the client file, no legal documentation was requested from the customer regardless of whether or not a pharmacist was present.
38. These are medicines sold by wholesalers or independent sales reps that do not have a marketing authorization (MA) in Ghana but do have an MA in other countries, particularly Nigeria (a nearby English-speaking country with close relations to Ghana). It also appears that some drugs that are not yet approved but are in the FDA approval process, or others that are no longer approved, may be sold. Finally, there have been several instances regarding the questionable origins of certain drugs or diagnostic tests, particularly during stockouts of the products in question in the country. For example, during some observations it appeared to us that coun-

terfeit Coartem had been circulating; this was subsequently confirmed to us at the same time (mid-2015) by studies conducted with the FDA in the framework of the Globalmed research program.

39. Beigbeder C., 2007, *Le "Low Cost": Un levier pour le pouvoir d'achat [Low Cost: A purchasing power lever].*; Rochefort R., 2008, *Un commerce pour la ville. Rapport au ministre du Logement et de la Ville [A Business for the city. Report to the Minister of Housing and Urban Affairs]*, Doc.fr.; Attali J., 2008, *Rapport de la commission pour la libéralisation de la croissance française: 300 décisions pour changer la France [Report of the Commission for the Liberalization of French Growth: 300 decisions to change France]*, Doc.fr.; *Rapport de l'Inspection Générale des Finances sur les professions non réglementées de 2013 [Report of the General Inspectorate of Finance on non-regulated professions in 2013]*; Competition Authority, Opinion no. 13-A-24 of 19 December 2013 on the functioning of competition in the distribution sector of medicinal products for human use in cities, p. 168.
40. These awareness campaigns, which were particularly active in 2008, 2009, and 2013, are available from E.Leclerc in the "History and Archives" section of its website: https://www.histoireetarchives.leclerc/photos/les-grandes-campagnes-de-communication/parapharmacie-et-pharamacie-les-campagnes-et-contre-campagnes, accessed February 2019.
41. See the July 21, 2009, law known as the HPST law (hospital, patients, health and territories) (Maurain, 2017), as well as National Assembly Amendment no. AS1487, presented by Mr. Mesnier on March 8, 2019. Great Britain is also experiencing this shift toward a new place for pharmacists in the health system (Mahalatchimy, 2017).
42. See Order no. 2012-1427 of December 19, 2012. The European Union has also recently restricted the scope of the French monopoly by removing products that were initially covered by it, such as pregnancy and ovulation tests or those for contact lens care and use (see Law no. 2014-344 on consumption adopted on March 17, 2014) (Debarge, 2017).
43. Which is legally possible (Article 9 of Order no. 13495 of December 28, 2006).
44. Proposals are regularly made by public health experts to institutionalize informal drug vendor activities (Goodman et al., 2007; Shah, Brieger, & Peters, 2011).
45. There are indeed divergent values in Europe and West Africa regarding the distribution of medicines: either the drug, whatever it may be, is perceived as a dangerous product that requires the supervision of a pharmacy professional (French and Beninese vision), or it is perceived as a basic necessity product that must be widely geographically accessible to potential patients (English vision, shared by a large part of Europe and in Ghana). Sweden is often reported as aligning with the French vision. After authorizing the sale of paracetamol in supermarkets in 2008, Sweden withdrew the authorization in 2015 because of the number of paracetamol-related poisonings, which had increased by 40% between 2009 and 2013 (Guerriaud, 2017).

## Reference List

Agblevor, E. A. (2016). *"I am now a doctor": Self-medication practices among households in Accra.* Unpublished master's thesis, University of Ghana, Legon, Accra.

Agblevor, E. A., Missodey, M., Arhinful, D. K., & Baxerres, C. (2016). Drugstores, self-medication and public health delivery: Assessing the role of a major health actor in Ghana. In *L'automédication en question : Un bricolage socialement et territorialement situé [Questioning self-medication: Tinkering in the social and territorial realm]* (pp. 202–209). (Conference proceedings). University of Nantes, France.

Anago, E., Djralah, M., Kpatchavi, A. C., & Baxerres, C. (2016). Pharmacies, vendeurs informels, centres de santé des villes et des campagnes : Interroger au Bénin l'automédication au regard de la formalité des circuits de distribution et des contextes géographiques [Pharmacies, informal vendors, urban and rural health centers: Questioning self-medication in Benin with regard to the formality of distribution channels and geographic contexts]. In *L'automédication en question : Un bricolage socialement et territorialement situé [Questioning self-medication: Tinkering in the social and territorial realm]* (pp. 210–217). (Conference proceedings). University of Nantes, France.

Anderson, S. (Ed.). (2005). *Making medicines: A brief history of pharmacy and pharmaceuticals*. London, UK: Pharmaceutical Press.

Arhinful, D. K. (2003). *The solidarity of self-interest. Social and cultural feasibility of rural health insurance in Ghana*. Doctoral dissertation, African Studies Centre, Leiden University, The Netherlands. Retrieved from https://openaccess.leidenuniv.nl/handle/1887/12919.

Arhinful, D. K., Sams, K., Kpatinvoh, A., & Baxerres, C. (2018). Complementary health care services by public, private for-profit and private not-for-profit providers: Understanding the multiplicity of biomedical care services in Benin and Ghana. In C. Baxerres, & C. Marquis (Eds.), *Regulations, markets, health: Questioning current stakes of pharmaceuticals in Africa* (pp. 138–147). (Conference proceedings). HAL, Ouidah, Benin. https://hal.archives-ouvertes.fr/hal-01988227.

Baxerres, C. (2013). *Du médicament informel au médicament libéralisé : Une anthropologie du médicament pharmaceutique au Bénin [From informal to liberalized drugs: An anthropology of pharmaceutical drugs in Benin]*. Paris, France: Les Éditions des Archives Contemporaines.

Brutus, L., Fleuret, S., & Guienne, V. (2017). *Se soigner par soi-même. Recherche interdisciplinaire sur l'automédication [Taking care of yourself. Interdisciplinary research on self-medication]*. Paris, France: CNRS Éditions.

Chauveau, S. (2005). Marché et publicité des médicaments [Drug market and advertising]. In C. Bonah, & A. Rasmussen (Eds.), *Histoire et médicament aux 19ème et 20ème siècles [History and medication in the 19th and 20th centuries]* (pp. 189–213). Paris, France: Éditions Glyphe.

Debarge, O. (2011). La distribution au détail du médicament au sein de l'Union Européenne: Un croisement entre santé et commerce [Retail distribution of drugs in the European Union: A cross between health and commerce]. *Revue internationale de droit economique*, XXV(2), 193–238.

Debarge, O. (2017). Le monopole pharmaceutique et le droit de l'Union européenne [The pharmaceutical monopoly and European Union law]. In A. Leca, C. Maurain, I. Moine-Dupuis, & G. Rousset (Eds.), *Le monopole pharmaceutique et son avenir [The pharmaceutical monopoly and its future]* (pp. 31–44). Bordeaux, France: LEH Édition.

Deville, C., Fecher, F., & Poncelet, M. (2018). L'assurance pour le renforcement du capital humain (ARCH) au Bénin: Processus d'élaboration et défis de mise en œuvre [Insurance for building human capital (ARCH) in Benin: Development process and implementation challenges]. *Revue française des affaires sociales*, *1*, 107–123. https://doi.org/10.3917/rfas.181.0107.

Faure, O. (2005). Les pharmaciens et le médicament en France au 19ème siècle [Pharmacists and medicines in France in the 19th century]. In C. Bonah, & A. Rasmussen (Eds.), *Histoire et médicament aux 19ème et 20ème siècles [History and medication in the 19th and 20th centuries]* (pp. 65–85). Paris, France: Éditions Glyphe.

Fouassier, E. (2017). Les fondements du monopole pharmaceutique: La logique sanitaire [The foundations of the pharmaceutical monopoly: The health logic]. In A. Leca, C. Maurain, I. Moine-Dupuis, & G. Rousset (Eds.), *Le monopole pharmaceutique et son avenir [The pharmaceutical monopoly and its future]* (pp. 45–57). Bordeaux, France: LEH Édition.

Gaudillière, J.-P. (2005). Une marchandise pas comme les autres. Historiographie du médicament et de l'industrie pharmaceutique en France au 20ème siècle [A commodity like no other. Historiography of medicines and the pharmaceutical industry in France in the 20th century]. In C. Bonah, & A. Rasmussen (Eds.), *Histoire et médicament aux 19ème et 20ème siècles [History and medication in the 19th and 20th centuries]* (pp. 115–158). Paris, France: Éditions Glyphe.

Goodman, C. A., Brieger, W., Unwin, A., Mills, A., Meek, S., & Greer, G. (2007). Medicine sellers and malaria treatment in Sub-Saharan Africa. *The American Journal of Tropical Medicine and Hygiene, 77*(6 Suppl), 203–218.

Guerriaud, M. (2017). Le monopole pharmaceutique français [The French pharmaceutical monopoly]. In A. Leca, C. Maurain, I. Moine-Dupuis, & G. Rousset (Eds.), *Le monopole pharmaceutique et son avenir [The pharmaceutical monopoly and its future]* (pp. 11–30). Bordeaux, France: LEH Édition.

Kamat, V. R., & Nichter, M. (1998). Pharmacies, self-medication and pharmaceutical marketing in Bombay, India. *Social Science & Medicine, 47*(6), 779–794.

Kpatchavi, A. C. (2012). Se soigner dans la rue : Les usages sociaux du médicament dans les quartiers périphériques de Cotonou (Bénin) [Treating yourself in the street: The social uses of drugs in the peripheral neighborhoods of Cotonou (Benin)]. *Cahiers du CERLESHS, 27*, 211–239.

Lanore, H. (2008). Dans un contexte de regroupement d'établissements de répartition pharmaceutique, comment répondre aux attentes des clients tout en tenant compte des contraintes économiques auxquelles est soumis le secteur ? [In a context of consolidation of pharmaceutical distribution establishments, how can customer expectations be met while taking into account the economic constraints facing the sector]. Unpublished State dissertation [Thèse d'Etat], Tours, Université François Rabelais, Tours, France.

Le Guisquet, O., & Lorenzi, J. (2001). *La distribution pharmaceutique en France [Pharmaceutical distribution in France]*, Paris, France: Elsevier.

Leca, A. (2017). La distribution des médicaments entre le service public et le marché, un équilibre à conserver mais à réaménager [The balance of drug distribution between public facilities and private markets: Retain but reorganize]. In A. Leca, C. Maurain, I. Moine-Dupuis, & G. Rousset (Eds.), *Le monopole pharmaceutique et son avenir [The pharmaceutical monopoly and its future]* (pp. 71–80). Bordeaux, France: LEH Édition.

Leca, A., Maurain, C., Moine-Dupuis, I., & Rousset, G. (Eds.). (2017). *Le monopole pharmaceutique et son avenir [The pharmaceutical monopoly and its future]*. Bordeaux, France: LEH Édition.

Lomba, C. (2014). Les grossistes de médicaments : Juste-à-temps et normes sanitaires [Drug wholesalers: Just-in-time systems and health standards]. In P. Fournier, C. Lomba, & S. Muller (Eds.), *Les travailleurs du médicament. L'industrie pharmaceutique sous observation [Drug workers. The pharmaceutical industry under observation]* (pp. 251–273). Toulouse, France: ERES.

Mahalatchimy, A. (2017), Le monopole pharmaceutique en Grande Bretagne [The pharmaceutical monopoly in Great Britain]. In A. Leca, C. Maurain, I. Moine-Dupuis, & G. Rousset (Eds.), *Le monopole pharmaceutique et son avenir [The pharmaceutical monopoly and its future]* (pp. 109–127). Bordeaux, France: LEH Édition.

Maurain, C. (2017). Une troisième voie… De la dispensation aux soins de premier recours [A third way… From dispensing to primary care]. In A. Leca, C. Maurain, I. Moine-Dupuis, & G. Rousset (Eds.), *Le monopole pharmaceutique et son avenir [The pharmaceutical monopoly and its future]* (pp. 95–105). Bordeaux, France: LEH Édition.

Senah, K. A. (1997). *Money be man. The popularity of medicines in a rural Ghanaian community*. Unpublished doctoral dissertation, University of Amsterdam, The Netherlands.

Shah, N. M., Brieger, W. R., & Peters, D. (2011). Can interventions improve health services from informal private providers in low and middle-income countries? A comprehensive review of the literature. *Health Policy and Planning, 26*(4), 275–287.

Sueur, N. (2018). *La maison Menier, de la droguerie au chocolat: 1816–1869. Aux origines de l'industrie pharmaceutique en France [The Menier company, from pharmacy to chocolate. 1816–1869. The origins of the pharmaceutical industry in France]*. Paris, France: L'Harmattan.

Van den Brink, H. (2017). Analyse critique des fondements du monopole officinal en France : la logique socio-économique [Critical analysis of the foundations of the pharmacy monopoly in France: The socio-economic logic]. In A. Leca, C. Maurain, I. Moine-Dupuis, & G. Rousset (Eds.), *Le monopole pharmaceutique et son avenir [The pharmaceutical monopoly and its future]* (pp. 95–105). Bordeaux, France: LEH Édition.

Van der Geest, S. (1987). Self-care and the informal sale of drugs in South Cameroon. *Social Science & Medicine, 25*(3), 293–305.

# 4 From depharmaceuticalization to drug abundance

## A social history of pharmaceutic regulations in Cambodia

*Eve Bureau-Point*

### Introduction

The first pharmaceutical medicines were introduced into Cambodia during the French protectorate (1863–1953). Representatives of colonial health services practiced the academic medicine developing in the West, delivered within a syncretic and pluralist medical system derived from Theravada Buddhism, Ayurveda, Chinese medicine, and animist theories (Chhem, 2001). The use of medicines imported from France and the practice of Western medicine were gradually incorporated into the existing medical offices. While pharmaceuticalization[1] of Cambodian society was taking hold in Indochina, Cambodia underwent a reverse process of "depharmaceuticalization,"[2] sparked by a succession of destructive wars and authoritarian regimes, exacerbated by the Khmer Rouge revolution (1975–1979). The entire pharmaceutical system was rebuilt. Most pharmacists were executed, and official production and distribution sites were destroyed. In this chapter, I will build on existing knowledge of the history of pharmaceuticalization/depharmaceuticalization in Cambodian society, using an approach that combines historic anthropology, the anthropology of objects and techniques, and medical anthropology. My analysis will specifically examine the "multiple regulations" that shape the structure of the pharmaceutical market in this specific context. Throughout the previous chapters, the concept of "multiple regulations," introduced by Mathieu Quet et al. (2018), goes beyond national and international regulations enshrined in legal documents and implemented by States and institutions and considers more alternative and informal regulatory models. As they explained, "the trajectories of pharmaceuticals are defined by alternative logistic regimes that must be explained and understood. The existence of such regimes depends upon multiple reasons: cultural representations, conflicts of need and availability, contradictions between regulation and marketing strategies, commercial initiatives, and so on" (p. 5). Looking at this issue through the lens of many sources of regulation offers an innovative theoretical framework to understand the diversity of social practices involved in regulating the circulation of medicines, whether such practices are driven by the State, healthcare professionals, distributors, or consumers. Social scientists researching health issues in the country have already highlighted historic and social aspects affecting the circulation of medicines in Cambodia (Bonnemain, 2008; Bourdier, Man, & Res, 2014; Crochet, 2001; Guillou, 2009; Ovesen & Trankell, 2007; Pordié, 2016). This chapter employs a historical perspective to expand on this research by presenting how the Cambodian pharmaceutical system is structured as well as the rules, practices, and adjustments—both formal and informal—that have been harnessed over time, in response to the exponential rise in the drug circulation in this context.[3]

## From the French protectorate to the 1990s: A historical overview of the pharmaceuticalization/depharmaceuticalization of Cambodian society

The primary mission of French colonial medicine was to provide medical care for soldiers and colonists. Colonized people's health was secondary and translated into prevention and vaccination programs to control the development of infectious diseases. The first pharmaceutical medicines were introduced in this context. Beginning in 1923, health officials in the pharmacy sector were trained at the Hanoi Faculty of Medicine (a 4-year program), and pharmaceuticals were only supplied by French pharmacists (Neou, 1999). There were four pharmacies, run by French pharmacists, all located in Phnom Penh. Health officers ran depots in the provinces. In her book on colonial medicine in Cambodia, Sokhieng Au points out that very few people sought biomedical consultations, but, in contrast, European pharmacopeia was a huge success (2011, p. 79). Laurence Monnais has documented the same finding for the Vietnamese situation (2014). Cambodia was noted for robust pharmaceutical manufacturing, producing over 400 specialties between 1940 and 1945 (Bonnemain, 2008).

After independence, under the reign of King Sihanouk (1955–1970), the first pharmacies directed by French-trained Cambodian pharmacists opened, along with the first local drug manufacturing companies. According to Seng Lim Neou, these pharmacists also held positions in the public sector (1999), a practice that endures today. Medicines continued to primarily come from France. Pharmacies were large companies that simultaneously managed imports and wholesale and retail sales. Health officers in pharmacy started to be trained at the Royal College of Medicine of Cambodia in the 1950s; after a 5-year program, the first graduates became pharmacists in 1962. Since these officers worked in cities, retired nurses were authorized to open pharmacy-depots in the provinces. Medicine distribution was carried out according to French law, which recognized the pharmacists' monopoly.[4] According to Seng Lim Neou, at this time in Cambodia, people bought medicines after consulting a physician who wrote a prescription (1999).

Starting in the 1970s, the political situation began deteriorating; the Lon Nol coup d'état and the collateral effects of the Vietnam War weakened the country. During the Khmer Republic of Lon Nol (1970–1975), described as plagued by corruption (Chandler, 1992), health services were overburdened by the war-wounded and refugees fleeing the fighting. Treatment options were limited despite massive aid from the United States (Guillou, 2009), and drug prices rose (Ovesen & Trankell, 2007). The country gradually fell under the Khmer Rouge (1975–1979), a radical Maoist communist regime based on an ideology promoting the purification of the Khmer people and an agrarian utopia aimed at self-sufficiency that resulted in the massacre of approximately one-quarter of the population. The intellectual professions, especially pharmacists and physicians, considered to be impure and contaminated by imperialism, were targeted first. Consequently, no more than 26 of the 150 trained pharmacists remained at the end of the Khmer Rouge regime (Neou, 1999). The health system, along with its workforce, was destroyed in order to create a new one. Biomedical scientists, such as Thiounn Thioeun, who was the Minister of Health under the Khmer Rouge, had joined the revolution before 1975. They trained their own medical staff ("*pet padevat*": *pet*, doctor; *padevat*, revolution). The study done as part of the Globalmed project was conducted in a former bastion of the Khmer Rouge, and the distribution actors who were interviewed there were primarily former Khmer Rouge health professionals who had been trained during the Democratic Kampuchea. Thus, the Khmer Rouge did not reject Western medicine as a whole; their priority was to limit dependence on the outside world and to produce drugs themselves. Its relationship to medicines shows this since Angkar[5] had appropriated inventory from pharmaceutical companies and pharmacies, and imported a few drugs from Thailand, China, and Hong Kong (Tyner, 2012). It created a drug importation company (the Ren Fung Company) and set up small local manufacturing (vaccines and penicillin) that produced finished products with questionable quality (Tyner, 2012). While the political project involved experimenting with traditional medicine[6] and establishing domestic production to become autonomous (Vilim, 2010, cited by Tyner, 2012), ultimately a two-tier medical system was put in place: one intended for Khmer Rouge cadres and armed combatants who received biomedical care and pharmaceuticals administered by staff trained in China, and the other one based on popular and traditional knowledge, that, according to Michael Vickery, applied to 90% of the population (1984). A factory to manufacture traditional medicines was set up in Phnom Penh, where production was supervised by the *kru khmaer*[7] and Chinese advisors (Tyner, 2012). Cooperatives to produce this same type of medicine were also found in the country's various districts (Guillou, 2009). These medicines were called *aarj tunsaï* by their consumers, Khmer for "rabbit droppings," because of their resemblance. Therefore, depharmaceuticalization was not absolute. In this context, it meant a drastic reduction in the pharmaceutical drug supply and the near-disappearance of actors working in pharmaceutical drug distribution (pharmacists and health officers) and designated places where they dispensed medicines (pharmacies and depots). Additionally, it reflected the establishment of a new production and distribution system that was less dependent on foreign countries and based on removing pharmaceuticals from their exalted position and replacing them with another episteme of care: traditional medicine.

The history of the Cambodian pharmaceutical system would soon take a turn. Pharmaceuticals were reintroduced massively and quickly, and "pharmaceutical anarchy" (Gollogly, 2002) took hold. After the Vietnamese intervention in 1979 that put an end to the Khmer Rouge regime and marked the debut of the People's Republic of Kampuchea under Vietnamese domination (1979–1989), everything was rebuilt. On the pharmaceutical front, the top priority was remedying the lack of human resources by implementing a rapid training system: 4 years of training for "auxiliary pharmacists," following the model used for the protectorate's health officers. These pharmacists were required to work in the public sector—in health facilities; supply, manufacturing, and distribution structures; or in the few "State pharmacies" that were opened under the auspices of the Ministry of Health. Three State factories were set up to revive local production. The Central Medical Store (CMS), created in 1992 (Neou, 1999), was responsible for supplying medicines to central, provincial, and municipal hospitals. These factories immediately faced problems with shortages of electricity, raw materials, and funding. In this generalized postcrisis context, marked by anomie and drug shortages, an informal sector emerged, managed by nonqualified personnel who "in the beginning, spread out their small quantity of medicines, sent by their families or friends abroad, on a scrap of mat or on little tables on the sidewalks or in markets" (Neou, 1999, p. 59). These vendors gradually organized themselves and then purchased medicines in Thailand (interviews with wholesalers, Phnom Penh, 2015). Medicines became consumer goods like any other, circulating outside the control of health professionals. Although access to care and medicines was officially limited to the public sector under this State socialism, the Ministry of Health, seeing the extent of these small businesses, "decided to group these merchants into formal shops and have them store their medicines on shelves" (Neou, 1999, p. 59). Courses covering basic pharmaceutical concepts were organized for them, and those owners who successfully completed the training program could be unofficially recognized by the State and attain the status of "blue pharmacy" (Neou, 1999, p. 59). This type of State-led adjustment serves as a reminder that States are also actors in implementing informal modes of regulation in response to the constraints of the situation.

A United Nations mission (United Nations Transitional Authority in Cambodia, UNTAC) was deployed in 1991 to ensure a return to peace. Although the Khmer Rouge were no longer in power, they were at war with the People's Republic of Kampuchea army until 1999, when the last Khmer Rouge, who until 1999 were entrenched in bastions, surrendered their weapons and joined the government through a "reconciliation" program. The 1990s would symbolize an intensification of exchanges with the outside world. To rebuild the country, the government opened its doors to international organizations and private companies. The pharmaceutical system was gradually liberalized. The main local production plants were privatized, the number of pharmaceutical companies[8] and the volume of medicines in circulation saw a steady rise, and the sources of medicines became diversified.

Pharmacists who until then were required to work in the public sector were authorized to open private pharmacies starting in 1989. According to Seng Lim Neou, an information program was developed by the Ministry of Health to explain the differences between legal pharmacies and informal blue pharmacies (1999). The public sector was rebuilt with foreign aid support. Medicine procurement was based on the essential medicines list.[9] According to the Ministry of Health, problems with stockouts in the public sector continued to arise, and supervision of the public distribution and storage system needed strengthening (2012). Thus, a public and private distribution system, dominated by the private sector,[10] (Neou, 1999) gradually took hold, and the need to establish laws regulating the organization and management of medicines became evident.[11]

## From 1990 to today: Constructing a new legal framework for drug circulation

Regulation followed French law until 1975, with two parallel systems, one public and one private (Neou, 1999, p. 109). Due to the years of war, the legal framework for drug circulation had changed very little. In 1994, a national agency for pharmaceutical regulation was created. It was the current Department of Drugs and Food (DDF), attached to the Ministry of Health. That same year, this department began registering medicines. The first pharmaceutical law, still in force today, was introduced in 1996. It sets the general rules for manufacturing and distribution. The pharmacists order would not be created until 2008. It is responsible by law to continuously ensure that the principles of morality, honesty, justice, and loyalty are properly and effectively applied to the pharmacist profession (royal decree, p. 120). Every pharmacy manager is required to register (cf. sub-decree of 2014).

In 1999, four licenses were created to regulate retail distribution: the first was for pharmacists (to open pharmacies); the second for assistant pharmacists (to open Depot-As); the third for retired health professionals (to open Depot-Bs); and the fourth license was for selling traditional medicines. Licenses for Depot-As and -Bs were created to address the lack of pharmacists in the country. The B licenses have not been issued since 2013, but anyone who had obtained one previously is allowed to use it until their retirement. As a result, we still find many Depot-Bs in Cambodia. Legally, the retail distribution system has been based on French law since the protectorate; it grants a monopoly to the pharmacist. However, not until the early 2010s when the government applied pressure did retailers routinely start registering with the Ministry of Health and applying for licenses (interviews with retailers and Ministry of Health representatives, 2015 and 2016). In addition, a nosocomial HIV outbreak caused by contaminated syringes in an informal private practice (Vun et al., 2016), uncovered in Battambang province at the end of 2014, resulted in the promulgation of a new decree to combat activity by non-qualified professionals and the circulation of "fake drugs."[12] Thus, this resulted in fewer informal retail outlets (Men, 2013); however, as we will see later in this chapter, licensees rarely conduct any oversight for medicines in their formal sales outlets, and informal practices are concealed within formal ones, as described in Ghana in the previous chapter.

Wholesale distribution, on the other hand, does not meet the standards either in France or in other former French colonies, particularly the francophone countries of West Africa—such as Benin and Côte d'Ivoire, discussed in previous chapters—where pharmaceutical legislation aligns closely with that of France. Wholesale distribution seems more liberalized in Cambodia, involving numerous pharmaceutical companies: 308 in 2015, compared to 7 in France and 5 in Benin. They are not legally bound, as in France, to each distribute all of the country's authorized medicines (interview with pharmacist, Phnom Penh, July 2015). Also, drug prices are regulated by the free market. Wholesale distribution in Cambodia more closely resembles the system in the English-speaking world, such as the United Kingdom, United States, and anglophone countries in West Africa like Ghana, to name a few. Thus, while France's imprint on the legal framework remains significant, various other influences have also shaped it.

It is also important to consider this legal framework through the regional dynamics in play since Cambodia joined the Association of Southeast Asian Nations (ASEAN) in 1999. The organization has established a free-trade zone between the ASEAN Free Trade Area (AFTA) countries aimed at eliminating customs duties, liberalizing the movement of goods and people, and harmonizing economic policies between member States. ASEAN is also taking initiatives to facilitate the circulation of pharmaceuticals between member States without compromising their quality, safety, or efficacy. To achieve this, ASEAN created the Consultative Committee for Standards and Quality (ACCSQ) in 1992 and a Pharmaceutical Product Working Group (PPWG) in 1999.[13] The member States meet regularly, with the 25th meeting held in 2018 in Vietnam. Efforts to harmonize pharmaceutical standards between member States are underway; however, as noted earlier, pharmaceuticals circulation is poorly regulated in the region, and the effects of ASEAN harmonization policies are often imperceptible. As a result, a considerable proportion of medicines circulate through nonofficial channels (Quet et al., 2018).

Falsified or substandard medicines pose a greater problem in developing countries where regulatory systems and their application are laxer (Quet, 2015). Thus, in Cambodia, the post-conflict context of anarchic drug circulation has fostered the circulation of falsified or substandard medicines, raising potential public health problems (Quet, 2015). In 2004, the situation analysis of the pharmaceutical sector in Cambodia identified that about 50% of medicines available on the market are not registered (Ministry of Health, 2004). Many falsified medicines in Cambodia are thought to be smuggled across borders from Thailand and Vietnam (Men 2013). During our study, some interviewees said that these medicines were primarily channeled across bilateral borders that only citizens of the two bordering countries could cross. Authorities exerted less control at these small border posts. Other informal entry points might include the Port of Sihanoukville, where ships come in, or even airports; however, our investigation did not allow us to examine these aspects in detail. Specific regulatory measures have been implemented in the country to address this concern. In 2005, an Inter-Ministerial Committee on Combating Counterfeit and Substandard medicines was created. The committee's mandate is to guide the fight against counterfeit and substandard medicines and illegal health services. According to the government and WHO, "a decline of the prevalence of counterfeit and substandard medicines appeared" (Ministry of Health, 2012, p. 16).

Contemporary State regulatory systems have been built through regional and international collaboration. As we will see in the rest of this chapter, their application depends, however, on other mechanisms, specific to the drug market, health professionals' practices, retail distribution actors, and the logics of consumers.

## The current Cambodian pharmaceutical market and its regulations

Although local production is on the rise,[14] actors in the distribution sector regularly call into question the quality of these products. One distributor that we interviewed had this to say about local products: "How do you explain that a blister pack of paracetamol costs 500 riels;[15] something is off here! These products have no ISO, no GMP, no analysis certificates" (Phnom Penh, March 2016). For the Ministry of Health, noncompliance with ASEAN Good Manufacturing Practice (GMP) standards hampers the development of the local market (Ministry of Health, 2012).

In Cambodia, most pharmaceuticals are imported. According to the DDF director, whom we interviewed in 2015, 70% of medicines arrive by boat, and when needed, by plane for emergencies (Phnom Penh, March 2015). While in 1994, 50% of distributed medicines came from France, by 2015, according to the DDF, that share had decreased to 7%, with most medicines now coming from Asian countries, as shown in the table below (see Table 4.1).

These transformations in medicine distribution in Cambodia should be interpreted in the context of the more globalized transformations affecting medicine production and the global drug market. Although pharmaceutical companies located in the Global North still play a central role in innovation, research, and intellectual property rights policy, the development of a market in some emerging countries has begun to disrupt the previously established order (Quet et al., 2018, also Introduction of this book). India and China have become major actors in the global drug market. The Indian pharmaceutical industry, which took off with the production and distribution of generic drugs, has become Cambodia's top

*Table 4.1* Medicine sources in Cambodia[16]

| | |
|---|---|
| Medicines from India | 31% |
| Medicines from Cambodia | 9% |
| Medicines from Thailand | 7% |
| Medicines from France | 7% |
| Medicines from Korea | 6% |
| Medicines from Vietnam | 5% |
| From other countries (Indonesia, China,[17] etc.) | 35% |

Source: Department of Drugs and Food Cambodia 2015, Author.

provider. Even though these official numbers inform us of the diversity of sources and their scale, they should, nevertheless, be interpreted with precaution since, as mentioned earlier, a high number of medicines are not included in national data, due to considerable informal pharmaceutical circulation.

Legally in Cambodia, an import license issued by the Ministry of Health is required for each drug or each of its formulations. Based on several interviews conducted with representatives of pharmaceutical companies, registration is expensive. Applicants must submit 120 samples, pay USD 1200, and wait two and a half years to obtain the license, which distributors sometimes call a "visa." As we observed during our study, there was still no electronic system to register medicines. In the eyes of some of our interviewees, this contributed to undermining the DDF's figures, and more generally, a lack of confidence in this registration system's effectiveness and the Ministry of Health's ability to test drugs. The registration process requires that medicines be tested at the national laboratory. On this topic, one company sales director confided to us: "At the national analysis laboratory, they don't have any means for testing medicines, no equipment, and they assume that a medicine registered in ASEAN, for example in Singapore or elsewhere, has been tested and, therefore, there is no need to do it. Registration is really a system to get funding" (Phnom Penh, October 2015).

During our conversations with semi-wholesalers[18] and retailers, we understood that both the private and public sectors were distributing imported molecules without a license, namely, molecules for which companies had no import permit. Several of our interviewees said: "Those who want to follow the law cannot. Some essential medicines are not registered." Morphine derivatives and anticancer molecules were cited the most. How is it possible that there is no official market for molecules that public health actors consider to be essential? Our interviewees' responses centered on economic arguments. Marketing these molecules would not be profitable enough for distributors. They explained that, especially in emerging countries, companies focus on distributing certain products. For example, the medicine market for chronic diseases would improve once health insurance was more widespread (interview with a distributor, Phnom Penh, April 2016). One importer-distributor told us: "In Cambodia, the population is young, so we mainly import products that target women and children" (interview with an importer, Phnom Penh, January 2016).

Also, the issue of "parallel imports"[19] came up regularly during our interviews with distribution actors. This refers to the importation of the same product by different distributors. These strategies—formal, if they are declared, informal if not—are described as tactics to spark competition and lower the market prices. One gave us the example of Sterimar®. While his company sold this product to retailers at USD 4.50, he saw the same product without a Cambodian Ministry of Health sticker[20] for USD 4 at a semi-wholesaler's. Speaking specifically about parallel imports, he noted: "It's not just a few products since it's enough that official distributors need to lower their prices!" (Phnom Penh, March 2016).

Criteria related to the market, above all, determine access to medicines. Importers complain about the rising number of importers and the increasingly fierce competition. The representative of one company explained: "The Cambodian market is saturated. It's hard to work; there are too many products circulating with no controls. The market is too free" (Phnom Penh, October 2015). Thus, in this context, many drugs with the same effects are on the market. A retail seller whom we met in Phnom Penh, for example, counted about 50 brands of paracetamol.

The investigation distinguished between three types of importers. Some are pharmaceutical companies that have opened branches in Cambodia. However, their policies differ. Two of them, encountered during the study, registered their products, then trained prescribers and promoted their products before going through a distributor for distribution. Other importers are importer-distributors. They register drugs from several pharmaceutical companies with the Cambodian government and distribute them to semi-wholesalers and retailers in the country's various provinces. During our study, three large distributors had acquired a large share of the drug market.[21] The third category of importers is the semi-wholesalers. They are primarily concentrated around the Olympic Market in Phnom Penh. Ninety-three pharmacies and pharmaceutical companies have been listed around this market (see Figure 4.1).

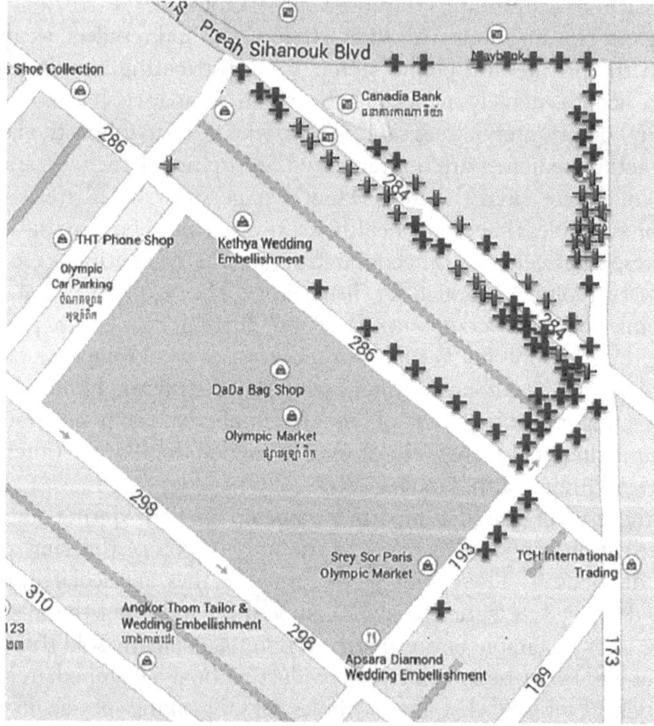


*Figure 4.1* Pharmacies and pharmaceutical companies in the Phnom Penh Olympic Market.

Source: © Phasy Res, 2015 (Research program Sorema)

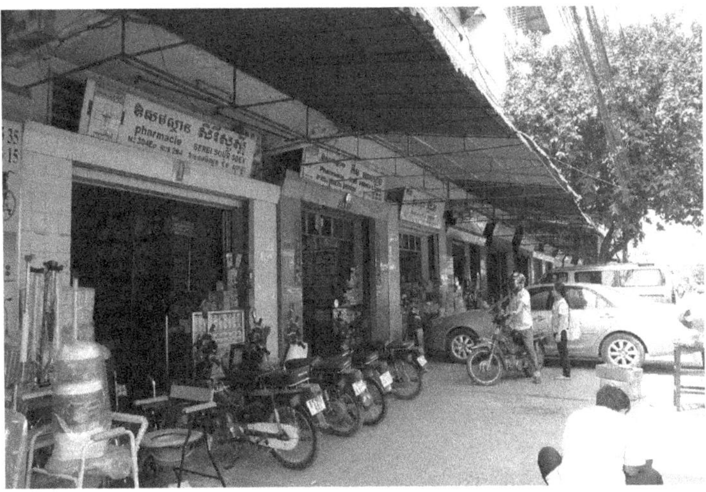


*Figure 4.2* Semi-wholesalers in Olympic Market, Phnom Penh.

Source: © IRD/Eve Bureau-Point, April 2015

Based on our interviews, these are small traders who sold small quantities of medicines around markets in the 1980s, and who gradually acquired these businesses and became official semi-wholesalers. Their shop fronts look like any other pharmacies. As with other types of businesses in Cambodia, the semi-wholesalers are in adjoining buildings in a single neighborhood.

Semi-wholesalers have developed a network of clients in all of the country's provinces since the reconstruction of the pharmaceutical market in the 1980s. For a long time, most wholesale transactions have been handled by these Olympic Market semi-wholesalers who use taxis to quickly supply various semi-wholesalers in the provinces. At the time of the study, they were distributing a large quantity of drugs throughout the country, but the arrival of formidable importer-distributors who distribute directly in the provinces began to change the flow of drugs and decreased their sales (interview with vendors in the Olympic Market, Phnom Penh, 2015). Nevertheless, we regularly heard: "You can find everything at the Olympic Market." Hence, they have maintained a large clientele.

Drugs are transported from the wholesalers to the retailers in boxes, loaded on small motorbikes and minivans that may or may not be refrigerated. It is important to remember that Cambodia is a tropical country where temperatures often exceed 30°C, while the instructions inserted in many medicines specify that they should be stored in conditions below 25°C or 30°C (see Figure 4.3).

Thus, with the liberalization of the economy, the drug market has become more complex. The number of actors and products requiring monitoring and testing has grown exponentially, each one implementing more-or-less legal accommodations to balance economic interests, practical considerations, and public health requirements. Subsequently, market forces led to an abundance, or even

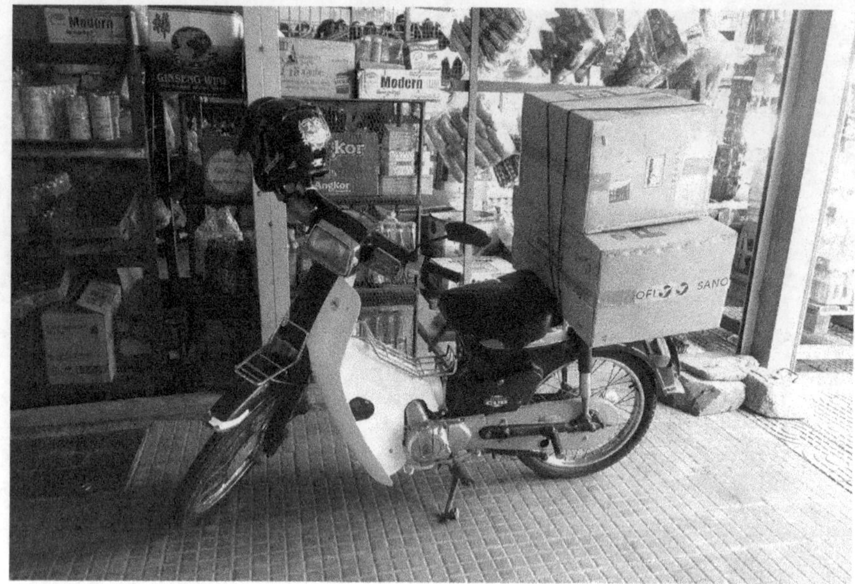


*Figure 4.3* Transporting medicines on motorbikes.

Source: © IRD/Eve Bureau-Point, April 2015

overabundance, of some therapeutic classes (analgesics, anti-inflammatories, antibiotics, etc.) to the detriment of others that are either rare or lacking, as illustrated elsewhere (Al Dahdah, Kumar, & Quet, 2018; Baxerres, 2013; Desclaux & Egrot, 2015).

## Regulations and deregulations affecting prescribers, retailers, and consumers

Reviewing the main drug supply sites used by families who were monitored in our study and my observations of interactions between distributers and consumwers, I will now describe the logics of distribution and access to medicines that facilitate or compromise the flow of drugs.

*Table 4.2* Main drug supply sites for families monitored during the study

| Medicine sheets | Pharmacies/ depots | Private consultation room | Public health facilities | Private clinics and hospitals |
|---|---|---|---|---|
| **Phnom Penh n=134** | 49 | 25 | 31 | 29 |
| **Battambang n=135** | 60 | 39 | 31 | 5 |

Our monitoring confirmed the Ministry of Health statistics (National Institute of Statistics, Directorate General for Health, & ICF International [NIS, DGH, & ICF], 2015). The majority of patients turn to the private sector, while the majority of medicines consumed by family members in the study were obtained in a pharmacy or pharmacy-depot (see above table 4.2). There are various reasons for the high number of visits to pharmacies and depots. First, contrary to the law, people can buy virtually any type of medicine without a prescription in these places. Vendors are rarely familiar with the official list of over-the-counter (OTC) drugs[22] and for the most part do not include them in their practices, with the exception of a small number of pharmacies that proliferate in cities and tourist areas (Phnom Penh, Siem Reap, Sihanoukville, and Kep), and the managers of which want to be known for applying best practices in pharmacy standards (presence of a pharmacist, air-conditioning, and prescription medicines only sold with a prescription). In 2016, we counted about 20 pharmacies of this type in Phnom Penh. Another factor why high numbers of consumers turn to the private sector: the public sector's failure to attract customers who want to treat everyday ailments. In fact, our study shows that public-sector drug distribution does not seem to meet patients' expectations. Various interviewees, from both urban and rural areas, used the following phrases: "there's only para [for paracetamol] at the health center," and "they don't have everything you need"; and "there are frequent stockouts," and "we have to go buy medicines in the private sector." People with the financial means generally avoid this sector or use it for very specific reasons: access to expensive medicines distributed for free (triple therapies for HIV or tuberculosis), a reproductive health follow-up visit, access to free treatments (for poor people with a fee-waiver card), vaccination, or use of an ambulance transport system in an emergency. However, in these facilities, patients see a health professional before being sent to the in-house pharmacy with a prescription. Access to medicines is under the control of health professionals. Yet, can we say that the public sector has greater control on drug circulation than the private sector does, as argued by a former Khmer Rouge cadre (Battambang province, December 2015)? Indeed, in the public sector, nurses in charge of pharmacy transactions fill out prescription and inventory registers in the private sector; whereas in the private sector, despite being a requirement, we have not seen any retail vendors record sales in registers. Nevertheless, drug circulation management in the public sector is regularly criticized. The Ministry of Health is sometimes at the center of health scandals involving fraud and embezzlement, as illustrated by the 2013 study conducted by the Global Fund to Fight AIDS, Tuberculosis and Malaria.[23] In addition, we were able to repeatedly find public-sector drugs, described as distributed solely through the public sector, on the shelves of private retail vendors.

Another accommodation has occurred since the 1980s during the reconstruction of the pharmaceutical system: pharmacies with no pharmacists and depots with no health professionals. This can be explained in different ways. In the rural area where we conducted our study, we noticed that the owners of these official retail shops were mostly nurses from the community health center. In parallel to their full-time activity in the public sector, these nurses have opened a private outlet and dispense medicines outside of their public work hours, but they sometimes do this during their public-sector shift. According to Ministry of Health data, low salaries have led to this dual practice (Ministry of Health, 2012). Public-sector health professionals do not earn enough to discourage them from working in parallel in the private sector. When health professionals were away from their private structures, we observed that their business remained open and that a nonqualified person from the socio-family network continued to conduct sales. Based on our observations and interviews in rural and urban areas, this fairly widespread phenomenon includes most health professionals in the public sector, whether in Phnom Penh or Battambang. In cities, it seems that the lack of pharmacists in pharmacies is explained less by unavailable human resources and instead by how unappealing pharmacists find working in a pharmacy. According to our interviews, most of these dissatisfied pharmacists seek jobs in international organizations or pharmaceutical companies, sectors that are substantially more rewarding. Contrary to the legal requirements taught at the university, the pharmacists we met in Phnom Penh explained that they "rent" their licenses to pharmacies or pharmaceutical companies in exchange for USD 100–150 per month. With a certain discomfort, they explained that they rarely set foot on the premises where they are officially responsible. This context of "pharmacies without pharmacists" was previously described by Ovesen and Trankell (2007). As noted in the study, the spread of this practice led the Ministry of Health to set up short-term training for drug vendors who are not officially authorized to sell pharmaceuticals to learn basic skills for medicine distribution in a broad range of outlets (pharmacies, Depot-As and -Bs). Some interviewees indicated that this training can be "purchased" and that not all drug vendors follow it, as underscored by Quet et al.; however, this does not mean that these drug vendors' practices are ineffective or dangerous (2018). Nonqualified vendors are also implementing strategies to ensure medicine quality and people's health. As pointed out by Quet et al., more often than not, these logics, along with others, make the practice "more functional" (2018, p. 15).

We noted that medicine distribution practices in private consultation rooms[24] are highly similar to those in pharmacies and pharmacy-depots. The doctors, nurses, midwives, and dentists who work there, along with other nonqualified vendors who replace them during their absences or assist them during peak times, take on the role officially reserved for pharmacists and gear their activities toward selling medicines. Health officials maintain that private consultation rooms may carry outpatient drugs for patient care; however, in practice, they have an arsenal of medicines that sometimes equals those of pharmacies and depots. Moreover, although they are not authorized to sell them, quite the opposite occurs: The staff at these facilities explained that the consultation, which rarely takes place, is free and the medicine is paid for. This is a prime example of a process of commodification of medicines. These professionals and laypersons distribute medicines as quickly as pharmacies and depots do, based on very limited conversations with patients. In 2012, this problem had already been uncovered in a Ministry of Health report: "this practice is not legal and the laws regarding separation of roles of prescribing and dispensing need to be enforced" (Ministry of Health, 2012). Again, this also does not mean that the practices are ineffective or dangerous. However, the habit of bypassing auscultation and avoiding direct contact with the patient—a practice that has been highlighted in various studies on health in Cambodia (Bureau-Point, 2016)—is considered to contradict the deontology of health professionals.

Other mechanisms help explain the high number of consumers who visit pharmacies, depots, and medical offices. Indeed, a patient's trust in a drug distributor is not based on the status of the locations and professionals but on the interpersonal relationship and the perceived efficacy of the treatment received. People generally have one or two preferred locations where they purchase medicines that they have chosen over time, based on their experiences there. A trusting relationship is established with the people who work there. Several factors explain why the sites' and professionals' status ultimately plays a minimal role in building trust. First, we mentioned that people hardly distinguish between private medical offices, pharmacies, and depots. The law has designated pharmacies and depots by green crosses and private clinics and consultation rooms by blue ones. However, in practice, the colors used do not always comply with these standards and seldom serve as a reference point for individuals to distinguish between these care or pharmaceutical distribution points. More generally, the coexistence of two color codes in popular perceptions in Cambodia partially explains why these color-coded crosses are inefficient: until recently, no distinction was made between green and blue.[25]

Moreover, although we found numerous unskilled drug vendors working in private medical offices, pharmacies, or depots, our interviews and observations in these structures revealed that clients think they are dealing with qualified health professionals who possess the medical expertise and proper pharmaceutical knowledge to meet their needs. Although clients rarely know the professional status of those who treat them, these individuals are all considered to be *pet* (a diminutive of *kru pet*: *kru*, master; *pet*, hospital, translated in English by "doctor" but used to designate all health professionals). Clients frequently call the people they meet in these various health-care points "*pet*." Health professionals often own depots or pharmacies, and vendors working with them who are generally from their socio-familial environment (a spouse, niece or nephew, cousin, son or daughter, or family friend) sell medicines with them. Regardless of their family status, they are perceived as *pet*, based on their somewhat remote relationship to biomedical knowledge. Several health professionals generalizing about their experience said with some irony: "When one family member is *pet*, the others become *pet* also." Consequently, in popular perceptions, retailers perform two jobs, providing both professional health consultations and medicines. Therefore, a consultation that does not result in dispensing medicine is generally perceived as useless.

High demand in pharmacies and depots must also be understood in the context of tactics developed by drug vendors and consumers to create a more practical context. One tactic is the practice of "*thnam psoam*." These distribution methods

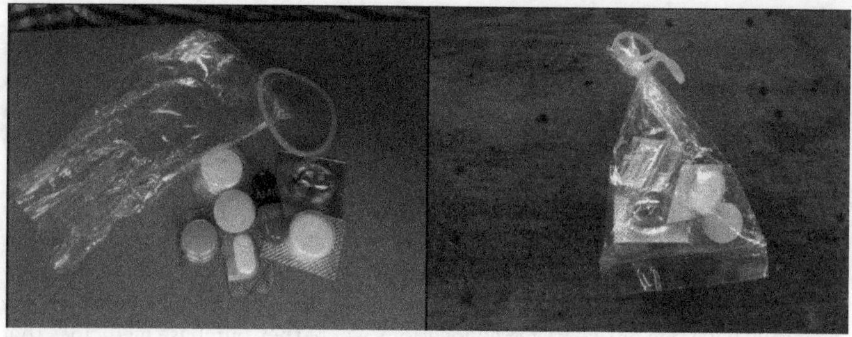

*Figure 4.4* Mixed medicines.
Source: © IRD/Eve Bureau-Point, April 2015

have advantages and disadvantages for both the vendor and the consumer, as we will see. Medicines, whether tablets or blister packs, are very rarely sold in their original packaging, but rather more often in bulk in clear plastic bags sealed with a rubber band and containing several doses (see Figure 4.4). In Khmer, these bags are called *thnam psoam*, or literally "mixed medicines." Frequently, vendors put two types of antibiotics, analgesics, or anti-inflammatories in one bag, usually corresponding to one dose. Rarely do vendors have a single type of medicine per bag. These bags are typically composed of three to eight different medicines, combining bulk tablets sometimes with blister tablets, the quantity, price, and colors of which vary depending on the vendor, client, urban or rural context, and health issue. Public health officers criticize this practice, particularly because it poses risks of overdosing.

The *thnam psoam* are sold and/or requested for certain categories of health problems, such as *pdassaï*,[26] toothache, stomachache, and diarrhea. Some retailers prepare bags in advance for these different pathologies but arrange their displays so that they are not very visible from outside the point of sale. They fear inspectors' visits or being reported by potential competitors, regulators of best pharmacy practices, and even researchers!

For vendors, the preparation of the *thnam psoam* allows them to unload the least expensive medicines (usually from Cambodia and India), even though from time to time, especially in cities, clients request *thnam psoam* with "French medicines," which may multiply the price by eight. It also allows vendors to meet their clients' demands, a key point in any business activity. Generally, vendors have repeat customers and know their preferences (whether or not they are interested in *thnam psoam*, preference for small or large *thnam psoam*, spending capacity for health care, preferred source of medicines, etc.), and passing clients whose preferences vendors try to guess based on their appearance (deducing purchasing power through clothing) and on their comments. Interactions between vendors and buyers are brief, and vendors manage with little direction from the patient to guide the treatment. From the vendor's viewpoint, one advantage of the *thnam psoam* is reducing the number of explanations; if the components were given separately, the vendor would have to explain each one to the consumer.

For most consumers, the *thnam psoam* guarantees a more effective treatment. "It's more effective to take the *thnam psoam* than one single medicine because when you're sick, there's always several health problems. So, there must be one medicine for each problem" (mother, Phnom Penh, February 2015). Local perceptions of efficacy dictate that the number of medicines should often be proportional to the number of symptoms. And consuming several medicines at the same time "helps you get better faster" (father, Battambang, March 2016). In addition, another advantage is that the consumer does not need to remember the dosage for each medicine, just the daily number of bags recommended by the vendor (Bureau-Point, Baxerres, & Chheang, 2020).

Client visits to private clinics and private hospitals,[27] which are under the responsibility of the Ministry of Health, were lower during the study monitoring. In these facilities, medicines obtained in clinics and private hospitals were prescribed by certified prescribers. Most clinics have either an in-house or an adjoining pharmacy, usually run by a family member of the owner, and patients have a strong incentive to buy their medicines from these facilities (see Figure 4.5 below).

Generally, our interviewees consider these places expensive because one must pay for both the consultation with a professional and for the medicines or because they are used to getting both services for one low price. Also, since they are located in urban areas, rural patients must cover transportation costs. Patients only consult them for serious problems requiring in-depth medical exams or specific equipment.

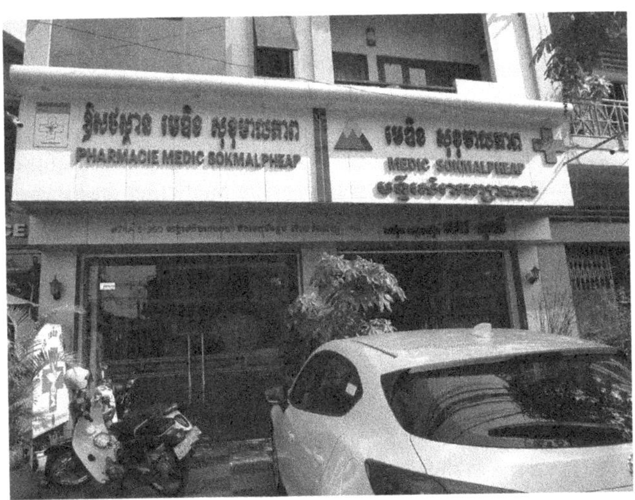


*Figure 4.5* Private clinic with an adjoining pharmacy.

Source: © IRD/Eve Bureau-Point, February 2016

These formal and informal practices of prescribers, retailers, and consumers highlight that, alongside today's State regulations that attempt to place tighter constraints on pharmacy practices, the three categories of actors described earlier play a significant role in the "multiple pharmaceutical regulations" outlined in the Introduction.

## Conclusion

This history of the structuring of the Cambodian pharmaceutical market and its excesses, which considers multiple sources of regulation, provides key contextual components to understand the circulation and consumption of medicines in contemporary Cambodia. It highlights several specific characteristics unique to the Cambodian case. The pharmaceutical system, having experienced a virtual return to "square one" with the Khmer Rouge revolution and various devastating political regimes that ensued, has been rebuilt in informal care delivery points, with traders, and health-care professionals who have undergone nonuniform, quick training that may or may not be recognized, in a context where State sovereignty is gradually being rebuilt.

This explanation of various stages of pharmaceuticalization/depharmaceuticalization, from the introduction of the first drugs during the French protectorate up until the neoliberal context of the 2010s, provides a detailed view of the friction caused by several forces. These include the State's indigence and its incomplete attempts to provide oversight, the influence of the region's producing countries (India) and regional regulatory systems (ASEAN), as well as the accommodations implemented by various actors involved all along the drug supply chain so that a medicine responds to each actor's economic, pragmatic, and/or cultural preferences.

When viewed as a market commodity embodying a means of boosting economic activity, drugs are easily caught up in financial stakes that are likely to contradict the rules governing biomedicine and public health. Numerous foreign investors, both Asian and European, were attracted by the opportunities offered by this market, which has few State controls. With their huge investments in Cambodia, with or without official support, the drug supply has grown exponentially, with an overabundance of some medicines and shortages of other molecules. The limited power of official pharmaceutical regulatory bodies and the market's incessant excesses empowers other, "bottom-up," regulatory modes implemented by the State representatives (blue pharmacies and training provided to informal vendors), drug distribution actors ("mixed medicines"), and patients (preferences, trust, and seeking efficacy).

## Notes

1. This concept refers to the rising volume of pharmaceutical drugs in circulation and their increasingly predominant place in society (Desclaux & Egrot, 2015).
2. I would like to thank Maurice Cassier who led the Globalmed team to this conceptualization of the situation in Cambodia during discussions at an internal project meeting in September 2016, held in Paris.

3. See the Introduction of this book for information about the data collection methodology for this study in Cambodia.
4. The pharmacist must supervise any drug transaction (importation or distribution) to ensure public health interests take precedence over economic interests.
5. A term that means "organization" in Khmer, often used under the Khmer Rouge regime to refer to the Khmer Rouge's revolutionary organization. Described as a mysterious, faceless authority, *Angkar* was a personified entity with a soul, feelings, and the capacity to act. People had to refer to *Angkar* as a protective and pure mother who must know everything.
6. Although there is no shortage of literature on *Kru khmaer* medicine ("*kru khmaer*": *kru*, master; *khmaer*, Khmer) (Crochet, 2000; Richman, Nawabi, Patty, & Ziment, 2010), there seems to be no specific literature on the composition of traditional medicines manufactured during the Khmer Rouge, except for a few examples cited here and there (Crochet, 2001; Tyner, 2012).
7. During the Khmer Rouge, according to Ovesen and Trankell (2010), the *Kru khmaer* were allowed to administer traditional medicines but not to recite mantras or make the offerings that usually accompanied care procedures. Any spiritual or religious component had to disappear.
8. In local use, the term "pharmaceutical company" refers both to local medicine manufacturing firms and medicine import-export and distribution companies. They have a special license from the Ministry of Health to import and export medicines.
9. This list was reissued seven times between 1995 and 2016.
10. In 2013, 80% of health-care services were delivered in the private sector (Men, 2013).
11. January 1990 working group reports in Phnom Penh on challenges in the pharmaceutical sector revealed this problem (Neou, 1999).
12. This concept covers very different phenomena: counterfeit drugs, defective drugs, and informal distribution (Baxerres, 2014; Quet, 2015).
13. https://asean.org/?static_post=accsq-pharmaceutical-product-working-group, accessed April 17, 2019.
14. In 2015, it accounted for 9% of the drug market (interview at the DDF, 2016).
15. The riel is the official currency of Cambodia; however, due to its weak value (4000 riels = USD 1, depending on the market rate), United States dollars have been in widespread use since the 1980s. Dollars are accepted everywhere and are the main currency used in cities and tourist provinces.
16. Based on official DDF data, only 5% of medicines that are formally distributed in Cambodia come from China. Today, the Chinese exportation of finished pharmaceuticals has been poorly developed, which, however, is not the case for its production of active ingredients, which it exports widely, including to India (Li, 2019).
17. Based on official DDF data, only 5% of medicines that are formally distributed in Cambodia come from China. Today, the Chinese exportation of finished pharmaceuticals has been poorly developed, which, however, is not the case for its production of active ingredients, which it exports widely, including to India (Li, 2019).
18. Semi-wholesalers purchase their supply from "pharmaceutical companies," sell wholesale or retail, and have a pharmacy license. They are not authorized to import, yet our interviews indicate they import products illegally, mostly from neighboring countries (Vietnam and Thailand). Sometimes these semi-wholesalers run an import company alongside their pharmacy.
19. Here, this term refers to importation of a product registered in another country, without the manufacturer's prior consent. Parallel imports of a patented product are assumed to be in compliance with the exhaustion regime of the manufacturer's national, regional, and international rights, once its product is marketed. After that point, it has no legal standing to oppose parallel imports.

20. Each registered product has a code beginning with KH on its packaging.
21. In order to prevent any form of publicity, these distributors' names have not been mentioned.
22. OTC drugs are pharmaceuticals that can be purchased without a prescription. The list of OTC drugs was established in 2009 in Cambodia.
23. https://www.theglobalfund.org/media/6814/oig_gf-oig-17-020_report_fr.pdf, accessed April 2019.
24. They are smaller than clinics and are the responsibility of municipal health departments (representative of the Physicians Council, February 2015).
25. According to several local sources, the color green did not exist for a long time. One health professional remarked: "Traditionally, we say that the rice fields or the trees' leaves are blue" (interview, Phnom Penh, March 2015).
26. *Pdassaïd* refers to a "nosologic popular entity" (Jaffré & Olivier de Sardan, 1999) generally translated by "flu" and "common cold"; however, Cambodians use the word *pdassaï* for different types of health disorders: runny nose, headache, sore throat, cough, fever, and sneezing.
27. Clinics are identified as having more than five hospital beds.

## Reference list

Al Dahdah, M., Kumar, A., & Quet, M. (2018). Empty stocks and loose paper: Governing access to medicines through informality in Northern India. *International Sociology*, *33*(6), 778–795.

Au, S. (2011). *Mixed Medicines. Health and culture in French colonial Cambodia*. London, UK: University of Chicago Press.

Baxerres, C. (2013). *Du médicament informel au médicament libéralisé : Une anthropologie du médicament pharmaceutique au Bénin [From informal to liberalized drugs: An anthropology of pharmaceutical drugs in Benin]*. Paris, France: Les Éditions des Archives Contemporaines.

Baxerres, C. (2014). Faux médicaments, de quoi parle-t-on? Contrefaçons, marché informel, qualité des médicaments… réflexions à partir d'une étude anthropologique conduite au Bénin [Fake drugs, what are we talking about? Counterfeits, informal market, drug quality … thoughts from an anthropological study conducted in Benin]. *Bulletin de la société de pathologie exotique*, *107*, 121–126. https://doi.org/10.1007/s13149-014-0354-9.

Bonnemain, B. (2008). Colonisation et pharmacie (1830–1962): Une présence diversifiée de 130 ans des pharmaciens français [Colonization and pharmacy (1830–1962): A 130-year diverse presence of French pharmacists]. *Revue d'histoire de la pharmacie*, *359*, 311–334.

Bourdier, F., Man, B., & Res, P. (2014). La circulation non contrôlée des médicaments en Asie du Sud-Est et au Cambodge [The uncontrolled circulation of drugs in Southeast Asia and Cambodia]. *L'espace politique*, *24* (3). https://doi.org/10.4000/espacepolitique.3220.

Bureau-Point, E. (2016). *Les patients experts dans la lutte contre le sida au Cambodge. Anthropologie d'une norme globalisée [Expert patients in the fight against AIDS in Cambodia. Anthropology of a globalized standard]*. Aix-en-Provence, France: Presses Universitaires de Provence.

Bureau-Point, E., Baxerres, C., & Chheang, S. (2020). Self-medication in the Cambodian pharmaceutical system in Cambodia, *Medical Anthropology*, p. p. 765–781. https://doi.org/10.1080/01459740.2020.1753726.

Chandler, D. (1992). *A history of Cambodia* (2nd ed.). Chiangmai, Thailand: Silkworm Books.

Chhem, R. K. (2001). Les doctrines médicales khmères: Nosologie et méthodes diagnostiques [Khmer medical doctrines: Nosology and diagnostic methods]. *Siksâcakr*, *3*, 12–15.

Crochet, S. (2000). L'invisible guérison: Notes d'ethnomédecine en milieu rural au Cambodge [Invisible healing: Notes on ethnomedicine in rural Cambodia]. *Aséanie*, 5, 13–39.

Crochet, S. (2001). *Etude ethnographique des pratiques familiales de santé au Cambodge [Ethnographic study of family health practices in Cambodiaa]*. Doctoral dissertation, Université Paris Nanterre, France. Retrieved from http://www.theses.fr/2001PA100211.

Desclaux, A., & Egrot, M. (Eds.). (2015). *Anthropologie du médicament au Sud. La pharmaceutica lisation à ses marges [Anthropology of medicines in the South. Pharmaceuticalization at its margins]*. Paris, France: L'Harmattan.

Gollogly, L. (2002). The dilemmas of aid: Cambodia 1992–2002. *The Lancet*, 360, 793–98.

Guillou, A. Y. (2009). *Cambodge: Soigner dans les fracas de l'histoire [Cambodia: Providing care in the clamor of history]*. Paris, France: Les Indes savantes.

Jaffré, Y., & Olivier de Sardan, J.-P. (1999). *La construction sociale des maladies: Les entités nosologiques populaires en Afrique de l'Ouest [The social construction of diseases: Popular nosological entities in West Africa]*. Paris, France: Éditions PUF.

Li, L. (2019, October). Captured between market and bureaucratic rules: State, health politics, and pharmaceutical industry in China. Paper presented at the Pharmaceuticals and Development in the Global South Research Workshop, Global Development Institute, University of Manchester, UK.

Men, C. R. (2013). *Safety of medicinal products in Cambodia: Assessment of the pharmacovigilance system and its performance*. Arlington, VA: Systems for Improved Access to Pharmaceuticals and Services.

Ministry of Health. (2004). *Situational analysis pharmaceutical sector in Cambodia*. Phnom Penh, Cambodia: Department of Drugs and Food.

Ministry of Health. (2012). *Pharmaceutical sector strategic plan, 2013–2018*. Accra, Ghana. Department of Drugs and Foods.

Monnais, L. (2014). *Médicaments coloniaux : L'expérience Vietnamienne, 1905–1940 [Colonial medicines: The Vietnamese experience, 1905–1940]*. Paris, France: Les Indes savantes.

National Institute of Statistics, Directorate General for Health, & ICF International (NIS, DGH, & ICF). (2015). *Cambodia demographic and health survey 2014*. Phnom Penh, Cambodia, and Rockville, MD: National Institute of Statistics, Directorate General for Health, and ICF International.

Neou, S. L. (1999). *Contribution à l'étude de l'évolution du système pharmaceutique au Cambodge [Contribution to the study of changes in the pharmaceutical system in Cambodia]*. Phnom Penh, Cambodia: University of Health Sciences.

Ovesen, J., & Trankell, I. B. (2007). Pharmacists and other drug-providers in Cambodia: Identities and experiences. In K. Maynard (Ed.), *Medical identities: Health, well-being and personhood* (pp. 36–60). Oxford, UK: Berghahn Books.

Ovesen, J., & Trankell, I. B. (2010). *Cambodians and their doctors. A medical anthropology of colonial and post-colonial Cambodia*. Copenhagen, Denmark: NIAS Press.

Pordié, L. (2016, June). Unstable pharmaceutical values. Drugs' distribution networks and practices in Cambodia. Paper presented at The Making of Pharmaceutical Values International Workshop, Paris, France.

Quet, M. (2015). Sécurisation pharmaceutique et économies du médicament. Controverses globales autour des politiques anti-contrefaçon [Pharmaceutical security and drug economies. Global controversies around anti-counterfeiting policies]. *Sciences Sociales et Santé*, 33(1), 91–116.

Quet, M., Pordié, L., Bochaton, A., Chantavanich, S., Kiatying-Angsulee, N., Lamy, M., & Vungsiriphisal, P. (2018). Regulation multiple: Pharmaceutical trajectories and modes of control in the ASEAN. *Science, Technology and Society*, *23*(3), 485–503. https://doi.org/10.1177/0971721818762935.

Richman, M. J., Nawabi, S., Patty, L., & Ziment, I. (2010). Traditional Cambodian medicine. *Journal of Complementary and Integrative Medicine*, *7*(1). http://dx.doi.org/10.2202/1553-3840.1194.

Tyner, J. A. (2012). State sovereignty, bioethics, and political geographies: The practice of medicine under the Khmer Rouge. *Environment and Planning*, *30*, 842–860.

Vickery, M. (1984). *Cambodia 1975–1982*. Boston, MA: South End Press.

Vun, M. C., Galang, R. R., Fujita, M., Killam, W., Gokhale, R., Pitman, J., … Vonthanak, S. (2016). Cluster of HIV infections attributed to unsafe injection practices. Cambodia. December 1, 2014–February 28, 2015. *Morbidity and Mortality Weekly Report*, *65*(6), 142–145.

# Part II

# Global and local markets of new antimalarials

This second section examines the construction of global and local pharmaceutical markets for the new artemisinin-based drugs invented in China in the 1970s and 1980s, and the rise of standardized herbal medicines, which have seen unprecedented momentum in Ghana since the mid-2000s. The globalization of new antimalarial drugs between Asia and Africa is based on the intermediation of international (World Health Organization) and global (global donor markets) health institutions, multinational firms, and Asian generic manufacturers, as well as on the initiatives of local producers and wholesalers, particularly in Ghana. The diffusion of these new antimalarial drugs, embedded in very different market systems in Ghana and Benin, is powerfully influenced by the distribution of drugs subsidized by global donors, which are confined to public distribution in Benin but available in the public sector and in a very large private market in Ghana. The markedly differing uses of these drugs in the two countries suggest that a variety of other antimalarials should be maintained in Benin. The Ghanaian policy of industrializing and standardizing herbal medicines is supported by administrative regulation that cooperates with traditional medicine organizations. The works presented here mobilize historical sociology, anthropology, and social epidemiology.

# 5 A new geography of pharmaceuticals

## Trajectories of artemisinin-based medicines

*Maurice Cassier*

Research in the geopolitics of medicines has focused on the emergence of copycat capitalism in countries in the global South since the 1970s, particularly in India and Brazil (Cassier & Correa, 2003; Chaudhuri, 2005). However, in this chapter, I would like to highlight the singular trajectories of artemisinin-based drugs—discovered and initially developed, industrialized, and tested in the People's Republic of China and in Vietnam—beginning in the early 1970s and 1980s. It is one of the rare, perhaps only, therapeutic classes of biomedicine to have been invented in a so-called emerging or "Third World" country, to use the vocabulary of that time. The chemist Tu Youyou of the Academy of Traditional Chinese Medicine, who was awarded the Nobel Prize for Medicine in 2015 for the discovery of artemisinin by hybridizing traditional pharmacopoeia and modern chemistry, entitled his lecture: "A gift from traditional Chinese medicine to the world."[1] What is less well known is that the most widely used treatment in the world since its inclusion on the WHO essential medicines list in 2002, artemisinin-based combination therapy (ACT), which combines artemether and lumefantrine (AL), was also invented by Chinese researchers.[2] This product was the subject of one of the first drug patents filed in China in 1990. The researchers subsequently established a partnership in 1991 with Ciba Geigy, now Novartis, to make it a global medicine. Chemist Zhou Yiqing was rewarded by the European Patent Office and the European Commission in 2009 for the invention of the first artemisinin-based fixed-dose combination therapy.[3]

The globalization of artemisinin-based medicines, i.e., the duplication of inventions, the spread of the industry, the creation of markets and uses in malaria-endemic countries, is unique in that it was not undertaken or controlled by Chinese scientific institutions and companies, but by multinationals (Novartis, Sanofi) and through the intermediary of WHO and humanitarian health organizations, especially Médecins Sans Frontières (MSF) (Balkan & Corty, 2009). The Special Programme for Research in Training in Tropical Diseases (TDR) a research group created in 1975 by WHO, the World Bank, and the United Nations Development Programme (UNDP) to accelerate the invention of new treatments for tropical diseases and compensate for the withdrawal of international laboratory R&D on these diseases, took an early interest in the Chinese researchers' work. TDR signed an initial research collaboration agreement in September 1979 with the

Shanghai Institute of Materia Medica.[4] In December 1980, the Secretary General of WHO, Halfdan Malher, who inspired the Alma Ata list of essential medicines and primary health policy, wrote to the Chinese Minister of Health and proposed organizing a Working Group on the Chemotherapy of Malaria (CHEMAL) seminar on artemisinin. This seminar was held in Beijing in October 1981, where it was decided that the resources for the program to develop artemisinin and its derivatives would be increased. In 1996, MSF pharmacists noted the arrival of artemisinin derivatives, presented as the result of "fortuitous analysis of traditional pharmacopeias" in the People's Republic of China (Trouiller, 1996). In 1999 and 2002, MSF published two articles of note in *JAMA* (Pecoul, Chirac, Trouiller, & Pinel, 1999) and *The Lancet* (Trouiller et al., 2002) highlighting the fact that the few innovations in the field of neglected diseases (1% of all compounds registered between 1975 and 1999) largely arose from the development of artemisinin derivatives. The authors note that these new drugs are produced and registered in China and marketed in Southeast Asia and Africa, an unusual geography for the invention, production, and marketing of medicinal products: "Although rare, examples of registrations exclusively within developing countries do exist–e.g., artemisinin derivatives for malaria developed and manufactured in China" (Trouiller et al., 2002, p. 2188). In 1999, MSF created the Drugs for Neglected Diseases Working Group (DNDWG) that brings together experts from scientific institutions in Brazil, India, Malaysia, the Harvard School of Public Health, MSF pharmacists, and TDR members, and is committed to developing two new fixed-dose ACTs: artesunate and amodiaquine (ASAQ) in France and artesunate and mefloquine (ASMQ) in Brazil (Cassier, 2008).

This unusual geography of therapeutic innovation, initiated in China and involving many scientific institutions and firms from Southeast Asia, India, Brazil, and Africa, can be explained by a few salient points. First is the public and common appropriation of the basic components of these drugs (artemisinin and its four derivatives with therapeutic usefulness: dihydroartemisinin, artesunate, artemether, and arteether), which were developed in China at a time when patents did not exist, so these molecules can therefore be legally copied and combined everywhere in the world. The second point concerns the public-private partnerships established through the intermediary of WHO or MSF, involving organizations from both the North and South and manufacturers of both trademarked and generic drugs, to support the R&D, manufacturing, and distribution of this class of drugs intended for low- and middle-income countries, particularly in Africa. The industrial geography is widespread: WHO drew up a list of pharmaceutical companies producing artemisinin-based medicines in 2006 (41 companies); the growth in this area was such that it had to reissue the list in 2007 (83 companies, 67 of which produced monotherapies and 16 ACTs), with companies distributed across several continents: Asia (China, India, Malaysia, Pakistan, Vietnam), Europe (Belgium, Denmark, France, Germany, Italy, Switzerland), and Africa (Cameroon, DRC, Ghana, Nigeria, Tanzania). Two factors led to a decrease in this wide-ranging production, most of it by generic companies: the reduction in monotherapy supply, as recommended by WHO and the Global Fund to Fight

AIDS, Tuberculosis and Malaria[5]; and the growth in ACT supply, which gradually became the norm in subsidized markets.[6] This dispersion of industrial supply coexisted with a concentration of economic value in two multinational companies, Novartis (marketing Coartem®) and Sanofi (marketing ASAQ), until the early 2010s, at which time Indian, and to a lesser extent Chinese, generic manufacturers impose their prices on the global donor market.[7]

While the artemisinin-based drug industry was globalizing, the cultivation of artemisia and the natural artemisinin extraction industry remained heavily concentrated in China and Vietnam, with a few spin-offs in East Africa and Madagascar.

In this chapter, I will examine four mechanisms behind the globalization of artemisinin-based drugs. The first section will analyze TDR's intermediation to organize both upgrading Chinese factories to international standards and globalizing these new treatments through agreements with foreign firms. The second section will focus on the globalization of the most widely used combination, AL, through a dual partnership between Novartis and Chinese inventors and producers on the one hand, and between Novartis and WHO on the other. The third section will look at the alliance between the Drugs for Neglected Diseases Initiative (DND*i*) and Sanofi to invent and market ASAQ, the second most widely sold ACT after AL. Finally, the fourth section will examine the manufacture of artemisinin-based medicines in Africa, which is the main region of consumption but where production is limited and intended for local markets.[8]

## The globalization of a Chinese invention: The intermediation of Tropical Diseases Research (TDR)

TDR was created by WHO in 1975 to accelerate the development of therapeutic innovations for tropical diseases, in a context of increasing resistance to existing malaria treatments and exhaustion of the proprietary model, which devotes few resources to these diseases. TDR uses its funding to establish research and industrialization partnerships between governments, academia, and industry (developing manufacturing and formulation technologies, performing clinical trials, bringing factories and products up to international standards, and so forth). TDR proclaims "the primacy of public interests"[9] through public-private partnerships and focuses on accessibility to treatment in developing countries. Its board represents recipient countries as well as donors, and it offers a prominent place to countries directly affected by these endemics. In 1975, TDR set up a group dedicated to malaria chemotherapy (CHEMAL).

The TDR archives show that WHO has been funding the initial research projects in China since 1979. Concerned about the rise in treatment resistance, WHO supports the work of Chinese researchers to speed the development of technologies for two promising artemisinin derivatives: artesunate and artemether.[10] Chinese institutions have already industrialized several artemisinin-based drugs that are registered in China, so WHO's goal is to bring Chinese laboratories and factories in line with international standards. Wallace Peters, who headed the CHEMAL committee on antimalaria drugs, points out the gap between the standards applied by China and international standards: "from the western regulatory point of view, there were big gaps in the Chinese toxicity and efficacy studies… but China wanted the drug sold and used, and was uncomfortable about TDR taking over this development work."[11] In March 1982, TDR notes the non-respect of Good Manufacturing Practice (GMP) standards: "the plant that is used to lyophilize the artesunate preparations does not conform to GMP."[12] TDR's collaborative research agreement specifically targets the "development of a standardized formulation of artesunate and artemether" (June 1982).[13] The account published by the Chinese inventors on the WHO collaboration emphasizes the work of bringing Chinese factories up to standards (pp. 88–89). Between 1979 and 1986, TDR financed several collaborative research agreements at the Shanghai Institute of Materia Medica, the Beijing Institute of Materia Medica, and the Shanghai Research Institute of Pharmaceutical Industry. The funding covered the purchase of scientific equipment, the development of new synthesis processes, and new techniques for analyzing molecules. TDR also subsidizes internships for Chinese researchers in laboratories in the United States and Europe: "Application form for research training grants for these two people will be sent to you shortly" (Scientific Working Group on Malaria Chemotherapy, December 1979); "I have been invited to visit the Netherlands by Professor B. B. Bremer of the Leiden University" (Shanghai Institute of Materia Medica, September 5, 1980). This same Chinese pharmacologist is pleased to be in contact with Hoffman Laroche: "Thank you for introducing me to Mr Fernex… The department of bioanalytical method of Hoffman Laroche New Jersey is very strong."[14]

Simultaneously with its research agreements with laboratories in China, TDR organizes the dissemination of work on artemisinin in laboratories in the North: "TDR helped to get researchers outside of China involved in artemisinin and get it on the research agenda" (Halfdan Mahler). TDR encouraged the Walter Reed Army Institute to grow artemisia and extract artemisinin in Mississippi. In 1986, the WHO Malaria Chemotherapy Research Group report identified two sources of raw materials for its own developments: "the acquisition of large quantities of artemisinin for conversion to arteether was facilitated by the generous gift of one kilogram of artemisinin from the government of China; other supplies were obtained from *Artemisia annua* grown in Mississippi, USA."[15]

In 1986, TDR also launched its own R&D line on one of the artemisinin derivatives, arteether, which it entrusted to the Dutch firm Artecef for industrialization. WHO itself even filed a patent on this molecule, the inventors of which are members of the CHEMAL research group, Arnold Brossi and Peter Buchs. The patent claims a novel synthesis of this artemisinin derivative, as well as a pharmaceutical composition comprising the product of this process and an excipient. The introduction of the patent refers to the long-standing use of artemisinin extracts in the "Republic of China" but does not reference the studies of Chinese researchers on this same derivative: "extracts of which have been used as an antimalarial preparation in the Republic of China for centuries" (EP330520, 1988).

The Chinese inventors' account illustrates their irritation: "only two years later, China discovered that WHO/TDR had signed an agreement with ACF Company in Holland to develop the ether derivative" (Jianfang, 2013, p. 111).

In the early 1990s, Rhône-Poulenc signed an exclusive agreement to distribute injectable artemether in Europe and endemic regions[16]; at the same time, TDR was communicating with Kunming Pharmaceutical Factory (KPF) to carry out preclinical and clinical studies of the drug and to implement GMP standards in the Chinese plant.[17] TDR hired two pharmaceutical consulting firms, one British and the other American, to visit the Kunming plant and make recommendations. Their audits corroborate the view that while the new factory, specially built by the Chinese, and the industrial equipment meet GMP standards, efforts should be made to improve the production and quality control procedures, especially technical documentation, which must accurately track production and control testing. Kunming was quite satisfied with the assistance it received to bring its new plant up to international standards. The WHO-appointed experts were able to conduct 10-day in-depth visits to the factory and were invited back by the Chinese. However, tensions arose in 1991 when WHO learned that China was preparing to deliver 20 million vials to Myanmar before the factory was GMP-certified and without informing WHO of this plan. In 1993, WHO and Rhône-Poulenc signed an R&D agreement to speed up registration of the drug in Europe and all endemic countries and to treat severe forms of malaria in those countries. In return for transferring its preclinical and clinical data for the product, marketed under the name Paluther®, WHO required that Rhône-Poulenc offers differentiated pricing for the public sector and that it provides oversight for the company's marketing as well as the therapeutic indication for severe forms of malaria. TDR was aware that the fixed price (USD 2 per vial) was unattainable for African countries: "the African public sector can support 10 cents per treatment, so even if the product is sold at cost, there is a need for donor financial support" (November 1992). In 1994, Rhône-Poulenc complained to WHO that it was discouraging the use of artemisinin-based drugs in Africa.[18]

WHO, and TDR in particular, therefore played a key role in supporting the spin-off of Chinese inventions and making them "global" medicines. Although this process benefits from the "public good" status of the basic components of these drugs, such status also leads to a loss of control by Chinese institutions over their industrial exploitation by foreign firms on the world market: "Our mistake was not to realize that publication of our data made that information public property, and it was lost to our control and claims of ownership" (Jianfang, 2013).[19] Above I described the tension between WHO and Chinese inventors over TDR's separate development of artemether in the late 1980s. This process of disappropriation is also facilitated by the barrier of manufacturing standards and clinical studies: "there are many commercial interests in this area of development outside of China… Unless the manufacturing issues can be successfully addressed, China will lose its competitive advantage to other companies outside of China who are able to manufacture certifiable products at lower cost" (TDR, September 1992).

Hence the TDR funded actions to implement GMP standards in Chinese factories. These plants have actually produced Paluther® for Rhône-Poulenc and are participating in a joint venture with Novartis to produce Coartem®.

Chinese firms have so far registered 26% of the WHO prequalified artemisinin-based medicines; Indian firms hold prequalifications for 50%.[20] However, the market share of Chinese firms is limited: in 2012, the sales of Guilin, the only prequalified Chinese manufacturer, represented 1% of the market in terms of the value of global donors. At the same time, Indian manufacturers captured 60% of the global ACT market,[21] due in part to earlier WHO certification. In 2013, Guilin supplied 5.5% of the ASAQ market compared to Sanofi's 90% (UNITAID, 2015). However, China supplies the majority of the active ingredients for these drugs, particularly artemisinin and artemether active pharmaceutical ingredients (APIs), including to India (Huang et al., 2016).

## The globalization of Coartem®: Agreements between Novartis, CITIC,[22] and WHO

Three-quarters of the global ACT market consists of the AL combination. Until 2008, Coartem®, produced and marketed by Novartis, accounted for 80% of the AL combination market, before falling to 12% in 2013 in the face of Indian prequalified generics. This combination is a Chinese invention, developed, clinically tested, and even patented in China in 1990. Novartis acquired the market through two main agreements: one with CITIC in 1991, without WHO intermediation, to complete the industrial and clinical developments and bring them in line with international standards; and the other with WHO in 2001, at Novartis' request in 2000, since WHO is the required point of entry for building and even administering this market.

The inventor of Coartem®, Zhou Yiqing, was one of the actors in the negotiations with Novartis and provides us with the justifications for this cooperation: "No Chinese pharmaceutical company was capable of introducing this medicine to the rest of the world. So I went to the Ministry of Science and Technology, which introduced me to China International Trust and Investment Corporation—CITIC—the only Chinese state enterprise at the time that was authorized to deal with foreign investors. With the State's approval and CITIC's help, we were introduced to Novartis."[23] Chinese researchers welcomed industrial cooperation with Novartis "because of their professionalism and eagerness to cooperate." The cooperation agreement included the reevaluation of the therapeutic combination using international standards: "Novartis requested both parties to repeat preclinical studies, clinical trials, and a complete review of all research data. The conclusion reached was that data of our initial experiments and studies coincided with the results of the repeat studies by an international research company" (Jianfang, 2013, p. 136). The registration dossier for Coartem® submitted by Novartis, which is in the WHO archives, consists of an amalgamation of Chinese preclinical and clinical data and data produced by the multinational company.[24] Recall that the AL combination was registered in China in 1992 and produced by two national companies, KPF and later the Zhejiang Xinchang Pharmaceutical Factory (Jianfang, 2013).

The first patent on the AL combination is co-owned by China and Ciba-Geigy: "In 1991, to help our team get patents around the world, Novartis established a partnership with the Institute of Microbiology and Epidemiology and Kunming's Pharmaceutical Corporation, through CITIC. Together we co-developed Coartem®" (Zhou Yiqing, WHO Bulletin, 2009). The seven inventors are all Chinese researchers with Zhou Yiqing as the primary inventor, and Ciba Geigy and the Chinese Institute of Microbiology and Epidemiology as the applicants. The international extension of this patent, through 2011 covered 52 countries, 15 of which are in Africa (including Egypt, Kenya, Morocco, Nigeria, and South Africa, which all host local pharmaceutical production). It should be noted that 17 African countries where Coartem® is registered were not covered by this patent (Benin, Burkina Faso, Côte d'Ivoire, Ethiopia, Gabon, Ghana Guinea, Madagascar, Mali, Mauritania, Mozambique, Niger, Senegal, Tanzania, Togo, Zimbabwe, and Zanzibar). Generic versions could therefore be legally produced or imported into these latter countries. Ciba-Geigy strengthened its patent portfolio in the 1990s and obtained full ownership without the Chinese institutions and in 1999 filed a patent on lumefantrine derivatives. In the 2000s, it obtained exclusive patent rights for Coartem® dispersible, developed in collaboration with the Medicines for Malaria Venture (MMV).[25] In 2014, Chinese inventors patented a new formulation of the combination: "preparation of artemether and benflumetol (or lumefantrine) compound fat emulsion for injection, and application of same for malaria treatment"[26]—that is, a sort of reappropriation of this medicine (patent coverage is however limited to China).

At the beginning of 2000, Novartis offered WHO a USD 1 pediatric Coartem® in endemic countries. The multinational company noted that very few countries had registered Coartem® at that time, and that adoption of the combination therapy would depend on the WHO's commitment: "What happened is that almost no government was interested in buying the drug. But then WHO changed the policy and we saw a change in behavior and some governments like Zambia for example placed some orders" (D. Vasella, Novartis, January 2007).[27] Furthermore, WHO refused to register Coartem® in 1999 on its list of essential drugs due to its high price (USD 4.5) compared to the antimalarial drugs used previously. It was also a new drug for which there was little feedback on its use. At the same time, WHO launched the Roll Back Malaria[28] initiative with the goal of reducing the incidence of malaria in Africa.

The agreement signed in May 2001 between WHO and Novartis aimed to complete the clinical data on the use of Coartem® and to set the price, which must not be at a profit when the drug is distributed in the public sector, and to establish the market. The agreement initially called for a Phase 4 clinical trial in three African countries to fill out data on Coartem® adherence, efficacy, and safety. The two partners agreed on co-ownership of the data from this trial, which was financed on a shared basis. WHO, via TDR, would also collaborate with Novartis to improve the drug packaging to increase patient compliance. This collaborative development work (Article 2: Collaborative development work)[29] helps justify Coartem®'s preferential price for the public sector, as public funds have been used for R&D.

This policy was discussed at a joint WHO/WTO (World Trade Organization) workshop in April 2001,[30] at the time when Pretoria's trial on South Africa's drug law was winding down.[31] Novartis participated in the workshop and presented the company's differentiated pricing and marketing strategy to develop the artemether/lumefantrine combination for two market segments: "The representative of a pharmaceutical company describes how a malaria drug, Coartem®/Riamet®, was designed from the beginning of the product's life, to be packaged, branded, registered, and priced differently for use in high- and low-income countries" (report cited, WHO-WTO, p. 16.). A provision in the Novartis/WHO agreement provides that WHO may perform audits of production costs to monitor the application of this price formulation. Such an audit was conducted in early 2003 and concluded that the price of USD 2.40 set by the agreement was lower than the observed production cost of USD 3.20 established by Deloitte, based on information provided by Novartis and without visiting the production plant located in China.[32]

One of the most important points of this agreement is that WHO will be in charge of constructing and administering this market: "WHO has agreed to sell and supply the product to Public sector agencies for such distribution on a not for profit basis" (Memorandum of Understanding, May 2001).[33] On the demand creation side, Article 5 of the agreement provides that WHO will review the registration of the AL combination in its list of essential medicines and its inclusion in its malaria treatment recommendations. Registrations that will promote the adoption of the new fixed-dose combination by States in endemic regions where resistance to chloroquine and sulfadoxine-pyrimethamine, the molecules used historically, are increasing. On the administration side of this market, WHO is setting up a mechanism for collecting purchase orders (Submission Form for Country Applying for Coartem®). A technical commission of five experts evaluates the procurement request forms. WHO does not advance funds for these purchases, which must be paid in advance by the requesting States. WHO also provides Novartis with demand forecasts for the next 6 months to plan industrial investments.

It can therefore be argued that this agreement formed and structured the market for public donors of ACTs while the Global Fund was in the process of being established (the WHO/Novartis agreement was signed in May 2001; the Global Fund was created in 2002). WHO in fact bore the cost of creating and administering this market, while attempting to avoid any marketing of the company: "WHO cannot allow the publication of material which provides a good public image for Novartis" (April 2002).[34] The WHO partnership and the creation of the Global Fund supported Novartis' commitment in a market considered to be unprofitable: "From the outset, Novartis was aware that in those regions where malaria is endemic there is a limited market in a commercial sense" (October 6, 2002).[35] Solvency, if not profitability, would be ensured by the growth of Global

Fund interventions: "While we provide Coartem® at cost, our efforts would be in vain without the Global Fund's financial aid allowing governments of malaria endemic countries to purchase the drug" (D. Vasella, Novartis CEO, April 2005).[36] Novartis will use its partnership with WHO to promote itself as a "corporate citizen" (corporate document referring to "corporate citizenship").[37]

Novartis had yet another reason for investing in the development of Coartem®: "it opened up the possibility of a cooperative venture with a group in China, which at the time was novel and of general interest" (October 2002).[38] The geography of Coartem® production was disclosed by Novartis at a meeting with WHO in November 2004:[39] a plant owned as a joint venture between Novartis and China that produced the artemether derivative as well as the AL combination in Beijing. The plant was certified to GMP standards. Upstream of this plant, Novartis must contract with Chinese growers for the cultivation of artemisia and with extraction plants for the raw material, natural artemisinin.

This production and distribution system for Coartem® was put to the test in 2004–2005 when it became clear that the supply of the drug could not meet the growth in demand from countries that had adopted the AL combination as a first-line treatment. As early as May 2004, WHO notified Novartis: "Both the WHO forecast and the recent analysis of the Global Fund indicate a probability of product shortage in 2005, where around 40–50% of the demand will not be met by Novartis unless the production capacity for 2005 is increased" (WHO letter to Novartis, May 20, 2004).[40] WHO urged Novartis to fund artemisinin extraction plants in Africa. To meet the strong growth in demand (10 million treatments in 2004, 60 million in 2005, 120 million in 2006), Novartis decided in 2005 to invest in the construction of a large-capacity plant in the United States[41] and temporarily collaborate with a plant in Switzerland to produce the artemether derivative to complement Chinese production. Novartis proposed passing on its capacity investments in the price of Coartem®, which WHO rejected.

Faced with this treatment shortage, which may have led some States to second-guess the adoption of ACTs, several lines of criticism emerged. MSF's Access to Essential Medicines Campaign blamed the company for the delay in investing in a program that was not profitable for it: "We had been sounding the alarm about the risk of shortages for several months, but Novartis paid little attention, because in reality it is not interested in this treatment. Novartis would never have been in this situation if the drug had been profitable" (JM Kindermans, November 23, 2004).[42] A Swiss NGO, the Berne Declaration,[43] challenged the "exclusivity" of the agreement between Novartis and WHO, which failed to ensure the supply of ACTs to African countries.[44] Not only did the Swiss firm fail to anticipate WHO's increased needs, but the agreement prevents the UN organization from sourcing from other producers of artemisinin-based combinations. The Berne Declaration wanted this monopoly dismantled through a two-pronged approach: WHO purchasing additional ACTs, and Novartis renouncing its patent in developing countries. In March 2005, WHO advocated opening the market to generics: "Current production levels of ACTs are insufficient to meet current needs and there is an urgent need to increase production… There are also only a limited number of producers. Generic substitution, stimulation of domestic production of quality generic medicines should not only increase production but also lead to lower prices through market competition".[45]

Novartis had a de jure and de facto monopoly on production of the AL combination and thus on the only fixed-dose ACT available at the time (Sanofi's ASAQ only came on the market in 2007). It was also the only prequalified ACT available for the global donor market. The 2001 agreement reiterated Novartis' ownership rights, via the patent co-owned with China, and did not consider the use of generics. However, this "public market under monopoly" described by Orsi and Zimmermann (2015) would open up without a patent dispute at the end of the 2005 shortage crisis. Initially, WHO began to consider opening up to generics in 2003.[46] Then Novartis, which had committed in the agreement to building a "corporate citizenship" image following the major crisis of the 2001 Pretoria trial, could not block the path to generics, even though its patents were valid until 2011. The multinational company was careful to cede its rights to China, co-owner of the patent for least developed countries (WHO/Novartis meeting November 26, 2004).[47] In 2005, the company announced a price reduction (USD 2.15), which was justified by the sharp increase in the scale of production. Finally, the 2001 agreement rightly developed Coartem® as a global public good based on the global donor market. Defending the monopoly was impossible. In 2008, Novartis still held 85% of the market, but by 2013, its share had dropped to 12%, and Indian manufacturers now have the lion's share.[48]

## The invention and globalization of ASAQ: Between humanitarian health and multinationals

In the early 2000s, the intervention of humanitarian medicine in the field of pharmaceutical R&D through the creation of the DND*i* led to a new geography of innovation and the ACT industry (Cassier, 2008). In 2002, MSF took over the WHO project to formulate two new fixed-dose combinations: ASAQ, to be developed in Bordeaux, France; and artesunate and mefloquine, to be developed by the public laboratory Farmanguinhos in Brazil (Kameda, 2014).[49] My focus here is on the development and industrialization of ASAQ, which occupies about one-quarter of the global donor market according to UNITAID, behind AL.

The FACT consortium[50] has entrusted development of the ASAQ formulation to the University of Bordeaux, supported by an R&D company spun off from the University, Ellipse Pharmaceuticals. It took the researchers 2 years to develop a stable formulation of the combination of the two components, ASAQ, which are difficult to hold together. Bordeaux received analytical technology developed by Mahidol University in Malaysia, which has been working on these molecules for many years: "We saw the transfer of the analytical method, for example between Malaysia and Bordeaux. This is a South-North transfer" (interview, Pascal Millet, University of Bordeaux, July 2016). The Universities of Oxford and Bordeaux assisted research centers in Senegal and Burkina Faso with ASAQ clinical trials.

Once developed, the technology was transferred free-of-charge to Sanofi for industrialization. Sanofi had also been working on a co-formulation of ASAQ, but without devoting sufficient resources and without success. In 2004, Sanofi approached the University of Bordeaux and DND*i*, and the multinational company was able to freely exploit the technology, which was not patented, and even enjoyed a period of exclusivity until the drug was prequalified by WHO (which occurred in 2008).[51] The invention, including the initial clinical trials, was therefore performed by a "non-profit R&D pharmaceutical laboratory" in the words of Yves Champey of MSF, and then industrialized by the multinational company. The latter was forced to adopt the public good model imposed by DND*i* (Bompart, Kiechel, Sebbag, & Pecoul, 2011). This public good model, defended by DND*i* as a means to promote access to medicines in resource-limited countries, is discussed by academic inventors who would have liked to file a patent, if only for the purpose of controlling the technology. However, it should be emphasized that DND*i* retains ownership of the data from the technology development and clinical trials it has funded and has the power to decide on further transfers and new production, which took place in East Africa beginning in 2011. Unlike the agreement between WHO and Novartis, the agreement between Sanofi and DND*i* embodies the strategy of technology sharing and spin-off: "DND*i* considers its products as public goods. It does not wish to profit from its new products and wants to share the knowledge it creates by transferring technologies to other researchers and manufacturers when required."[52] Here, however, DND*i* is the inventor and sets the intellectual property policy.

Sanofi decided to locate the industrial production of ASAQ in one of its subsidiaries in Morocco, a decision that had a significant impact on the country's pharmaceutical industry. Sanofi-Maphar, located in Casablanca, was already assembling the ASAQ combination in co-blister pack form in the early 2000s. Implementation of the fixed-dose technology developed in Bordeaux began in 2004, with the assistance of the Bordeaux inventors (Bertin Pharmaceuticals). The transfer operation was especially delicate because the technology did not originate from Sanofi's internal R&D department. The establishment of ASAQ production was accompanied by several simultaneous investments in the Casablanca plant: (1) investments to modernize equipment: ASAQ's technology involved the purchase of new machinery to produce a two-layer drug; (2) investments to create a logistics platform to export the product, which was intended for endemic countries, mainly in Africa; and (3) investments to raise the standards of the plant in order to obtain WHO prequalification. Establishing ASAQ manufacture in Morocco was part of Sanofi's strategy to extend its reach into markets it considered "emerging" and to have production close to endemic regions of sub-Saharan Africa (interview, Director of the Sanofi-Maphar plant in Casablanca, May 2016). It should be noted that the economy of this local production had limitations: (1) the Casablanca plant imported the active ingredients for amodiaquine from India and for artesunate from Italy, produced semisynthetically by Sanofi; and (2) the boxes of ASAQ produced in Casablanca were sent to France before being shipped back to the African markets, for reasons of financial consolidation within the company: "The finished product of ASAQ was not distributed directly from Morocco; instead it was transferred to France for onward distribution" (WHO inspection, November 2016).[53]

The installation of the ASAQ production facility in Morocco had two significant local impacts. First, replicating a technology as complex as ASAQ, which involved transfer from Bordeaux to Casablanca via a German R&D company that did the preindustrial testing, required the creation of local industrial expertise and knowledge between 2004 and 2008, until the drug was prequalified by WHO. The industrial teams in Casablanca then had to overcome a real production crisis in 2011–2012, as the Global Fund was setting up a new system of subsidized markets, the Affordable Medicine Facility-malaria (AMFm), which will be discussed in the next chapter, and which resulted in strong growth in demand for ASAQ. The production process had to be adapted to address recurring problems of artesunate underdosing, which generated waste and reduced yield at a time when Sanofi was the sole supplier of ASAQ in fixed-dose combinations. The production and development teams at the Moroccan plant and in the group in France, at Ambarès near Bordeaux, were mobilized for many months to stabilize the process and the product: "The 2011 crisis put us back almost a year" (interview, quality engineer, Casablanca, May 2016).

Second, obtaining WHO prequalification for ASAQ, a condition for marketing the product on global donor markets, required extensive internal documentation of production and quality control operations, in close collaboration with Sanofi's central services in Paris. This work of coding and recording data led to changes in the plant's industrial culture, according to the statements by Sanofi managers in Paris and Casablanca. Obtaining ASAQ prequalification by the Casablanca

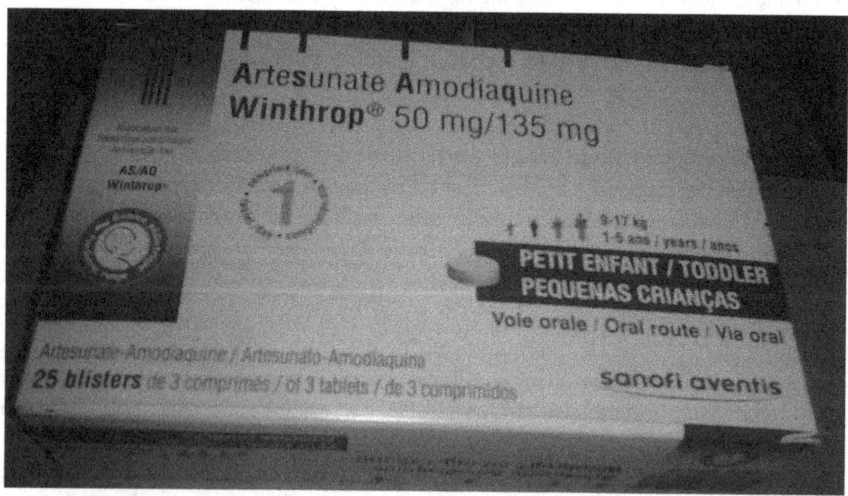


*Figure 5.1* A box of ASAQ Winthrop produced in Casablanca and photographed in the warehouses of the Central Purchasing Office for Essential Medicines in Cotonou.

Source: © IRD/Stéphanie Mahamé, Cotonou, June 2014

plant also helped to further progress pharmaceutical regulation in Morocco: the country established a bioequivalence center in 2016, and the bioequivalence standard for generic drugs is promoted by law.

Sanofi enjoyed a de facto monopoly on the market for the fixed-dose combination of ASAQ until 2013: "In 2012, Sanofi accounted for approximately 98% of ASAQ volumes procured. Between June and November 2012, six more FDC ASAQs became prequalified from two manufacturers (Ipca Laboratories Ltd and Guilin), however, these still represent very small portions of the market" (UNITAID, 2015). Sanofi was protected by the temporary exclusivity clause granted to it by DND*i* until 2008, as well as by the late publication of the formulation developed in Bordeaux (in 2011). Indian manufacturers were able to copy the technology from several sources: by reverse engineering the combinations that had been marketed since 2007 or by referring to the 2011 publication of the technology in the *Malaria Journal*. Moreover, they benefited from an incidental disclosure of the industrial process during a training session given by WHO, according to Sanofi's malaria manager (interview, Paris, February 2016). In any case, competition from Indian and Chinese generics became very strong from 2014 onward: production at the Casablanca plant in 2015 was half of what it was in 2013, falling from 100 million treatments in 2013 to 50 million in 2015 (Cassier, 2016). In 2017, Sanofi sold the majority of Maphar's shares in Casablanca to Eurapharma, a long-standing pharmaceutical distribution group in Africa, a subsidiary of CFAO.[54] This can be viewed as a strategy of increased exports to African markets as well as a withdrawal by Sanofi in the face of low margins compared to its high-profit therapeutic areas (cancer and diabetes).

## Making artemisinin-based medicines in Africa? DND*i* transfers ASAQ technology to Tanzania

In the early 2000s, several local producers of artemisinin-based drugs emerged in Africa, in the form of monotherapies, free combinations, or co-blister packed combinations. The lists of producers drawn up by WHO in 2006 and 2007, aimed at encouraging manufacturers to turn away from monotherapies to produce combinations, show local generics production in Cameroon, Ghana (three firms), Nigeria, the Republic of Congo, and Tanzania. Chinese companies also established firms that produced ACTs (in Côte d'Ivoire, for example, to produce AL). African producers appear to face several barriers: (1) a technological barrier, particularly in mastering the technology of the ASAQ fixed-dose combination[55]; (2) the barrier of product certification standards: no African firms had thus far obtained WHO prequalification, which limited their products to local markets and prevents them from reaching global donor markets[56]; and (3) competition from subsidized products distributed on private markets through financing mechanisms such as the AMFm in the early 2010s, which had the effect of crowding out local firms, if only temporarily (Pourraz, 2019). However, local production for this therapeutic class intended for local and regional markets does exist (see Chapter 6).

I wish to focus here on the singular trajectory of the ASAQ technology that DND*i* decided to transfer to a laboratory in Tanzania, Zenufa. As soon as Sanofi's production was installed and certified by WHO in 2009, DND*i* embarked on a process of technology transfer to another producer in Africa. The foundation's goals were to ensure an open market, to distribute production as close as possible to the endemic regions, and to secure supplies. In 2009–2011, DND*i* commissioned a study to evaluate the production capacities of several laboratories in Africa. After considering an agreement with a Nigerian firm, initially of interest to Sanofi, DND*i* opted for a firm from the Democratic Republic of Congo based in Tanzania, the Zenufa Group.[57] Sanofi was henceforth excluded from the transfer process and the managers of the Casablanca plant now identify Zenufa as a potential new competitor. Potential, because the Tanzanian plant only started the WHO prequalification process in July 2016 and is still not on the list of prequalified combinations. This transfer operation is no less remarkable: (1) the DND*i* Foundation has scrupulously followed its policy of nonexclusive exploitation of its invention and encouraging local production in Africa; (2) although the technology has not been patented, the DND*i*, which conducted the R&D, does own and control the technological and clinical data for the development work, which it transmitted to Zenufa to file the ASAQ registration files; and (3) it was the inventors of the technology in 2002 and 2003 in Bordeaux who carried out the technology transfer operations in Tanzania. They visited Zenufa no less than 11 times to teach the technology to the operators, supervise the purchase and installation of equipment, and conduct tests on the first batches: "We had to do a lot of work on Good Manufacturing Practices (GMP) and on our quality reference materials, both for technology and especially for documentation; everything about documentation, traceability, we helped them quite a lot with that"; (4) more than a mere transfer of technology, this was a true industrial recreation of the plant, including the purchase of new equipment, the introduction of two-layer technology, training of technicians and operators,

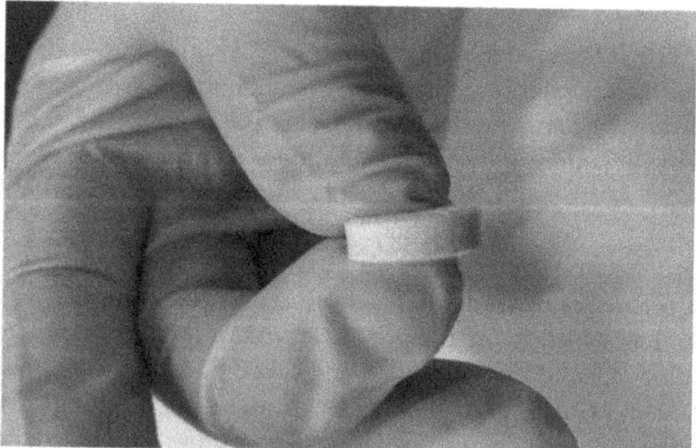

*Figure 5.2* Two-layer tablet of ASAQ produced in Tanzania.

Source: © DNDi

implementation of production data documentation, and so forth, in a context of a high turnover of technicians, often Indian, who are in charge of management; and (5) in October 2016, a few months after the ASAQ prequalification file was submitted, the Zenufa group was bought out by Catalyst, an investment fund with a strong presence in East Africa, adding uncertainty to the project. If WHO accepts Zenufa's ASAQ prequalification dossier, it would be the first factory in Tanzania to obtain this international standard.[58]

## Conclusion

The geography of artemisinin-based drug innovation and industry is uniquely distributed; originally developed in China, it was subsequently globalized through WHO, humanitarian medicine, and the multinational pharmaceutical companies Novartis and Sanofi. Dissemination was encouraged by the public and common good status of the basic molecules, which were legal to duplicate and combine. This resulted in the dispersion of manufacturing companies and a multiplicity of products, which WHO attempted to rationalize in the early 2000s to eliminate monotherapies that were potential sources of drug resistance, recommending the manufacture of combinations, increasingly at fixed doses. Patent claims on the first fixed-dose combination of AL, in China in 1990 and then internationally through co-ownership between Ciba Geigy and China in 1991, did not prevent the market from opening in 2005, when Novartis production capacity proved inadequate. Exclusive rights could not stand in the way of generics once these medicines had been constructed as global public goods. More generally, the market monopolies of Novartis and Sanofi fell victim to price competition from India's large, certified generic manufacturers.

Although Chinese inventors lost control of their inventions because they had not been patented and because of the standards barrier that separated them from world markets, Chinese researchers and industrialists continued to play an important role: part of Novartis' Coartem® production was located in Beijing; Chinese factories account for a predominant share of the production and exportation of active ingredients (85% of the world market, mainly with artemisinin and artemether APIs)[59]; 85%–90% of the extraction capacity of natural artemisinin is located in China.[60] China defended the economy of natural artemisinin against the market for semisynthetic artemisinin developed by the Bill and Melinda Gates Foundation and Sanofi, which sold its plant. Chinese researchers continued to develop new ACTs such as dihydroartemisinin-piperaquine; prequalified Chinese products represent one-quarter of WHO-certified products; and the market share of Chinese finished pharmaceutical products, which was very limited in the early 2010s, is trending upward (Huang et al., 2016). While most drugs in this therapeutic class are used on the African continent, modest local production there remains disconnected from international markets. The technology transfer organized by DND*i* in Tanzania illustrates the possibilities of raising the industrial standards of a factory in Africa for a very modest transfer cost, and the 2019–2021 Sino-African cooperation plan includes the transfer of pharmaceutical technology.

## Notes

1. Tu Youyou, Institute of Chinese Materia Medica, China Academy of Chinese Medical Sciences, Beijing, China. Nobel lecture, 31 pages.
2. AL still accounts for 75% of the market today (UNITAID, 2015).
3. "Non-European countries: Zhou Yiqing (China) for his antimalaria drug based on a herbal agent, which has been instrumental in saving hundreds of thousands of lives" (European Inventors of the Year, 2009).
4. TDR archives T16-181-M2-61, WHO Geneva.
5. The Global Fund to Fight HIV/AIDS, Tuberculosis and Malaria was created in 2002 at the urging of the United Nations to raise funds to combat these diseases. It is not a UN agency, but a nonprofit foundation that works closely with WHO. Most of its funds (93%) come from government grants, with the remaining 7% from private foundations and industry.
6. Malaria Medicines Landscape (UNITAID, 2015).
7. Chapter 6 of this book discusses the shift from Novartis and Sanofi originator medicines to Indian generics.
8. See the introduction of the book for more information on the data collection methodology.
9. Making a Difference: 30 years of Research and Capacity Building in Tropical Diseases, WHO, 2007.
10. This cooperation is documented in both the TDR archives at WHO and in the book edited by the Chinese inventors (op. cit.) translated by Keith Arnold, who was one of the first Western researchers to take an interest in artemisinin on behalf of the Roche Foundation.
11. "Making a Difference," WHO, op. cit.
12. TDR archives T 16-181-M2-83
13. TDR archives T 16-181-M2-83.
14. Archives T16-181-M2-61.
15. "The Development of artemisinin and its derivatives." Report of the Scientific Working Group on the Chemotherapy of Malaria, Geneva, October 6–7, 1986, 30 pages.
16. The injectable form of artemether was tested in China as early as 1978 and approved for production from 1987. Kunming Pharmaceutical Corporation still markets this formulation today under the brand name Artem.
17. TDR archives M20-372-5.
18. This is reminiscent of the controversy raised by MSF about the delay in WHO recommendations for introducing artemisinin-based medicines in Africa (Balkan & Corty, 2009). Up to the early 2000s, WHO stressed the price barrier to deploying these new medicines in Africa: "The substantially higher cost of ACTs is probably the major obstacle to the implementation of this strategy, especially in sub-Saharan Africa. As a public health measure, subsidies could be justified, but assurance is needed that financial mechanisms will be sustainable" (The use of antimalarial drugs. Report from an informal consultation, WHO, 2001).
19. In recent years, Chinese lawyers have been defending filing patents on isolated compounds from traditional Chinese medicine, which makes it possible to control the inventions and to organize royalty returns to the sources of these patents (Xiating, 2011).
20. See List of Prequalified Medicines for Malaria, WHO, 2020.
21. Malaria Medicines Landscape (UNITAID, 2015).
22. China International Trust and Investment Corporation, a public company created in 1979.

23. Ancient Chinese anti-fever cure becomes panacea for Malaria. An interview with Zhou Yiking, Bulletin of the World Health Organization, volume 87, no. 10, October 2009, pp. 743–744.
24. The same amalgamation of Chinese clinical data and Rhône Poulenc data can be found for the Paluther® registration.
25. MMV was created in 1999 by development funding from Switzerland, Great Britain, and Germany, together with funding from the World Bank and the Rockefeller Foundation. MMV in some respects takes over from TDR for developing and industrializing new antimalarial drugs through Product Development Partnerships between academia and industry. Since 2015, MMV has also managed the two ACTs invented by DND*i*, ASAQ, and ASMQ.
26. Patent WO2014/180011A1, filed by Xi'an Libang Pharmaceutical Co., Ltd.
27. RBM archives M50 372-3, WHO, Geneva.
28. Roll Back Malaria is a consortium for coordinating public and community health actions to combat malaria. It was created in 1999 by WHO, the World Bank, UNDP, and UNICEF. It brings together a wide variety of partners: governments, multinationals, generic manufacturers, associations, universities, foundations, etc.
29. Memorandum of Understanding between Novartis Pharma and WHO, May 23, 2001: M50 372-3.
30. Report of the Workshop on Differential Pricing and Financing of Essential Medicines, WHO and WTO Secretariats, Norwegian Ministry of Foreign Affairs, World Health Council, April 8–11, 2001, 31 pages.
31. Cassier M, 2002, Propriété industrielle et santé publique, [Industrial property and public health], *Revue Projet*, No. 270, 47–55.
32. RBM archives M50-370-21.
33. RBM archives M50-372-3.
34. M50-372-3.
35. M50-372-3.
36. Novartis: New Study Finds Coartem® (Artemether-Lumefantrine) is the Most Effective Malaria Treatment in Areas of High Resistance to Conventional Anti-Malarials, Novartis, April 26, 2005.
37. M50-372-3: WHO: Clearance of documents submitted by Novartis, September 25, 2003.
38. Yale Initiative on Public-Private Partnerships for Health, October 6, 2002, M50-372-3.
39. Coartem® Demand and Supply Planning Meeting, November 26, 2004, Novartis Pharma Basel, M50-372-3 and M2-441-84.
40. Archives M50-370-21.
41. WHO & Novartis meeting on Coartem®, August 31, 2005.
42. Un médicament antipaludisme qui marche mais qui manque [An antimalarial drug that works but is in short supply], *Libération*, December 2, 2004.
43. The Berne Declaration was founded in 1968 with the idea of establishing more equitable relations between Switzerland and developing countries. In 2016, the Berne Declaration changed its name to Public Eye. https://www.publiceye.ch/en/media-corner/press-releases/detail/berne-declaration-becomes-public-eye.
44. "Les pays africains font les frais de l'accord problématique de Novartis avec l'OMS [African countries bear the brunt of Novartis' problematic agreement with WHO]," April 25, 2005.
45. Malaria Control Today, WHO, March 2005, p. 26.
46. Improving the affordability and financing of ACTs, WHO, 2003.
47. Archives M50-372-3.
48. Malaria Medicines Landscape (UNITAID, 2015).
49. This Brazilian technology was later transferred to Cipla in India.

50. The Fixed-Dose Artesunate Combination Therapies (FACT) consortium was established in 2002. Its coordinator was Jean René Kiechel, a former pharmaceutical industry executive who became project manager at DND*i*.
51. Sanofi would market ASAQ under two brand names: one for public markets, Asaq Winthrop®, at a price fixed by the agreement (USD 1 for adults and USD 0.50 for children), and the other, Coarsucam®, for private markets, with a free price. The private market quickly closed, and Sanofi stopped production of Coarsucam®.
52. "Pragmatic and Principled: DND*i*'s Approach to IP Management," IP Handbook of best practices, Jaya Banerji and Bernard Pecoul, 2009, 7 pages.
53. WHO Public Inspection Report, Maphar Laboratories, Morocco, 12 pages.
54. This society is also discussed in Chapters 1 and 2 of this book.
55. See the ASAQ crisis that occurred in Ghana in 2004–2005, which is well documented in Jessica Pourraz's dissertation, 2019.
56. "Kenya is also a country who produces Artemisia and artemisinin, but due to the stringent WHO prequalification standards is precluded from local manufacturer of prequalified ACTs," Health Minister, Artemisinin Conference, Nairobi, January 14–16, 2013. However, three Kenyan-based manufacturers have registered eight prequalified ARVs.
57. Zenufa is introduced in "Pharmaceutical Manufacturing Decline in Tanzania: How Possible is a Turnaround to Growth?" (Tibandebage, Wangwe, Mackintosh, & Mujinja, 2016).
58. On the African continent, 7 laboratories have registered 17 medicines prequalified by WHO (including Maphar in Morocco for three formulations of ASAQ). The other laboratories are located in Egypt, Kenya, and South Africa.
59. India and North America are the main importers of Chinese artemisinin-derived APIs (Huang et al., 2016).
60. Malaria Medicines Landscape (UNITAID, 2015).

## Reference list

Balkan, S., & Corty, J.-F. (2009). Paludisme: Les résistances traitées par une médiation sud-sud [Malaria: Resistances treated through South-South mediation]. In J.-H. Bradol, & C. Vidal (Eds.), *Innovations médicales en situations humanitaires. Le travail de Médecins sans Frontières [Medical innovations in humanitarian situations. The work of Médecins Sans Frontières]* (pp. 135–153). Paris, France: L'Harmattan.

Bompart, J., Kiechel, J.-R., Sebbag, R., & Pecoul, B. (2011). Innovative public-private partnerships to maximize the delivery of anti-malarial medicines: Lessons learned from the ASAQ Winthrop experience. *Malaria Journal, 10*, 1–9. https://malariajournal.biomedcentral.com/articles/10.1186/1475-2875-10-143.

Cassier, M. (2008). Une nouvelle géopolitique du médicament (1980–2005) [A new geopolitics of medicine (1980–2005)]. In A. Flahaut, & P. Zylberman (Eds.), *Des epidémies et des hommes [Epidemics and humans]* (pp. 101–109). Paris, France: La Martinière.

Cassier, M. (2016, June). Between financial capitalism and humanitarian concerns: Value, price and profits of hepatitis C antivirals and artemisinin-based combinations therapies for malaria. Paper presented at the international workshop: The Making of Pharmaceutical Value: Drugs, Diseases and the Political Economies of Global Health, Paris, France.

Cassier, M., & Correa, M. (2003). Patents, innovation and public health: Brazilian public sector laboratories' experience in copying AIDS drugs. In J.-P. Moatti, B. Coriat, Y. Souteyrand, T. Barnett, J. Dumoulin, & Y. A. Flori (Eds.), *Economics of AIDS and access to HIV/AIDS care in developing countries. Issues and challenges* (pp. 89–107). Paris, France: ANRS.

Chaudhuri, S. (2005). *The WTO and India's pharmaceutical industry: Patent protection, TRIPs and developing countries*. New Delhi, India: Oxford University Press.

Huang, Y., Li, H., Peng, D., Wang, Y., Ren, Q., & Guo, Y. (2016). The production and exportation of artemisinin-derived drugs in China: Current status and existing challenges. *Malaria Journal, 15*(365), 1–8. https://doi.org/10.1186/s12936-016-1422-3.

Jianfang, Z. (Ed.). (2013). *A detailed chronological record of project 523 and the discovery and development of qinghaosu (artemisinin)*. K. Arnold, & M. Arnold (Trans.). Houston, TX: Strategic Book Publishing and Rights Co. (Original work published 2006).

Kameda, K. (2014). Needs-driven versus market-driven pharmaceutical innovation: The consortium for the development of a new medicine against malaria in Brazil. *Developing World Bioethics, 14*(2), 101–108.

Orsi, F., & Zimmermann, F. (2015). Le marché des antipaludéens: Entre régulation et défaillance [The antimalarial market: Between regulation and failure]. *Mondes en développement, 170*(2), 21–40.

Pecoul, B., Chirac, P., Trouiller, P., & Pinel, P. (1999). Access to essential drugs in poor countries: A lost battle? *JAMA, 281*(4), 361–367. doi:10-1001/pubs.JAMA-ISSN-0098-7484-281-4-jsc80337.

Pourraz, J. (2019). *Réguler et produire les médicaments contre le paludisme au Ghana et au Bénin : Une affaire d'Etat ? Politiques pharmaceutiques, normes de qualité et marchés de médicaments [Regulating and producing malaria drugs in Ghana and Benin: A State affair? Pharmaceutical policies, quality standards, and drug markets]*. Doctoral dissertation, Ecole des Hautes Etudes en Sciences Sociales, Paris, France. Retrieved at http://www.theses.fr/2019EHES0014.

Tibandebage, P., Wangwe, S., Mackintosh, M., & Mujinja, P. (2016). Pharmaceutical manufacturing decline in Tanzania: How possible is a turnaround to growth?. In M. Mackintosh, G. Banda, P. Tibandebage, & W. Wamae (Eds.), *Making medicines in Africa: The political economy of industrializing for local health* (pp. 45–64). London, UK: Palgrave Macmillan.

Trouiller, P. (1996). Recherche et développement pharmaceutique en matière de maladies transmissibles dans la zone intertropicale [Pharmaceutical research and development in the field of communicable diseases in the intertropical area]. *Cahiers Santé*, 6, 299–307.

Trouiller, P., Olliaro, P., Torreele, E., Orbinski, J., Laing, R., & Ford, N. (2002). Drug development for neglected diseases: A deficient market and a public-health policy failure. *The Lancet*, 359(9324), 2188–2194.

UNITAID. (2015). *Malaria medicines landscape*, Geneva, Switzerland: World Health Organization.

Xiating, S. (2011). New problems of intellectual property during innovation of traditional Chinese medicine, *World Science and Technology, 13*(3), 466–469.

# 6 Clashes between subsidized and private ACT markets

## When administrative, Global Health, and marketing regulations collide

*Carine Baxerres and Jessica Pourraz*

The World Health Organization's (WHO) international recommendation to use artemisinin-based combination therapies (ACTs) in the mid-2000s spurred pharmaceutical innovations. Initially driven by two multinational firms based in the West—the Swiss Novartis and the French Sanofi-Aventis—and their partnership with universities and/or transnational actors (WHO and Drugs for Neglected Diseases *initiative* [DND*i*], respectively),[1] production of these artemisinin-based combinations has increased both in the Asian countries that produce generics and in Africa. Numerous ACTs, combining different molecules with artemisinin derivatives, the use of which may or may not be recommended by WHO, have been put on the market in a variety of ways in countries affected by malaria. National pharmaceutical regulations for these drugs vary, depending on whether or not they are included in malaria treatment lines in various countries; the criteria for granting Marketing Authorizations (MAs) issued by regulatory authorities; and their actual technical, material, and human resources. Global Health actors working in malaria control, primarily the Global Fund and the President's Malaria Initiative (PMI)[2] for the situations we studied, or Chinese development aid for example in others (Sams, 2016), clearly influence trends in these markets by making ACT available in the countries. By supplying specifically from a few pharmaceutical firms, these Global Health programs support the distribution of certain products that have international certifications. To deal with their dominance over the markets, competing companies are organizing themselves to promote their own ACTs as well.

This chapter discusses these pharmaceutical production and distribution trends and their logics as manifested in Benin and Ghana. Using inventories, we conducted of ACTs sold in formal pharmaceutical distribution facilities (private pharmacies; over-the-counter [OTC] medicine sellers; pharmaceutical depots; public, private, and mission health centers—see Introduction of this book), we will begin by presenting the supply of these medicines in the two countries. Then, we will analyze the composition of these ACT markets to show how directors of the pharmaceutical companies at the source of this supply capture market share by maneuvering between the administrative and Global Health regulations implemented by national and transnational actors and the marketing regulations developed by the firms themselves.[3]

## ACT supply in Benin and Ghana

### *Subsidized ACTs from European firms and major Asian generics producers*

Although in theory the lack of patents on ACT component molecules allows for a competitive market to develop between companies, in actuality Novartis held a virtual monopoly until 2008, when Sanofi-Aventis, in partnership with DND*i*, obtained WHO prequalification (Lantenois & Coriat, 2014) for its co-formulation of ASAQ Winthrop®, previously marketed as a co-blister combination (artesunate + amodiaquine).[4] Novartis' virtual monopoly within subsidized markets is due to the fact that, beginning in 2001, it was the only company marketing Coartem®, a fixed-dose combination of artemether and lumefantrine (AL), prequalified by WHO. To ensure accessibility for all countries in Africa, WHO signed an exclusive 10-year agreement with this company to supply public markets with Coartem®, at a price of USD 2.40 per adult treatment (Orsi & Zimmermann, 2015).[5] In 2005, the Global Fund signed agreements with the Indian generics manufacturers Ajanta and Cipla to encourage them to produce fixed-dose combinations of AL. Novartis responded beginning in 2006 with an initial price decrease for Coartem® (Singh, 2018). Thus, between December 2008 and December 2009, the global market for subsidized ACTs expanded with these WHO-prequalified AL combinations produced by the Indian companies Ajanta and Cipla, joined later by Ipca. Because combining artesunate and amodiaquine (ASAQ) in the same tablet posed much greater technical challenges, it was not until 2012 that the Indian firm Ipca prequalified its co-formulated ASAQ, followed by the Chinese company Guilin in that same year, then by the Indian companies Ajanta in 2013 and Cipla in 2014 (Orsi, Singh, & Sagaon-Teyssier, 2018).

At the time of our studies between 2014 and 2016, subsidized ACT found in the public sector in Benin and Ghana was, for the most part, purchased by PMI and the Global Fund.[6] It was manufactured by two European multinationals—Novartis and Sanofi-Aventis—and by two Indian companies manufacturing generics, Ipca and Cipla. With the Global Fund and PMI supply policy conditional on the purchase of ACT certified through WHO prequalification, the sources do not vary between Benin and Ghana. In both cases, Coartem® manufactured by Novartis is by far the predominant medicine, which is mostly found in health centers and public hospitals.

In Benin, subsidized ACTs are only available in the public sector and are purchased primarily by PMI. Only the pediatric formulations of ACT, which are distributed via an intermediary—*relais communautaires*, community health workers assigned mostly in rural areas through specific public health programs—are purchased by the Global Fund and to a lesser extent by UNICEF. At the time of our study, a treatment using subsidized ACT cost between CFA 150 and 600 (between EUR 0.22 and 0.91), depending on the patient's age and weight. The national policy provides for free treatment for children under 5 years. In Ghana, subsidized ACT, primarily purchased with Global Fund donations, has also been distributed in the private sector since 2010 through the mechanism of the Affordable Medicines Facility-malaria (AMFm), a pilot program developed in eight countries through Roll Back Malaria,[7] a public-private partnership, and implemented and managed by the Global Fund. Through a co-financing mechanism, AMFm pays 95% of the price of ACT provided by the six companies with whom the Global Fund negotiated an 80% price reduction (Davis et al., 2013). The Global Fund fixes the price at which manufacturers must sell ACT to first-line buyers—namely, private wholesaler-importers—so the ACT cost for them is 5% of the negotiated price, since the Global Fund pays the other 95%. ACT from AMFm is sold in Ghana for 1.5 Ghanaian cedis (GHC), equal to just under USD 1, while the price of ACT produced by a local company, Danadams, for example, ranges between GHC 3.40 and 5.40, or two to three times more. The AMFm aims to promote ACT use while decreasing their cost in order to increase their accessibility and availability in the public sector, but more particularly in the private sector. In addition to being distributed in public health centers, subsidized ACTs are also available in private health centers, pharmacies, and from OTC medicine sellers. This results in locally produced ACTs co-existing with imported ACTs, some with WHO prequalification, on private Ghanaian markets.

The AMFm opened the subsidized ACT market to more Asian firms, making these drugs available on the private market. ACTs subsidized through this initiative are manufactured by the Swiss and French multinationals, Novartis and Sanofi-Aventis, by Indian generics producers (Artefan® from Ajanta Pharma, Lumartem® from Cipla, AL from Ipca) and one Chinese producer (Arsuamoon® from Guilin). AMFm has thus proven very useful in helping these companies, which already do business across the globe, to grow and increase their activities. At the end of the AMFm's 2-year pilot phase, the mechanism became the Private Sector Copayment Mechanism (PSCM) in 2014 and was offered in all countries supported by the Global Fund. The seven PSCM manufacturers remained the same as during the AMFm, with the addition of two Indian generics producers: Strides Arcolab Limited, which manufactures Combiart®, and MacLeods with Lumiter® (see Figure 6.1 below).

Deployment of the AMFm and later the PSCM in Ghana made it possible for Asian ACTs to capture much larger shares of the subsidized market than in Benin, where neither the AMFm nor the PSCM had been implemented. However, during the PSCM, the number of first-line buyers purchasing ACTs decreased to 15 compared to 31 during the AMFm. Funding for Ghana was largely revised downwards to USD 20 million in 2014 and to USD 10 million for both 2015 and 2016, compared to USD 28 million for the single year of 2011 at the time of the AMFm (Anadach Group, 2012). Decreases in funding and in the number of buyers under the PSCM probably did not allow ACTs from Strides Arcolab Limited and MacLeods to capture as much of the market share as their competitors who were already firmly established through the AMFm. The price of subsidized ACTs also increased slightly under the PSCM. At the time of our study, the treatment price was between GHC 1 and 6, or between about USD 0.2 and 1.2, depending on the patient's age and weight.

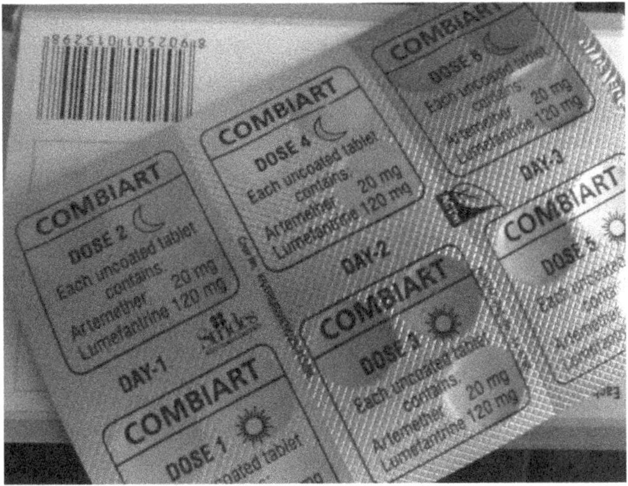


*Figure 6.1* The artemether-lumefantrine produced by Strides Arcolab Limited.

Source: © IRD/Moïse Djralah, Comè, September 2015

While these mechanisms enable wide distribution of Asian and European ACTs, they also caused local firms in Ghana to suspend ACT production. During the AMFm, these firms found it much more profitable to be a distributor than to manufacture their own ACT since first-line buyers only had to pay 5% of the Global Fund negotiated price and could therefore earn much higher profit margins than local producers.[8] In this sense, the AMFm is a substantial public subsidy for the private distribution sector. The Ghanaian Ministry of Health used this argument to encourage Ghanaian companies, most of which are also importers and distributors, to participate in the AMFm as first-line buyers (Pourraz, 2019). The PSCM is limited to a 3-year period that is not renewable in Ghana. Once the supply of subsidized ACTs in the private sector was stopped in 2016, coinciding with the end of our field study, local companies could once again consider producing ACTs to recapture the share they previously held in the private domestic market.

### *Unsubsidized ACTs from Asian, African, and European companies*

Through observations conducted in 2007, we have highlighted elsewhere that before subsidized ACTs were available in Benin and Ghana, different combinations from Indian or Ghanaian manufacturing were already offered at a slightly higher price in the chemical shops (today's OTC medicine shops) in Ghana (at around USD 2.5), while ACTs produced by European or Asian companies were only available at higher prices (about EUR 6) in private pharmacies and public health centers in Benin (Baxerres, 2013a). Another study, conducted in 2012 when the mechanisms implemented by the Global Fund (AMFm then PSCM) had just been launched in Ghana, shows that a comparable range of ACTs was distributed at that time in the retail private sector in the two countries. Whether under a trade name or International Nonproprietary Name (INN), 41 ACTs were counted in Benin, compared to 55 in Ghana; the difference is due to the fact that at the time, there were five Ghanaian companies, the products of which were not available in Benin. With the exception of these companies, the same producers (mainly Asian but also European and African) supplied the private sector in the two countries (Baxerres, Egrot, Houngnihin, & Le Hesran, 2015).

Two or 3 years later, according to our Globalmed studies, the ACT market had changed significantly in both countries. Benin offered a much higher number of products with a broader range of types of combinations than Ghana. During our inventories in both public and private distribution sites, we counted 49 different ACTs[9] in Benin, compared to 22 in Ghana (see the table 6.1 below). Several of them were only distributed in one of the two countries: 41 ACTs sold in Benin were not available in Ghana, and 12 ACTs distributed in Ghana were not found in Benin. Comparing the list of MAs for ACT, provided at that time by national pharmaceutical regulation officials, the Food and Drugs Authority (FDA) in Ghana and the Directorate of Pharmacies, Medicine, and Diagnostic Investigations (DPMED) in Benin, indicated that there were 71 ACTs in Benin compared to 42 in Ghana.[10] Furthermore, Benin offered eight different types of artemisinin-based combinations, compared to three in Ghana; we will return to this aspect later in the chapter. The prices of these drugs varied depending on the brands in the two countries. An unsubsidized adult treatment sold in the private retail market in Benin, ranged between CFA 1425 and 4660, or between about EUR 2 and 7. In Ghana, the price of an adult ACT treatment varied in the private sector, for both subsidized and unsubsidized ACTs, from GHC 3.5 to 36.24, or approximately USD 0.7 to just over USD 7, depending on the brands and distribution sites.[11]

The source of unsubsidized ACTs differed for the two countries. While the majority of companies were also Indian, there were more Indian companies in Benin (25 versus 10, according to our inventories); the same was true for European

*Table 6.1* Evolution of the ACT markets in Benin and Ghana

| | *Benin* | *Ghana* |
|---|---|---|
| Number of ACTs distributed in 2012 | 41 | 55 |
| Number of MAs for ACTs in 2014 | 71 | 42 |
| Number of ACTs distributed in 2015 | 49 | 22 |
| Number of combinations in circulation in 2015 | 8 | 3 |
| Sources of ACTs in 2015 | 25 Indian, 13 European, 7 Chinese, 4 African | 10 Indian, 4 European, 2 Chinese, 5 African |

Source: Authors.

companies (13 in Benin versus 4 in Ghana) and Chinese companies (7 in Benin versus 2 in Ghana). African companies were nearly equal (5 in Ghana, 4 in Benin). By contrast, African companies in Ghana were almost all local (four out of five),[12] while in Benin, these medicines came from companies in other francophone countries (Côte d'Ivoire, Democratic Republic of the Congo, and Togo).[13] Despite the challenges posed by the AMFm described earlier, Ghanaian local production nevertheless slightly changed the structure of the ACT market in this country. Surprisingly, only 14 ACTs had a common MA in both countries. These were primarily products from European companies and large Asian generic manufacturers positioned on the subsidized markets. As for Indian companies, other than the 6 main ones mentioned earlier, 14 were doing business in Benin and not in Ghana, and 9 were in Ghana but not in Benin.

Of course, these figures do not illustrate the varying influence of these different companies in terms of distribution volumes or sales. The work of Fabienne Orsi and her collaborators highlights that 2012 was a major turning point for subsidized ACT markets (Orsi et al., 2018; Orsi & Zimmermann, 2015). As noted earlier, Novartis was the only company producing a WHO-prequalified ACT until 2008, but the tides began to turn with the arrival of Sanofi that year. Between December 2008 and December 2009, the market saw the addition of three ACTs produced by the Indian companies Ajanta, Cipla, and Ipca, which had obtained WHO prequalification for their AL. The arrival of Indian competitors gradually put an end to the Novartis monopoly. In 2012, ACTs from three Indian companies represented 67% of the volume purchased for the public sector with subsidies from the Global Fund in Africa (Orsi et al., 2018).[14] As part of the Globalmed program, our research at the crossroads of qualitative and quantitative approaches also gives some indications of the respective weight of various firms in the private markets in 2015 and 2016. Data collected during an ethnography conducted with two wholesalers in Okaishie in Accra highlight that Indian companies (six of them) and to a lesser extent Chinese companies (two) have an especially strong presence. They account for over 80% of ACT sales for these wholesalers. Novartis, for its part, with its subsidized and unsubsidized Coartem®, accounted for 14% of ACT sales.[15] The Indian firms with products being not subsidized accounted for 27% of ACT sales. Products from the two Indian companies in question were each distributed exclusively by a single Ghanaian wholesaler. One of these two wholesalers was also a drug manufacturer. By contrast, as noted earlier, local companies were virtually absent from ACT sales (3.5). In Benin, based on sales data collected over 2 months during our ethnographies in two pharmacies in Cotonou and one pharmacy and one pharmaceutical depot in the Mono department, even though only unsubsidized ACTs are distributed there, Novartis accounted for just over 7% of sales and Indian and Chinese companies just over 65% (55% and 10.1%, respectively), with European products making up the remainder.

In the next section, we analyze the role of national and transnational actors involved in regulating subsidized markets. Then we will look at private markets and attempt to analyze the weight of economic actors who invest in them and the marketing strategies they deploy.

## Market competition and sharing

### *Intertwining administrative and Global Health regulations*

#### *The construction of subsidized ACT markets by Global Health actors*

Understanding the presence of ACTs produced by Novartis, Sanofi-Aventis, Ajanta, Cipla, and Ipca in public health facilities and, beginning in 2010, in a portion of the Ghanaian private sector is explained by how the global ACT market is constructed. Similar to markets for other drugs made available to countries through Global Health programs (antiretrovirals, tuberculosis drugs, contraceptives, etc.), this market is governed by a triptych of biomedical, technical, and financial norms defined by WHO and transnational actors (Global Fund, PMI). The pharmaceutical industry producing these medicines is closely aligned with the directions taken by international public health policies and the Global Health actors that fund them (Fournier, Lomba, & Muller, 2014). WHO plays a decisive role as prescriber (Orsi & Zimmermann, 2015) by defining the reference treatment and developing technical standards by publishing usage recommendations and guidelines, as well as through the Essential Medicines List that it published for the first time in 1977 and updates regularly.

WHO is also involved in the quality certification process for ACTs through its prequalification department (Lantenois & Coriat, 2014). WHO prequalification requires that production sites comply with good manufacturing practice (GMP), requiring companies to invest significantly in applying their standards and ensuring that the generic drugs they produced are similar to the reference drug. It also requires them to conduct very expensive bioequivalence studies, though these differ depending on where they are conducted. This means international financing conditioned on the purchase of WHO-prequalified ACTs favors those pharmaceutical companies with the means to obtain prequalification, namely, multinationals and the large Asian generics producers, at the expense of local companies. Thus, in 2017, out of the total 46 antimalarial drugs approved worldwide through WHO prequalification, nearly half (n = 21) were produced by Indian companies, 13 by other Asian companies, and 12 by Western multinationals (Singh, 2018).[16] For African producers, WHO prequalification acts as a barrier to entry to subsidized markets and contributes to a hierarchy of markets and generics producers. The normative system, conveyed here by Global Health actors who hold the power to include or exclude, becomes a regulatory tool for markets that knew how to mobilize manufacturing actors from the North and the main generics producers in the South to their advantage. This system leads to a certain type of ACT being available in the public sector as well as in the private Ghanaian market, via the AMFm and then the PSCM. The effects of this regulation in private markets differ from those observed in the public sector where most ACTs are sold at a very low cost and even provided free of charge to some categories of the population such as young children in Benin. However, by imposing a sale price on private intermediaries, the AMFm and the PSCM are imposing a form of regulation in the Ghanaian private sector; in this case, it is economic and runs counter to Ghanaian market rules that encourage the law of supply and demand and free competition between economic actors. Ghana, unlike Benin, does not regulate drug prices. Yet, the fact that ACTs from the AMFm and PSCM are sold at a much lower price than their competitors and that distribution intermediaries can earn a comfortable margin on these products contributes to the AMFm's, and later the PSCM's, ability to crowd out other ACTs from the market that could circulate. This was also the case in the Beninese informal market where retailers only distributed AMFm-subsidized ACTs (Baxerres et al., 2015).

When the PSCM ended in 2017, the Global Fund set out to evaluate pharmaceutical production capacities in Africa in order to be able to procure drugs locally.[17] USAID, one of the United States development aid agencies in the health sector, is also part of this new trend but contributes directly to implementing GMP standards for pharmaceutical manufacturing units, for example, in Nigeria to source some drugs locally.[18]

WHO prequalification does not, however, replace registering drugs by national regulatory authorities. Firms must also comply with a country's national regulations for registering and distributing their product in both the public sector and private markets.

### *State regulation: Between public health concerns and business interests*

While WHO prequalification can guarantee a drug's quality, it cannot exempt the manufacturer, or any other distributor, from requesting an MA in the countries where it hopes to distribute the product. Regulators issue MAs based mainly on the information provided by manufacturers and contained in a dossier, which constitutes a written representation of the drug (Hauray, 2006). By requiring companies to produce numerous documents and to verify the efficacy and safety of their treatments, the MA is a remarkable form of State control (Urfalino, 2007). Benin and Ghana are equipped with regulatory systems, although very different (see Chapter 1), allowing them to conduct drug registration, control, and certification activities to assess their quality and safety before these drugs are distributed to the public. As State monopolies through their national regulatory authorities, these activities are the most traditional way to regulate drugs, what Jean-Paul Gaudillière and Volker Hess (2013) describe as administrative regulation.[19]

In Benin and Ghana, the steps for granting an MA are quite similar: from the submission to the analysis of the pharmaceutical dossier, the process focuses on technical aspects like security, safety, and efficacy, as well as the health products' therapeutic value. In both cases, these technical aspects of the dossier are reviewed by a group of experts, and analyses are conducted in laboratories on drug samples provided by the requesting company. In Ghana, a report of an FDA-Ghana inspection is added to the dossier, unlike in Benin where the DPMED does not conduct inspections of foreign drug manufacturing sites (see Chapter 1). Expert evaluations, quality control test results, and inspection results (in Ghana) are also added to the dossier, which is reviewed by a committee which must decide whether to register the medicine in the country for marketing.

Nevertheless, differences emerge between the two national regulatory authorities' practices.[20] In Benin, in the case of one molecule that was already widely available on the market and had no treatment advantages, experts responsible for evaluating the MA applications were asked to compare the pharmaceutical's suggested pre-tax price to the prices of drugs that are already available.[21] Even though in theory the suggested price must be lower for the MA to be issued, our observations show that this criterion is usually not included. This promotes the addition of products on a market that is already widely saturated by the number of available drugs.

By contrast, in Ghana, there are no criteria limiting the number of me-too drugs.[22] More liberal approaches adopted by Ghanaian health officials for pharmaceutical registration, and distribution should logically have led to a much greater number of MAs issued for ACTs than in Benin, the health officials of which claim to promote a more controlled pharmaceutical distribution system with greater administrative oversight. However, the actual number of MAs issued in Benin and Ghana shows a very different reality. As discussed earlier, comparing lists of MAs for ACTs revealed 71 different ACTs in Benin versus 42 in Ghana. Benin also offered a much greater variety of combination types than Ghana. In addition to the AL combination recommended as first-line treatment by national policy and ASAQ recommended in some specific cases (PNLP, 2005), six other combinations were available in Benin that were not subject to any usage recommendations from WHO or the National Malaria Control Program.[23] However, this is not the case of Ghana, which, beyond AL, which is also the most common ACT, distributed ASAQ and dihydroartemisinin-piperaquine (DHPP), all three of which are recommended by the national policy for malaria control (Ministry of Health, 2010). The fact that the FDA in Ghana restricts ACT registration to the three combinations that are officially recommended by national treatment guidelines limits the number of MAs, and allows companies that only produce these combinations to penetrate private markets. This control is further strengthened by the AMFm and the PSCM, which only allow the distribution of these three types of ACTs on the private market. It also limits the number of new combinations and inhibits competition on a market that, in Ghana, is not regulated by the State per se but governed by the law of supply and demand.[24] In the public sector, the Global Fund and PMI are forced to buy only those ACTs recommended by national policies, again limiting the types of combinations available in public health facilities. Various regulatory methods deployed around ACT availability, whether supported by Global Health programs or by States, contribute to an intertwining of national and global institutional regulations.

The alignment of FDA registrations of ACTs with the National Malaria Control Program recommendations highlights the FDA's reliability in Ghana (see Chapter 1). It underscores how public health interests were prioritized over commercial logics and the desire to promote appropriate ACT use expressed by Ghanaian regulatory officials. Although more liberal overall, the Ghanaian private ACT market is ultimately much more regulated than in Benin, where the ACTs registered by the DPMED are not aligned with the combinations recommended by the national policy. Therefore, no fewer than 50 different ACTs are available for sale in a single Beninese pharmacy. This is not the case in Ghana, where pharmacies are not required to distribute the majority of drugs authorized in the country: only six to seven different ACTs are usually available there. Add to this the AMFm regulatory system, the operations of which, as illustrated in the previous section, "have 'cleaned' the market up of any other ACTs that could have circulated" (Baxerres et al., 2015, p. 151).

The situation is reversed, however, when looking at a therapeutic class that is unregulated by transnational actors, such as anthelmintics, which have lower public health stakes than the management of malaria. There were 23 MAs for drugs consisting of albendazole or mebendazole in Benin compared to 57 in Ghana.[25] This observation corroborates the hypothesis that unlike in Benin, the private ACT market in Ghana is regulated both by aligning registrations with national policy recommendations and by Global Health initiatives, namely, the AMFm and PSCM, which limit the availability of some ACTs to a specific drug category.

Lastly, it is important to highlight another form of national regulation active in Ghana but not (or minimally) in Benin. Ghana is one of the rare sub-Saharan countries to have implemented, in 2003, a universal health insurance program, the National Health Insurance Scheme (NHIS), which has actually been effective (Blanchet, Fink, & Osei-Akoto, 2012). The list of drugs reimbursed by the NHIS is a way to encourage health practitioners to prescribe these medicines rather than nonreimbursed drugs. By setting the prices and type of drugs that it reimburses, the NHIS also plays a key role in the drug regulatory system in private markets, even though in Ghana, as we have seen, prices and various intermediaries' profit margins are not set by national authorities. Health insurance systems and their decisions about which drugs to reimburse and at what price also shape pharmaceutical markets (Gaudillière & Hess, 2013) and play an important role in regulation, on a national scale in Ghana, which intertwines with the systems described earlier.[26]

Both in Ghana and Benin, ACT markets are governed by a jumble of regulations stemming from both national institutions and Global Health actors. To penetrate markets, pharmaceutical companies are forced to adapt their strategies to the features of the institutional and regulatory environment where they operate (Singh, 2018).

## *Market regulation and economic actors' business strategies*

As noted, the institutional regulations developed by national and transnational actors play the most vital role in subsidized ACT markets. In the unsubsidized private sector, however, market forces are the biggest driver, above and beyond institutional regulations for market authorization. These forces are developed by the economic actors: manufacturing companies and distributors.

### *When European and "big" Asian generic companies want to have it both ways*

First, companies that produce the WHO-prequalified ACTs discussed earlier also develop strategies for unsubsidized private markets. Whether based in the West or in Asia, they all offer unsubsidized ACTs sold in private pharmacies in both countries and by OTC medicine sellers and health centers in Ghana. They play on both sides of the field, so to speak, and thus profit from the market hierarchy created by the systems of norms and standards described earlier with regards to WHO prequalification. Some of these companies sell their unsubsidized products under the same trade name as their subsidized ACT. Novartis, for example, sells Coartem® in both types of markets but with different packaging: in a blister pack with illustrations for the subsidized market and a sturdy individual box with no illustration for the unsubsidized private market. Despite being identical to the blister pack, this second product is not sold at the same price and is perceived much differently.[27] In local terms, it is called "original coartem," sold at GHC 25 in Ghana and CFA 4085 in Benin (or just over EUR 6), absolutely not perceived in the same way as the "coartem ACTs," costing thanks to AMFm GHC 4 and CFA 600 (or less than EUR 1). Novartis' market shares have soared in the two countries. The same is true for Cipla, the Indian company, which sells its AL drug under the same name (Lumartem®) but at different prices for the public and private markets. For some authors, "this behavior indicates the firm strategy to gain legitimacy" (Singh & Orsi, 2018, p. 48). Other companies sell their product under an INN in the subsidized markets and under a trade name in unsubsidized markets. These trade names may vary from one country to another. Ipca, for example, sells subsidized AL, but markets it as Laritem® in Benin and Lumarex® in Ghana for the private market at higher prices (around EUR 4). Sanofi sells ASAQ Winthrop® in subsidized markets and Coarsucam® at nearly CFA 4000 in private pharmacies in Benin. Some companies sell one ACT combination for subsidized markets and another for unsubsidized markets. Still, other companies develop a strategy for private markets in one country even though they are only there through subsidized markets in another. The Indian firm Strides Arcolab, for example, sells its subsidized Combiart® in Ghana for less than GHC 1.5 (under USD 1) and the same drug only in unsubsidized markets in Benin for nearly CFA 3000 (EUR 4.5). These differing configurations around products' commercial names and INNs and their presence on specific markets all reveal the marketing strategies firms cleverly developed based on national contexts and targeted market segments. Sudip Chaudhuri discusses how multinational pharmaceutical companies develop a "dual-brand strategy," which "enables them to be present not only in the price-insensitive segment of the market but also in the price-sensitive segment" (Chaudhuri, 2016, p. 108). Firms must also consider any transnational regulations in place, which in this case include the presence or lack of AMFm and subsequently PSCM initiatives in private markets.

For this last reason, as noted earlier, some European companies, the ACTs of which are not prequalified by WHO, are present on the unsubsidized private markets in Benin but not in Ghana; examples include the French Bailly Creat and Medicale Pharmaceutique, the Belgian Dafra Pharma, the Swiss Mepha and Nyd Pharma, and the German Denk Pharma. The greater number of European companies represented in Benin is due to its private sector's continued reliance on France and Europe for pharmaceutical supplies (Baxerres, 2013a). These companies often specialize in generic drugs. Many of them do not manufacture but distribute internationally; they are central procurement offices that purchase products they then repackage with their brand and resell in several countries, especially in Africa.

### *When small and medium Indian and Ghanaian companies take back market share*

Indian companies that make ACTs with no WHO prequalification also develop business strategies to conquer private markets in Benin and Ghana. The Indian industry is described worldwide as the "pharmacy of the developing world," making Africa the destination receiving the second highest amount of its pharmaceutical exports, after North America.[28] The Indian generics industry accounts for 20% of the global generics supply and generates over 50% of its total sales revenue by exporting to nearly every country in the world (Singh, 2018). It is the world's third largest producer of pharmaceuticals (Horner & Murphy, 2018). Apart from the "big" Indian generics producers with the financial and technical capacities to integrate into the highly regulated markets of the North or subsidized ones elsewhere, there are many small and medium Indian firms that earn a significant part of their income in the "semi-regulated markets" in Asia and Africa (Singh, 2018, p. 29; Chaudhuri, 2016).[29] Some specialize exclusively in these markets, or even in a single country, as discussed earlier. Indian companies develop various strategies. Sauman Singh has proposed a categorization of the three different "entry modes" that they use to integrate into markets of other countries, each one having advantages and disadvantages: (1) exports, (2) contractual agreements (licensing, franchising, management contract), and (3) production in countries targeted by joint ventures or through acquisition of a firm in the country of establishment. For marketing operations required for exportation, the Indian firm can go through an Indian intermediary (indirect exports), go through its own channels, or by using one or more local intermediaries (direct exports). "To reduce uncertainty, firms start their international activity through indirect export to countries where the perceived psychic distance is small. That is, they select countries which are comparatively well known and similar regarding business practices, education, industrial development, and other factors" (Singh, 2018, p. 18–19). This echoes our previously published observations: generics from India were introduced to West Africa by anglophone countries, particularly beginning in the 1970s in the fellow Commonwealth countries of Ghana and Nigeria, before becoming part of markets in francophone countries later, but in dramatic fashion, beginning in the late 2000s (Baxerres, 2013b).

Sauman Singh uses the pharmaceutical market in Mali to underscore how Indian firms were introduced into francophone countries in Africa exclusively through exports. This also occurred in Benin, the pioneering country in West Africa until 2012 when it was overtaken by other countries. Indian firms must use wholesale-distribution services operating in Benin that all distribute the same products at the same price (see Chapters 2 and 3). "Concerning Sub-Saharan Africa, market entry through export is further facilitated by the prevailing free trade regime as most countries do not impose tariffs on imports of finished formulations. Exporting allows Indian firms to take advantage of their low-cost domestic production. Also, it is a low-risk entry mode and does not necessitate a firm to undertake direct investment in host countries which is costlier, and firms risk losing the capital if the foreign market engagement fails" (Singh, 2018, p. 153). Chapter 1 examined joint ventures and acquisitions in the country of establishment and showed that the regulatory and fiscal conditions in francophone West African countries are not conducive to setting up local manufacturing plants.

Penetration of pharmaceutical markets is more diversified in anglophone countries, as our studies have shown in Ghana. In addition to conventional exports, Chapter 1 highlights several Indian joint ventures or acquisitions of local firms. Examples of this include the locally established firms Unichem Industries Limited, Eskay Therapeutics Limited, and Pharmanova Limited. Contract agreements are also used to penetrate markets; we saw some contracts between Indian firms and private Ghanaian wholesalers, sometimes with exclusivity clauses for the firm's product or products. It is said locally that wholesalers have "the monopoly" on such and such a product. "Contract manufacturing" is another type of agreement; in this case, the Ghanaian wholesaler has an Indian firm manufactured product under its own brand. We observed several cases of ACTs produced through contract manufacturing in Ghana, especially when the PSCM was beginning to lose its efficiency. One private Ghanaian wholesaler explained: "I came with the concept of AL, artemether lumefantrine; the SS means single strength, that will be 20/120mg. And then I have DS, which is double strength, 40/240mg; and then I have the Forte, which is the 80/480mg. I started the registration of these in 2013. And it was done in 2014. And I started this because we realized that the AMFm was not going to be sustainable. So, if the AMFm initiative is not going to be sustainable, then it means after AMFm, after the private sector co-payment mechanism, there will be a gap. (…). So strategically, I decided to bring mine in case the Global Fund was not interested in continuing. Or in case they are not adequately funded, and then we will still have efficacious antimalarials to still give to our people. (…). Not too expensive. I am selling mine for 8.00 cedis, while the Global Fund one is selling for 4.50. (…). For the start, from 2010, it didn't make business sense to import antimalarials, but now it makes a lot of business sense…" (interview, Accra, March 15, 2016). Some Ghanaian wholesalers who had invested during this time in contract manufacturing with Indian firms to distribute ACTs also use packaging that quite closely resembles that of subsidized ACTs (see Figure 6.2 below).

Ghanaian wholesalers are then responsible for promoting the products. These contracts are beneficial for both the Indian and Ghanaian parties. "The primary advantage of Indian firms is their low-cost production abilities, but they lack market information, distribution channel and human resources for product promotion in host countries. Local operators, on the other hand, are well aware of the specificities of their home country market. They possess assets in the form of local marketing and distribution networks, market intelligence and can easily access local labor market. Further, they are familiar with regulatory frameworks, have connections in government offices and know the right approach to get things done" (Singh, 2018, p. 157). Thus, some unsubsidized ACTs produced in India for which the Ghanaian wholesaler has exclusive rights and has developed a very effective promotion campaign capture substantial market share. This is the case for Lonart®, manufactured by a medium-sized Indian firm, Bliss GVS, and distributed in Ghana exclusively by one of its largest wholesalers working in the country, Tobinco (see Figure 6.3 below).[30]

With the end of AMFm and the PSCM's reduced efficiency, most of the Ghanaian manufacturing firms went back to focusing on ACTs, but lagged

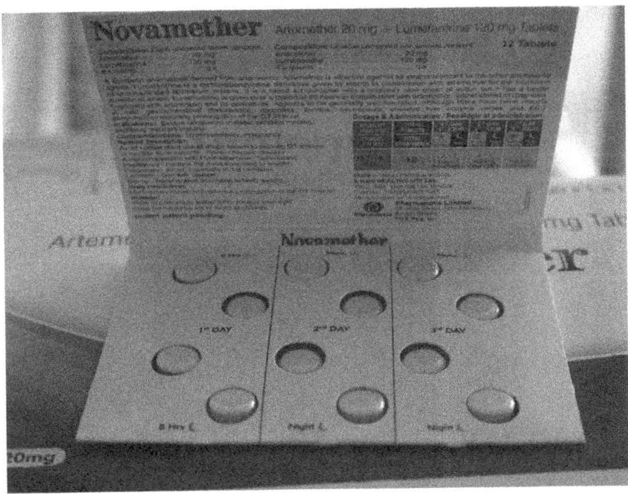


*Figure 6.2* ACT produced in India for exclusive distribution in Ghana by Pharmanova.

Source: © IRD/Carine Baxerres, Accra, November 2015

behind the contract manufacturing wholesalers because of the time needed to restart their ACT production chains and the difficulty in repositioning themselves on the markets (finding distributers, capturing market shares). In 2016, the company Entrance, for example, registered Lufart®, an AL combination, and began to develop another DHPP-based ACT. Some of these firms, like the wholesalers mentioned earlier, also used packaging similar to that of subsidized ACTs. Producers and wholesale distributors are not the only forces involved here. Retailers and consumers also participate in the market regulation of drugs when they choose to buy one ACT instead of another, in relation to the social stratification of pharmaceutical markets. Chapters 10 and 11 discuss this issue, looking at the market as a whole.

## Conclusion

Beyond the most traditional form of pharmaceutical regulation administered by the States, we have highlighted how other ways ACTs are regulated become intermingled in Benin and Ghana: the "global mode" of regulation, developed by Global Health actors (Pourraz, 2019) and the market mode, which contribute in their own way and jointly to shaping pharmaceutical markets. Each regulatory way has corresponding specific combinations of practices, values, and logics, thus underscoring various rationales underpinning the process of drug management (Gaudillière & Hess, 2013). Investigating pharmaceutical regulation in the countries of the Global South through the prism of ACTs requires considering both

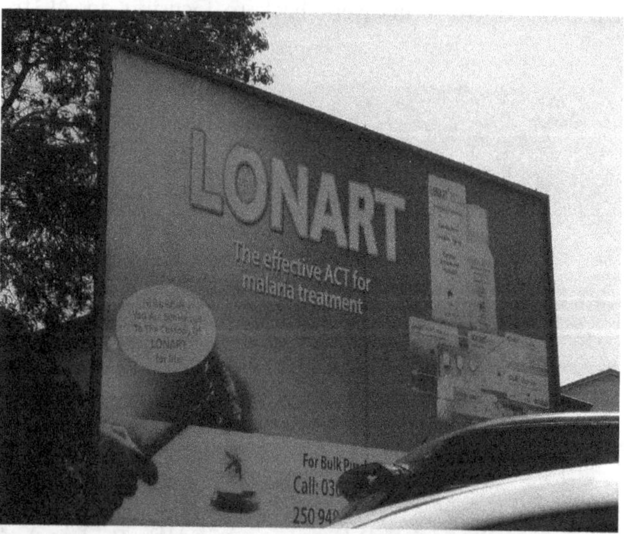


*Figure 6.3* Advertising roadside billboard photographed in Accra.

Source: © IRD/Carine Baxerres, Accra, November 2015

the role of the States as well as the weight and effects of Global Health programs, industrials, and actors in private distribution. In the following chapters, we will see how prescribers and individual consumers of drugs also participate in structuring these markets.

Global Health programs appear to play a considerable role in structuring pharmaceutical markets in the Global South for the subsidized products used to treat priority health issues (AIDS, tuberculosis, malaria, contraceptives, etc.), including in countries where pharmaceutical distribution is generally largely liberalized, as in Ghana. In response, Asian generics manufacturers, local African firms, and European firms—large and small—deploy marketing strategies to conquer private unsubsidized markets. These firms are linked in such efforts by retailers who offer consumers the ACT "that they need" based on their socioeconomic status. In Ghana, local wholesalers, who are in stiff competition with each other, play a significant role in the structuring of the ACT markets. In particular, they strongly promote the ACTs produced by small and medium Indian firms for which they have the exclusive sales rights or for which they contract out manufacturing for themselves. Firms, the drugs of which are not prequalified by the WHO and the products of which are not subsidized by Global Health actors, play these economic market-sharing games to capture substantial shares.

As Mathieu Quet and his collaborators have pointed out regarding the "Regulation Multiple" in South-East Asia—"confronted as it is with multiple realities and real-world practices" (Quet et al., 2018, p. 2)—this chapter highlights how various layers of regulation governing ACT markets stack up on each other and create drug hierarchies. The regulations implemented by Global Health actors are intertwined with national regulations for malaria (recommended combinations) and, more broadly, pharmaceutical markets (issuance of MAs).[31] Moreover, market regulations are also at work: companies' commercial strategies include attractive packaging and invented trade names, which may change by market segment and targeted country or remain steady and unchanging to further establish their reputation. Sometimes these various regulations conflict with each other, as regularly demonstrated in the court cases between pharmaceutical companies and States.[32] This was not the case at the time of our studies for the situations we have described, where these regulations appear to have adapted quite well to each other in the end.

## Notes

1. For more about these partners, see the previous chapter. The role of the DND*i* is to develop new treatments for neglected maladies. Novartis is presented as the largest pharmaceutical multinational and Sanofi is the fourth largest (Chaudhuri, 2016). By transnational actors, we mean the various types of extra-national actors currently working on public health issues in so-called "Southern" countries: bilateral institutions (the various cooperation services) and multilaterals (World Bank, Global Fund); non-governmental organizations (NGOs); foundations; and public-private partnerships (see Baxerres & Eboko, 2019).

2. The Global Fund is a multilateral initiative to fight AIDS, tuberculosis, and malaria created in 2001 by the Secretary-General of the United Nations, Kofi Annan. The President's Malaria Initiative (PMI) is a United States bilateral development program created by President George Bush in 2005.
3. For information on these different modes of regulation, refer to the Introduction of the book.
4. Prequalification guarantees the generic's quality and similarity with the reference medicine. This quality standard for medicines is certified by WHO each time for each company/product pair.
5. For more details about this agreement, refer to the previous chapter.
6. The World Bank and UNICEF also work in Benin, but to a much lesser degree.
7. Ghana, as well as Kenya, Madagascar, Niger, Nigeria, Tanzania, Uganda, and Cambodia, participated in the AMFm pilot phase between 2010 and 2012. The Roll Back Malaria (RBM) partnership, which brings together UNICEF, the United Nations Development Programme, and the World Bank, was created in 1998 by the WHO Director-General at the time, Dr. Harlem Gro Brundtland, with the goal of implementing a coordinated global response to the fight against malaria.
8. The estimated profits on ACTs for first-line buyers range from USD 0.63 to USD 0.92 per treatment sold (Pourraz, 2019).
9. Here we have considered both the marketing name (INN or trade name) and the producer. The different dosages proposed by the companies based on the patient's weight are not incorporated into these figures.
10. Thus, there is a difference between the issued MAs and the actual products distributed in the country.
11. Based on fluctuating currency exchange rates, the euro is generally slightly higher than the dollar (EUR 1 ≈ USD 1.15). Quoting the prices in euros for Benin and in dollars for Ghana, as is the practice in these two countries, highlights how each of these financial, and by extension, cultural contexts have an impact in Benin and Ghana, respectively.
12. The fifth African company was located in Senegal. The ACTs produced in Ghana were Camosunate® and Danmether® by Danadams; Globartem® and Gloderp® by African Global Pharma; Artifran® and Asumod® by Phyto Riker GIHOC; and Malar-2® by Ernest Chemists. During our field studies in Ghana and in addition to the inventories conducted at the start of the research, we also found Lumether® by Kinapharma and Lumenate® by Pharmanova, two firms that were also local.
13. The only pharmaceutical company located in Benin, Pharmaquick, did not produce ACT; Chapter 1 has more on this company.
14. The countries covered in this study are Central African Republic, Côte d'Ivoire, Ethiopia, Gambia, Kenya, Mozambique, Namibia, Nigeria, Rwanda, Sao Tome and Principe, Sudan, Tanzania, Uganda, Zambia, and Zimbabwe.
15. These figures should be interpreted with caution. They are based on sales volumes rather than price analysis and are not representative of the Ghanaian market since they only come from two wholesalers. Moreover, Ghanaian wholesalers differ significantly from one another in terms of products distributed and sales (Baxerres, 2018). One of the two wholesalers in our ethnographies, for example, was the exclusive distributor of one of the ACTs produced by an Indian company, which meant its sales were overrepresented.
16. These figures include different dosages for each medicine.
17. In collaboration with the Federation of African Pharmaceutical Manufacturers Associations (FAPMA), the Global Fund held a consultative meeting in June 2017 with manufacturers and technical partners based in Africa to discuss the status of local pharmaceutical production capacities and opportunities. A survey was launched to help the Global Fund Supply Department assess African producers' ability to

supply essential medicines. For more information, see the Consultative Meeting Presentations: https://www.theglobalfund.org/media/6582/psm_2017-06-globalfund-fapmameeting_presentation_en.pdf, accessed March 2, 2020.

18. USAID supports numerous African producers through the Promoting the Quality of Medicines project. The United States bilateral agency would no longer require WHO prequalification as a condition. Its purchasing department, with its own quality assurance system, implemented its own quality assessment criteria for drugs (source: interviews with USAID supply managers, October 2017, Geneva).
19. These authors adopt John Pickstone's concept of "Ways of Knowing" and identify five "ways of regulating drugs": administrative (government interventions), which is the most traditional way; professional (scientific societies); industrial (firms); public (civil society); and juridical (law professionals, legal associations).
20. We conducted an ethnographic study of the drug committees that oversee the technical evaluation of the applications and issuance of MAs covering several days at the DPMED in Benin and the FDA in Ghana. We analyzed the decision-making process and highlighted the evaluation criteria and differences in regulatory practices between national authorities.
21. The price of drugs in Benin is set by the State (see Chapters 2 and 3).
22. The term "me-too" "means a substance developed to penetrate a niche market already occupied by a similar specialty, without providing any new profits" (Hauray, 2006, p. 147).
23. The Beninese national policy recommends the use of ASAQ in the event of unavailability or intolerance to AL and for children under 6 months. In addition to AL and ASAQ, we found the following combinations in Benin: dihydropterin + piperaquine; dihydroartemisinin + sulfadoxine-pyrimethamine; artesunate + sulfadoxine-pyrimethamine; artesunate + mefloquine; sulfamethoxypyrazine + artesunate + pyrimethamine; and artemisinin + naphthoquine. Until 2006, WHO recommended the use of four combinations that could be used as first-line treatments for malaria: AL, ASAQ, artesunate-mefloquine (ASMQ), and artesunate-sulfadoxine-pyrimethamine (ASSP) (WHO, 2001, 2006). The DHPP combination was added later (WHO, 2015).
24. The AMFm program was strongly criticized by PMI and USAID representatives who opposed any form of subsidies for the private sector. From their perspective, AMFm had introduced a way to regulate the private market, which should be regulated solely by the rules of free competition. On this topic, see also Baxerres et al. (2015).
25. Source: inventory, conducted in June 2019, of drugs containing albendazole and mebendazole, distributed in pharmacies in Cotonou for Benin and the MA list of products containing albendazole and mebendazole provided by the FDA in Ghana in 2015.
26. However, Ghana's NHIS is facing a host of problems, as we will see in Chapters 9 and 10.
27. The different perceptions that consumers have about drugs based on their trade name and their brand are explored in Chapter 11.
28. Indian companies in particular hold a central place in the global fight against AIDS, tuberculosis, and malaria (Singh, 2018).
29. There are 3000 pharmaceutical firms in India and over 10,000 legal manufacturing units belonging to them (Cepuch & Ashalhani, 2018).
30. One of Tobinco's tactics was running very effective advertisements for Lonart® on Ghanaian television and roadside billboards: A mosquito is tried in a court of law, and the judge hammered his gavel as a box of Lonart® appeared.
31. Negotiations and power games between national and transnational actors are interesting to study. Revolving instead around the transnational actors' advantage, they nevertheless highlight the States' leeway and the procedures implemented to (re)conquer their sovereignty (Baxerres & Eboko, 2019; Pourraz, 2019; Pourraz, Baxerres, & Cassier, 2019).

32. See the 2001 lawsuit filed by 39 pharmaceuticals against the Government of South Africa regarding antiretroviral drugs (Whyte, Van der Geest, & Hardon, 2002); those against the Swiss company Novartis and the Indian government in 2007, 2009, and 2012 on the Indian law on patents and its application for Glivec®, a cancer drug produced by the firm (Chaudhuri, 2013) and, more broadly, the confrontations between the State and the pharmaceutical companies in India and Brazil (Cassier, 2013).

## Reference list

Anadach Group. (2012). Sustaining affordable co-paid ACT retail prices over 12–24 months, Early considerations from Ghana.

Baxerres, C. (2013a). *Du médicament informel au médicament libéralisé : Une anthropologie du médicament pharmaceutique au Bénin [From informal to liberalized drugs: An anthropology of pharmaceutical drugs in Benin]*. Paris, France: Les Éditions des Archives Contemporaines.

Baxerres, C. (2013b). L'introduction différenciée des génériques entre pays francophones et anglophones d'Afrique de l'Ouest: Une illustration de la globalisation du médicament à partir du cas du Bénin [Differentiated introduction of generics between French-speaking and English-speaking countries in West Africa: An illustration of the globalization of drugs based on the case of Benin]. *Autrepart*, 63, 51–68. https://doi.org/10.3917/autr.063.0051.

Baxerres, C. (2018). D'intermédiaire informel, devenir détaillant, grossiste puis producteur pharmaceutique : les trajectoires « vertueuses » des hommes d'affaires du médicament au Ghana [From informal intermediary to becoming a retailer, wholesaler, and then pharmaceutical producer: The "virtuous" trajectories of drug businessmen in Ghana]. In C. Baxerres, & C. Marquis (Eds.), *Regulations, markets, health: Questioning current stakes of pharmaceuticals in Africa* (pp. 30–40). (Conference proceedings). HAL, Ouidah, Benin. https://hal.archives-ouvertes.fr/hal-01988227.

Baxerres, C., & Eboko, F. (Eds.). (2019). Global health: Et la santé ? [Global health: And health?]. *Politique Africaine*, 4, 156.

Baxerres, C., Egrot, M., Houngnihin, R., & Le Hesran, J.-Y. (2015). Dualité de l'accès au médicament en Afrique de l'Ouest : Les ACT entre large distribution et consommation sous surveillance [Duality of drug access in West Africa: ACTs between wide distribution and consumption under surveillance]. In M. Badji, & A. Desclaux, (Eds.), *Nouveaux enjeux éthiques autour du médicament en Afrique. Analyses en anthropologie, droit et santé publique [New ethical issues around drugs in Africa. Analyzes in anthropology, law, and public health]* (pp. 141–158). Dakar, Senegal: L'Harmattan.

Blanchet, N., Fink, G., & Osei-Akoto, I. (2012). The effect of Ghana's National Health Insurance Scheme on health care utilization. *Ghana Medical Journal*, 46(2), 76–84.

Cassier, M. (2013). Pharmaceutical patent law in-the-making: Opposition and legal action by States, citizens and generics laboratories in Brazil and India. In J.-P. Gaudillière, & V. Hess (Eds.), *Ways of regulating drugs in the 19th and the 20th centuries* (pp. 287–317). Hampshire, UK: Palgrave Macmillan.

Cepuch, C., & Ashalhani, A. (2018, September). UHC, Access and Good Quality Medicine. Paper presented at Medicine Quality & Public Health Conference, Oxford, UK.

Chaudhuri, S. (2013). The larger implications of the Novartis Glivec judgment. *Economic and Political Weekly*, 48(17), 10–12.

Chaudhuri, S. (2016). Can foreign firms promote local production of pharmaceuticals in Africa?. In M. Mackintosh, G. Banda, P. Tibandebage, & W. Wamae (Eds.), *Making medicines in Africa: The political economy of industrializing for local health* (pp. 103–121). London, UK: Palgrave Macmillan.

Davis, B., Ladner, J., Sams, K., Tekinturhan, E., de Korte, D., & Saba, J. (2013). Artemisinin-based combination therapy availability and use in the private sector of five AMFm phase 1 countries. *Malaria Journal, 12*(135), 9. https://doi.org/10.1186/1475-2875-12-135.

Fournier, P., Lomba, C., & Muller, S. (Eds.). (2014). *Les travailleurs du médicament. L'industrie pharmaceutique sous observation [Drug workers. The pharmaceutical industry under observation]*. Toulouse, France: ERES.

Gaudillière, J.-P., & Hess V. (2013). General introduction. In J.-P. Gaudillière, & V. Hess (Eds.), *Ways of regulating drugs in the 19th and the 20th centuries* (pp. 1–16). Hampshire, UK: Palgrave Macmillan.

Hauray, B. (2006). *L'Europe du médicament. Politique, expertise, intérêts privés [Europe of drugs. Politics, expertise, private interests]*. Paris, France: Presse Sciences Po.

Horner, R., & Murphy, J. T. (2018). South–North and South–South production networks: Diverging socio-spatial practices of Indian pharmaceutical firms. *Global Networks, 18*(2), 326–351.

Lantenois, C., & Coriat, B. (2014). La « préqualification » OMS: Origines, déploiement et impacts sur la disponibilité des antirétroviraux dans les pays du Sud [WHO "prequalification": Origins, deployment, and impacts on antiretroviral availability in Southern countries]. *Sciences Sociales et Santé, 32*(1), 71–99.

Ministry of Health. (2010). *Standard treatment guidelines* (6th ed.). Accra, Ghana.

Orsi, F., & Zimmermann, F. (2015). Le marché des antipaludéens: Entre régulation et défaillance [The antimalarial market: Between regulation and failure]. *Mondes en développement, 170*(2), 21–40.

Orsi, F., Singh, S., & Sagaon-Teyssier, L. (2018). The creation and evolution of the donor funded market for antimalarials and the growing role of Southern firms. *Science, Technology & Society, 23*(3), 1–22.

PNLP. (2005). *Politique nationale de lutte contre le paludisme et cadre strategique de mise en œuvre [National malaria control policy and strategic framework for implementation]*. Cotonou, Benin.

Pourraz, J. (2019). *Réguler et produire les médicaments contre le paludisme au Ghana et au Bénin : Une affaire d'Etat ? Politiques pharmaceutiques, normes de qualité et marchés de médicaments [Regulating and producing malaria drugs in Ghana and Benin: A State affair? Pharmaceutical policies, quality standards, and drug markets]*. Doctoral dissertation, Ecole des Hautes Etudes en Sciences Sociales, Paris, France. Retrieved at http://www.theses.fr/2019EHES0014.

Pourraz, J., Baxerres, C., & Cassier, M. (2019). La construction des politiques pharmaceutiques nationales à l'épreuve des programmes de santé globale. L'approvisionnement des médicaments contre le paludisme au Bénin et au Ghana [The construction of national pharmaceutical policies able to stand the test of global health programs. Antimalaria drug supply in Benin and Ghana]. *Anthropologie et Développement*, 48–49, 169–192. https://doi.org/10.4000/anthropodev.706.

Quet, M., Pordié, L., Bochaton, A., Chantavanich, S., Kiatying-Angsulee, N., Lamy, M., & Vungsiriphisal, P. (2018). Regulation multiple: Pharmaceutical trajectories and modes of control in the ASEAN. *Science, Technology and Society, 23*(3), 485–503. https://doi.org/10.1177/0971721818762935.

Sams, K. (2016, July). La Chine et « la meilleure façon de faire » : La circulation des médicaments à base d'artémisinine aux Comores [China and "the best way to do it": The circulation of artemisinin-based medicines n the Comoros]. Paper presented at the Fourth African Studies Meeting in France, Paris.

Singh, S. (2018). *Entry and operation strategies of Indian pharmaceutical firms in Africa under the dynamics of markets and institutions*. Doctoral dissertation, Aix-Marseille University, France. Retrieved at http://www.theses.fr/2018AIXM0238.

Singh, S., & Orsi, F. (2018). The market for artemisinin-based combination therapies and the new era of "market makers." In C. Baxerres, & C. Marquis (Eds.), *Regulations, markets, health: Questioning current stakes of pharmaceuticals in Africa* (pp. 42–52). (Conference proceedings). HAL, Ouidah, Benin. https://hal.archives-ouvertes.fr/hal-01988227.

Urfalino, P. (2007). Introduction au dossier Médicaments et sociétés, enjeux contemporains [Introduction to the drugs and societies dossier, contemporary issues], *Annales HSS*, *2*, 269–272.

WHO. (2001). *Antimalarial drug combination therapy: Report of a WHO technical consultation*. Geneva, Switzerland: World Health Organization.

WHO. (2006). *Guidelines for the treatment of malaria*. Geneva, Switzerland: World Health Organization.

WHO. (2015). *Guidelines for the treatment of malaria* (3rd ed.). Geneva, Switzerland: World Health Organization.

Whyte, R. S., Van der Geest, S., & Hardon, A. (2002). *Social lives of medicines*, New York, NY: Cambridge University Press.

# 7 When the pharmaceutical system creates persistent attachments or new appropriations of drug molecules

## Divergent ACT distribution and use in Benin and Ghana

*Carine Baxerres, Kelley Sams, Daniel Kojo Arhinful, Jean-Yves Le Hesran*

The recommendation by the World Health Organization (WHO) to use artemisinin-based combination therapies (ACTs) as first-line treatment for malaria dates back to 2001 for Southeast Asian countries where the parasite (*Plasmodium falciparum*) had developed an intolerable resistance to the antimalarial drugs used up to that point (chloroquine, sulfadoxine-pyrimethamine [SP], and mefloquine) (Souares, 2007). After several years of lobbying orchestrated by the nongovernmental organization Médecins Sans Frontières (Doctors Without Borders), in 2006, this recommendation was applied to Africa, the continent most affected by the disease (Balkan & Corty, 2009).[1] Prior to this, as early as 2004, the Global Fund to Fight AIDS, Tuberculosis and Malaria had been promoting the use of ACTs in Africa; in that year, without waiting for an official WHO recommendation, the Ministries of Health in Benin and Ghana decided to change their recommendation for first-line treatment of malaria. In Benin, the health authorities adopted the artemether-lumefantrine (AL) combination, promoted by an agreement signed in 2001 between WHO and the Novartis company (see Chapter 5), despite scientists' preference for another combination (artesunate-mefloquine). Ghana first chose the artesunate-amodiaquine combination (ASAQ), later adding AL to its recommended treatment following the "ASAQ crisis" caused by a local industrialist, due to the technological limitations of Ghanaian industry, shortcomings of the regulatory authority, and the State's refusal to financially support drug manufacturers at the time (Pourraz, 2019).

Institutional, industrial, political, and economic stakes were already emerging in the countries' decisions to adopt ACT and in their choice of drug molecules. Benin and Ghana are very close geographically and have quite comparable epidemiological contexts for malaria.[2] In this chapter, we will see how the combination drugs on the market in the two countries are screened through the local pharmaceutical system before being made available to consumers.[3] Therefore, although consumers perceive the disease in a fairly similar way, as we will see, they actually use ACTs in very different ways. Moreover, when these drugs are introduced into countries, they do not arrive "tabula rasa." ACTs have to compete with the multitude of other pharmaceutical products available, whether for malaria or other illnesses, not to mention herbal medicines, which will be discussed in the next chapter. This chapter will highlight how the ties that bind individuals to pharmaceutical molecules—through attachment, rejection, or appropriation—are primarily constructed through existing legislation and pharmaceutical distribution methods. The anthropology of medicine has been studying the relationships between individuals and industrial products since the 1980s (Van der Geest & Whyte, 1988). Initially, researchers looked primarily to local culture to understand these links, studying how such medicines were incorporated into medical traditions based on frameworks other than biomedicine. Later works included economic, political, and health system organization elements in the analysis (Desclaux & Egrot, 2015; Petryna, Lakoff, & Kleinman, 2006). Our work is from this second perspective. In this chapter, which draws its strength from the combination of qualitative and quantitative studies and the comparison between two countries, we will highlight the importance of structural factors over cultural factors.[4]

## *Palu, malaria, hwevó, abun, tanvio, atikéssi*: Benin and Ghana share similar popular perceptions of the disease

A fairly extensive anthropological literature on malaria has highlighted the discrepancies that exist between this biomedical entity and people's perceptions of it, as they associate it with various popular nosological entities (Jaffré & Olivier de Sardan, 1999). The terms *sibidu* and *sumaan ndiig* have long been used in Senegal, *atikéssi* and *hwevó* in Benin, and *koom*, *weogo*, and *sagba* in Burkina Faso, and these various French-speaking countries also use the term *palu* (from *paludisme*, or malaria in French) (Baxerres, 2013; Bonnet, 1986; Faye, 2009; Kpatchavi, 2011). These various popular entities do not strictly align with the biomedical entity of "malaria," although in some aspects they may be similar. The differences between them concern the manifestations or first symptoms of the disease (which are much broader in popular perceptions), the etiological agents (which go far beyond the mosquito alone), and the potential severity of the disease (much lower in popular perceptions, where it is often trivialized because of its frequency and the many cases that spontaneously resolve). However, studies have shown that these popular perceptions can change significantly over time under the influence of health professionals and public health awareness campaigns (Baxerres et al., 2021; Faye, 2009).

In Benin, we have observed a kind of biomedical normalization of perceptions of *palu* since our first fieldwork in 2005 (Baxerres, 2013), which was much more evident in the city of Cotonou than in the rural Mono department. In contrast to our previous study, the term *palu* is now used there almost exclusively to refer to headaches, fever, vomiting, body aches, chills, fatigue, loss of appetite, and the yellow color of eyes and urine[5]; this aligns with the symptoms described in biomedicine for uncomplicated malaria. Use of the term *palu* has gained over *hwevó* (meaning "sun" in Fon, the primary language spoken in Cotonou), and this latter term was only rarely mentioned in interviews. However, in the Mono department, in addition to *palu*, the terms *hwecivio* (in the Pedah language) and *hwecivoè* (in Sahouè), both of which also mean "sun," *tanvio*, which means "mouth" or "bitter saliva" in Pedah, and *atikéssi*, which means "water from the root of the tree" in Ouatchi, are frequently used for similar symptomatology and etiologies.[6] Perhaps related to this terminology, the symptoms mentioned by individuals here are broader than those stated in Cotonou, and include stomachache, "dirty stomach" (diarrhea), heavy eyes, red eyes, bitter taste in the mouth, heavy head, not being active, not being oneself, being sad, sleeping poorly, and having nightmares.

In Cotonou, it appears that popular perceptions more readily accept mosquitos as the causative agent for *palu* than in the previous study. This was routinely stated by respondents in the qualitative study, and 9 of the 15 mothers of Cotonou families only cited the mosquito as the cause of *palu*. "It's mosquitoes, nothing else causes malaria, it's mosquitoes. If I am tired one day and I lie down on the ground, you know that mosquitoes will eat the children and me, if you don't pay attention and surrender yourself to the mosquitoes, they spit dirty things into your body" (mother of a "poor" family, Cotonou, February 2015). Most of the Mono respondents and six of the Cotonou mothers also referred to other causes, described in our previous study: sun and heat; other elements to which people are exposed (rain, coolness, cold, wind, the Harmattan wind, dust, impurities in food, food that is inappropriate for the person, being dirty); difficulties in life (hard and intense work, worries, thinking too much, getting angry, needing to move around, and not getting enough sleep).

In both urban and semirural contexts in Benin, individuals stress that there are two kinds of *palu*, one more serious than the other. This gradation existed at the time of our previous study in Cotonou, and we explained it by the influence of biomedical perceptions of "uncomplicated malaria" and "severe malaria." It seems that this influence has increased, at least in conversations where *malaria* is linked to potential death, which was not the case in our previous study. "That *hwecivio asì*, that's what causes the fever and is what we were talking about. *Hwecivio asú*, it turns your eyes yellow, even the palms of your hands, everything turns yellow, and when you open your eyes, you'll see that it's yellow. That's when we talk about *hwecivio asú* and that's the dangerous one… It's not good, if you don't get help quickly for that, it often leads to death"[7] (father in a "middle-class" family, Mono department, December 2015).

In Ghana, contrary to what we found during our initial field investigations,[8] popular perceptions associated with the English term "malaria" are similar to those in Benin. Yannick Jaffré and Jean-Pierre Olivier de Sardan highlight the "resonances," "similarities," and "overlaps" at work in the popular nosological entities that are active in the countries of West Africa (Jaffré & Olivier de Sardan, 1999, p. 8). In Accra, perhaps because of the more concentrated use of English in the area compared with rural areas, *malaria* was usually referred to by its English term, even when speaking in local languages. In the semirural research site, Breman Asikuma, *malaria* was also referred to in Fanti as *abun* (meaning "green," which could refer to the color of vomit) in households from all three socioeconomic categories. *Abun* was described by one mother to be synonymous with fever. "We call it *abun*...it is also the same [as fever]... both of them are the same. Sometimes we call it *atridii*[9] in Twi" (mother, "middle-class" family, November, 2014).

Although there were some differences between rural and urban areas concerning the conceptions of etiology and symptoms of *malaria*, with more of a tendency toward a biomedical definition of the disease in Accra, in both the semirural and urban research sites, the popular definition of *malaria* was much broader than the biomedical entity. As expected, *malaria* was often associated with fever, but this was not the only symptom described by respondents. Like in Benin, the presence of *malaria* or *abun* was indicated by more than—and sometimes without—an elevated body temperature: it also meant experiencing chills, weakness, bitterness in the mouth, loss of appetite, or body pain. One respondent stated, "If the malaria comes into you, you'd realize that all your joints would be aching, and you can't do anything. If you have to pick something up off the ground it would be a problem for you. Also, your mouth would be bitter, and you won't be able to enjoy any taste from the food you eat, no matter how much you eat" (mother, "poor" family, Breman Asikuma, July, 2015). Other symptoms, seen to indicate by themselves the presence of *malaria* or *abun*, were also cited, for example, Anthonia[10] (mother, Accra, "wealthy" family) stated that her lips and tongue would often turn white when she was infected. Mr. Tetteh stated that, in addition to weakness and body pains, *malaria* "makes your eyes yellow, and you wouldn't be able to eat; and when you urinate, it would be very deep yellow... Also it makes your joints weak and also headaches" (grandfather, "middle-class" family, Breman Asikuma, March 2016).

The perceived etiologic agents of *malaria* in Ghana described by interlocutors were more diverse than in Benin, proving the dynamism of popular *malaria* perceptions. While most mothers interviewed in research households of Cotonou cited mosquitos as the sole cause of *palu*, in Ghana, mosquitos were cited as only one of several factors that were responsible for the symptoms that accompanied *malaria*. Some interlocutors explained their perception of *malaria* as a condition caused by a multitude of variables: "Mostly they say mosquitos cause malaria but I don't totally agree. Maybe you would be bitten by mosquitos, but as you do hard work, and you have poor eating habits or you don't eat well, you often get malaria. At the times I got malaria, I was not eating well, I mean like you go somewhere to work the whole day without eating, you see you would be excessively tired and it would cause malaria" (father, Breman Asikuma, "wealthy" family, March 2016). This very broad perspective on the factors that provoke disease was echoed by rural interlocutors like Mary, "[Malaria is] caused by the sun, sometimes mosquitos too, also from the food we eat… from the water we drink. Also if you travel, you don't have a house to sleep inside, so you would have to sleep outside and bad air can cause [it]" (mother, Breman Asikuma, "poor" family, February 2015). Excess oil consumption and eating poorly were also cited as provoking the disease. The idea that heat or sun exposure, as in Benin, could cause *malaria* or its related symptoms was especially salient in lower socioeconomic status households, in both the semirural and urban research sites, and when respondents were discussing cases with high fever. Often, sunshine was described as working in tandem with mosquitos to provoke the disease, as explained by Gladys "Fever is brought about by sunshine. When the sun shines like that, and mosquito bites someone that increases fever. Mosquitoes bring fever, but the main cause of fever is sunshine and the mosquitoes add the malaria" (mother, Accra, "poor" family, January 2015).

In both semirural and urban areas, *malaria* was perceived as a common and simple illness to routinely self-treat with medications at home. Many interlocutors explained that reoccurring *malaria* infection was an expected part of life, classified with other routine illnesses, and that it was no reason to panic. Franck, for example, stated that, when one feels certain symptoms, "you know it's your malaria which is showing up… for malaria in Africa what I can say is that whether you like it or not you would get malaria (…). The way I see it no matter what you do, you would still get it" (father, Breman Asikuma, "poor" family, March 2016). While this regularly occurring, simple *malaria* was mainly treated at home, as in Benin, several interlocutors described the existence of another more serious version of the disease that required treatment at a health facility. Judith described when her 15-year-old son suffered from this version of *malaria*, "[He had] the serious one and I took him to Our Lady of Grace Hospital here in Asikuma… He was hot, and he became very high and aggressive. I remember he attacked me, held me so that I could not escape. I had to call people to help grasp him and take him to the hospital" (mother, Breman Asikuma, "middle-class" family, January 2015).

Various popular nosological entities that may be associated with the biomedical entity "malaria" in Benin and Ghana cover a variety of vague, nonspecific symptoms that occur frequently in daily family life among both children and adults. They are part of the normal course of events. These popular nosological entities are generally seen as benign, although people are aware of possible complications. In the contexts studied, they constitute active entities that people know how to identify and treat.[11] Several authors in Africa have pointed out that when people think they have "malaria," they turn first to the private and informal pharmaceutical distribution sectors and do not initially visit health facilities (Kamat & Nyato, 2010; Kangwana et al., 2011; ACTwatch[12]). We will therefore look at how the pharmaceutical distribution systems in these countries are critical to understanding the use of the "new" malaria treatments, ACTs, which had been officially recommended in Benin and Ghana when we began our field studies a decade ago.

## Divergent ACT distribution and use between the two countries

Although these popular nosological entities are perceived in relatively similar ways in Benin and Ghana, individuals have quite different access to ACTs to treat them.

In Benin's pharmaceutical system, public and private distributions are clearly dissociated[13]; as a result, subsidized, inexpensive ACTs (CFA 150–600 or EUR 0.22–0.91 per dose, depending on the patient's age and weight) were distributed only through the public wholesaler (the Central Purchasing Office for Essential Medicines and Medical Consumables, or CAME[14]) and public health centers at different levels of the health pyramid (national reference hospitals, district hospitals, district and commune health centers, and isolated maternity units). Subsidized ACTs were not available in private pharmacies or pharmaceutical depots. Only unsubsidized ACTs were available in these locations, with the price for an adult dose ranging between CFA 1425 and 4660 (about EUR 2–7) depending on the product. Pharmaceutical company representatives did not make prescribers working in private clinics and health centers aware of the use of these subsidized products, as is done for other products available in private pharmacies.[15] In Benin, private health facilities are not authorized to sell medicines; the professionals who work there write prescriptions that their patients then bring to pharmacies or depots.

In Ghana, however, private distribution actors are a considerable force, and the public and private sectors are closely intertwined. Subsidized ACTs were available not only in public and private health-care facilities but also through the many private wholesalers (nearly 600 companies) as well as all private retailers, which includes both pharmacies and the numerous OTC medicine sellers, which number more than 10,000 nationwide.[16] They are promoted by representatives of manufacturers and wholesalers to prescribers in both the public and private sectors. In Ghana, these subsidized ACTs have also been the subject of a very effective communication campaign by the National Malaria Control Program, the malaria department of the Ministry of Health, using a green artemisia leaf logo on all boxes of medicines.

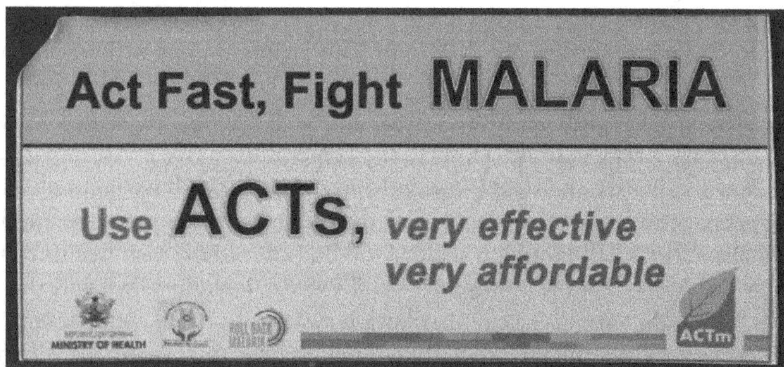


*Figure 7.1* Sticker from the subsidized ACTs promotional campaign showing the green leaf logo.

Source: © IRD/Carine Baxerres, Accra, January 2014

At the time of our surveys, subsidized ACTs were priced at 1–6 Ghanaian cedis (GHC), or USD 0.2–1.2, depending on the patient's age and weight. The price of unsubsidized adult ACTs ranged from GHC 3.5 to 36.2 (USD 0.7 to just over USD 7.00), depending on the brand and distribution site.[17]

These differences in drug distribution result in individuals in Benin and Ghana adopting very different appropriation and use of ACTs, both subsidized and unsubsidized.

In Benin, the situations in the city of Cotonou and the department of Mono diverge significantly. In the latter, our qualitative studies show that people used very little ACT on their own, in self-medication.[18] Of the 15 families we surveyed, only 2 "middle-class" and 1 "poor"[19] family had self-medicated with ACTs. The vast majority of ACTs consumed by families in Mono department were prescribed by public health facilities, rarely private, or through community outreach workers.[20] Subsidized ACTs with the green-leaf logo, widely distributed in Ghana,[21] were informally crossing borders and ending up in informal markets in Benin (Baxerres, Egrot, Houngnihin, & Le Hesran, 2015). But because subsidized ACTs are not prescribed by private health professionals or promoted by private retail distributors in Benin, individual demand for the green-leaf products is low. In this way, the formal pharmaceutical system also influences demand seen by informal vendors.

The situation in Cotonou was significantly different. With the exception of "poor" families, who consumed few or no ACT for self-medication, "middle-class" families and especially "wealthy" families all self-medicated with ACTs at one time or another, both for children and adults. This practice is in line with popular perceptions of *palu*, and as such may seem abusive to physicians. For example, one "wealthy" mother had taken an ACT "because she had headaches and a cold" (bimonthly monitoring, Cotonou, August 2015). An ACT was given to a 1.5-year-old boy from a "middle-class" family "because he wasn't eating well" (bimonthly monitoring, Cotonou, October 2015). Some families also self-medicated with ACTs to prevent *palu*.[22] "Every three months, I treat the children, symptoms or no symptoms (…), every three months I buy *palu* drugs. I get para, amoxi and an antimalarial, very often ACTs, which I give them and then I deworm them" (mother of a "wealthy" family, Cotonou, December 2014). It may be that these ACT-based self-medication practices are gradually adopted from the most to the least advantaged families and from the cities to the countryside. More radically, it is possible that the practices observed 6–9 years after these drugs became available may be considered an issue of non-appropriation by the least advantaged families. Indeed, the parents of some "wealthy" or "middle-class" families in Cotonou were only familiar with ACTs to treat *palu* in their children. "I think that ACT existed before my children were born. The first time they got *palu*, I bought ACT. They prescribed it to us at the hospital" (mother of a "middle class" family of four children, aged between 1 and 9 years, Cotonou, December 2014). In contrast, many of the "poor" families living in Cotonou never even mentioned these treatments.

In Ghana, regardless of socioeconomic status, individuals were very familiar with ACTs, strongly appropriated these drugs, and self-medicated with them frequently. ACTs were widely used in both urban and semirural research sites to treat *malaria* by adults and children. This treatment was generally perceived very positively.[23] In the household monitoring, 25 of the 30 families reported that someone in their household had taken ACTs during the monitoring period. In both settings, this was reported by households in all three of the socioeconomic categories. Most of these ACTs were obtained from OTC medicine shops and pharmacies and used in self-medication or following the recommendations of the medicine seller. In interviews, many respondents expressed a desire to avoid the waiting time and hassle of seeking care at a health facility.

Apart from treating *malaria* and *abun*, in both Breman Asikuma and Accra, many interlocutors described using ACTs regularly to treat ailments such as headache or fever, either from the stock of medicine that the household already possessed or from a nearby drugstore (OTC medicine shops or pharmacy in urban Accra). For example, in one semirural "wealthy" family, members regularly consumed ACTs bought from the local drugstore for *malaria* prevention, and teenage daughter Agnes reported once taking three tablets of ACT to treat a headache. Another example of this broad use of ACTs was also reported by Rabiatu, the mother of a "poor" family in urban Accra, she said that anytime her husband is "feeling a bit hot or not feeling well he goes to buy the ACT medicine" (interview, April 2015).

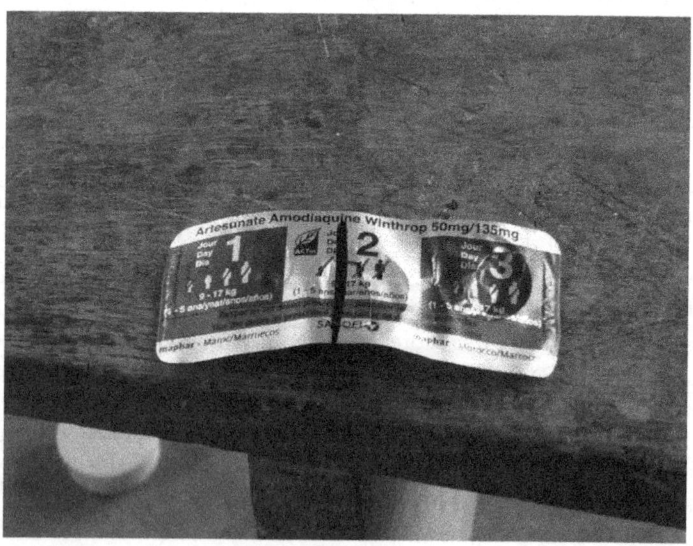


*Figure 7.2* Blister pack of an ACT monitored during the study in a family in Ayipey.

Source: © IRD/William Sackey, Ayipey, May 2015

Previous success of a treatment was often cited as a reason to try this type of treatment again for a new illness episode. Individuals also described imitating the prescription patterns of health centers or hospitals. Young children received the bulk of medication that was recorded during monitoring visits. These were often given based on past success with the medication, such as when Berenice (mother, "middle-class" family) bought Winthrop ASAQ tablets (subsidized ACT) from the pharmacy for Perpetual (age 5) after she started showing her "usual symptoms of malaria" (vomiting and signs of a cold) (monitoring visit, Accra, August 2015). Some interlocutors also reported relying on recommendations from drugstore attendants, for example, when the local drugstore recommended Ipca AL (subsidized ACT) to respond to Godwin's (age 2, "poor" family) symptoms; "his urine was very yellow, he couldn't play with the other kids, and his body was very hot" (monitoring visit, Breman Asikuma, October 2015).

Quantitative data from the population surveys we conducted in 2016 and 2017 in about 600 households in urban and rural areas in the two countries clearly show a difference in how families treat *palu* or *malaria*. In Benin, ACTs are not often used as first-line treatment. They account for only 21% of self-administered pharmaceutical treatments for *malaria* in Cotonou and 28% in the Mono department. However, if we include herbal treatments that are taken alone and not in combination with commercial products, this percentage drops to 10% in rural areas and 19% in Cotonou (Damien, Baxerres, Apetoh, & Le Hesran, 2020).

In Ghana, families use ACTs much more frequently. These drugs account for 77% (in rural areas) and 90% (in urban areas) of the pharmaceutical products taken as self-medication for *malaria*. Yet, as in rural Benin, families' exclusive use of herbal remedies should also be taken into consideration, as this accounts for nearly 40% of cases in both the city of Accra (38%) and in rural areas (37%). In addition to "homemade herbal teas," in Ghana, we also find a significant healthcare phenomenon in the form of "standardized herbal medicines," which are sold in OTC medicine shops and pharmacies alongside commercial treatments.[24] This phenomenon is more prevalent in urban areas. In fact, 55% of the herbal products consumed in Accra for *malaria* are "standardized herbal medicines" versus 33% in rural areas. The next chapter of the book is devoted to this issue.

## A variety of antimalarial drugs and attachments to them

ACTs do not arrive in either country as unknown entities. In addition to herbal medicines, people's daily lives are already peppered with commercial molecules that they use against *palu*, *malaria*, *hwevó*, *abun*, *tanvio*, *atikéssi*, and so forth, molecules to which they are more or less attached depending on their socioeconomic status, their place of residence (urban or rural), and above all the national contexts.

In Benin, antimalarial molecules that predate ACTs are well known to consumers. Some lump them together into a single category they call "quine-quine," indicating they view these drugs as having similar effects. However, most people perceive differences between chloroquine, Nivaquine® (even though this is a trade name for chloroquine), and quinine. Chloroquine is well known because of its longstanding promotion in public health for the treatment and prevention of malaria.[25] After the *P. falciparum* parasite developed significant resistance to this molecule beginning in the late 1990s, health authorities began recommending other antimalarial drugs. However, our surveys show that chloroquine was still used by several of the families questioned; to treat and primarily to prevent the popular nosological entities mentioned previously. This was true for more than half of the families we followed in the Mono department, regardless of their socio-economic status; it was also the case for "poor," "middle-class," and "wealthy" families living in Cotonou. Our quantitative survey of the general population showed that nearly 10% of households used chloroquine as their first-line treatment for *palu*, both in urban (8.8%) and rural (9.2%) areas.

Quinine tablets were also used for curative and sometimes preventive self-medication by several "poor" and "middle-class" families living in Cotonou and, to a lesser extent, the Mono department. Our quantitative survey found that nearly 30% (28.8%) of families reported using quinine for curative self-medication in Cotonou, compared to only 4.5% in the Mono department. SP, which was initially recommended by the Ministry of Health and WHO as a replacement for chloroquine in the presumptive treatment of uncomplicated malaria and used since the early 2000s in intermittent preventive treatment of malaria during pregnancy, is also used in curative self-medication, more frequently in Cotonou than in Mono, by both adults and children. Several of the families interviewed, including "middle-class" and "wealthy" families, used SP before switching to ACTs. Our quantitative survey revealed that 7% of families living in Cotonou reported using SP for *palu*, but this drug was not reported by families living in the Mono department.

For several families, these various antimalarial drugs might be used interchangeably; they might sometimes use one and sometimes the other. Thus, for the same person, some *palu* might require ACTs, while for others, SP or quinine is sufficient. This was the case of a "middle-class" family living in the Mono department. Two of the four children in this family, aged 4 years and 12 months, had taken ACTs for *palu*, after a health center prescribed this medicine for the first child, and again a few days later for the second. The mother of the family had brought them for a consultation because she was particularly concerned about the children's symptoms. This was actually the only biomedical consultation sought out by this family in more than a year of research; usually this family gave their children Nivaquine to treat *palu*.

Finally, in addition to antimalarial molecules, several other commercial products were used in Benin as curative or preventive self-medication against the popular nosological entities described earlier. We also found that at times no antimalarial drug was combined with these other molecules. This was especially the case in the Mono department for all socioeconomic categories and was true for "poor" families living in Cotonou. The therapeutic classes used were analgesics (paracetamol, paracetamol combined with caffeine, Aspirin®, Efferalgan®), anti-inflammatories (ibuprofen, diclofenac), vitamins (iron, foldine), sometimes antibiotics (cotrimoxazole, amoxicillin, ampicillin), and antihelmintics

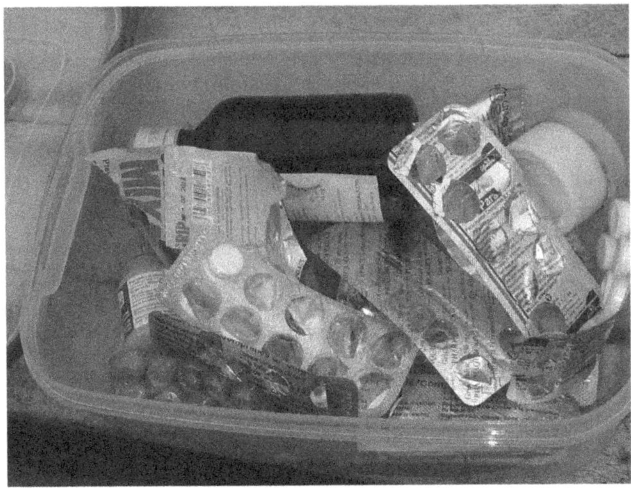

*Figure 7.3* Home pharmacy of a family living in the Mono department.

Source: © IRD/Emilienne Anago, Mono Department, November 2014

(albendazole, mebendazole). Paracetamol was the clear leader.[26] When resistance to chloroquine became a problem, public messaging communicated its lack of effectiveness, but this may have resulted in discrediting all antimalarial drugs among those who cannot afford ACT. "Later they said that if children have a fever and you use Nivaquine, it's no good. A doctor told me that the fever increases; that's why I don't use Nivaquine anymore and I prefer paracetamol" (mother of a "wealthy" family, Mono department, February 2015). Quantitative surveys show that these commercial products, used without antimalarial drugs, represent 27.5% of the pharmaceutical treatments used in self-medication for *malaria* in Cotonou and 58.5% in Mono.

In Ghana, our quantitative surveys show that antimalarial drugs other than ACTs (chloroquine, amodiaquine, quinine, or SP) are used very little, both in rural and urban areas (only 7 out of 600 households reported using them). Many respondents through qualitative interviews referred to chloroquine or quinine as "old medicines" that were no longer used. Commercial products other than antimalarial drugs were also much less commonly used than in Benin, especially in Accra where they represented only 6.4% of cases. In rural areas, they still accounted for 20% of the pharmaceutical drugs taken. "Blood tonics" were used to prevent illness and in combination with *malaria* treatment. These blood tonics comprised nutritional supplements such as "B'co" (containing multiple B vitamins), multivitamins, or iron supplements. Other medications used in Ghana were similar to those used in Benin, including cotrimoxazole (for stomach problems), vermifuge, cough syrups, Efpac® (paracetamol, aspirin, caffeine), and "para" (paracetamol). In Ghana, the fact that subsidized ACTs are extremely well distributed—reaching every corner of the country, through public but most especially through the very numerous private actors in pharmaceutical distribution—results in a very different landscape from that of Benin. Other commercial products to treat *malaria* lack such broad distribution in Ghana, thus limiting popular perceptions about them.

In Benin, however, popular perceptions have developed about the gamut of antimalarial molecules, related to an individual's socioeconomic status and the molecules that are within their financial reach. Chloroquine, Nivaquine®, and the "quine-quines" are perceived as old drugs and associated with the past by the "middle-class" and "wealthy" families of Cotonou who regularly self-medicate with ACTs. "Chloroquine, quinine, Nivaquine, that was it… those were very common at the time against *palu*. I used them all, especially when I was with my parents. We took them to prevent *palu*, mother gave them to us" (mother of a "wealthy" family, Cotonou, March 2015). This is also the case for "wealthy" families in the Mono department. Chloroquine (Nivaquine®), and quinine is also often described in interviews as causing numerous side effects. For chloroquine, people often mentioned ringing in the ears ("it clogs the ears too much," "it kills the ears"), itching, allergies, and harmful effects on the eyes. For quinine, side effects in addition to those mentioned earlier include dizziness, fatigue, weakness, difficulty sleeping, headaches, stomach problems, and joint issues. Their very bitter taste is also often pointed out as a reason why some people reject them. These side effects are most often described by those who have "embraced" ACTs.[27] Thus, for all other Beninese who cannot afford to self-medicate with ACTs or who believe they do not need ACTs for the *palu* they have at the moment, and despite the fact that these compounds are not or are no longer officially recommended as first-line treatment for malaria, quinine, and even chloroquine, continues to be widely used.[28]

## Conclusion

In Benin and Ghana, we see two quite different, almost opposing, landscapes for the distribution and use of ACTs, despite the fact that these countries are very similar geographically, socioculturally, and in terms of health.

The simultaneous presence of different antimalarial treatments in Benin—quinine, ACTs, SP, and even chloroquine—in the consumption habits of families is surprising. At first glance, it may seem to underscore how much time is needed for individuals, families, and health professionals to become familiar with and accept new therapeutic protocols. Therapeutic recommendations pile up, change regularly, and, in the case of malaria, are different for children, pregnant women, and other adults, which certainly makes it difficult for both patients and caregivers to understand and become comfortable with them. Recommendations are not simply erased as the next one arrives but are associated in individual and collective memory.

However, the comparison with Ghana highlights the elements that influence these persistent attachments or new appropriations of molecules. It is not just people's perceptions of medicines and their knowledge and understanding of the disease; in fact, the most significant factor seems to be the country's existing pharmaceutical system, the way in which various drugs are actually distributed to people and at what price.[29] We believe people's confidence in one compound or another develops on the basis of these structural factors (Brhlikova et al., 2011; Egrot, 2015; Hamill et al., 2019), as we saw in surprisingly different ways in Benin and Ghana. In the end, these are the elements that determine whether a pharmaceutical compound is abandoned, persists, or becomes integrated into individuals' lives (Fainzang, 2001; Gregson, 2007).[30]

The different situations in the two countries clearly raise questions for public health. Will the broad use of ACTs in Ghana as self-medication, usually without a confirmed malaria diagnosis, lead to parasite resistance to these combinations? Conversely, in Benin, where they are less widely used as self-medication, is there a lower risk of resistance to ACTs emerging? If these questions are relevant in such close geographical areas with highly permeable borders, we are faced with a public health dilemma: a wide distribution and possibly inappropriate use of ACTs that could lead to resistance problems; or a more limited, more appropriate distribution, but also a significant risk of treating actual cases of malaria with ineffective drugs that are no longer recommended for the disease or even inappropriate drugs (Baxerres et al., 2015).

These biological considerations are important and need to be taken into consideration. However, our studies also show that how a country's pharmaceutical system functions appears to have a considerable impact on how consumers at the end of the distribution chain use drug compounds. In countries with limited or intermediate resources, such as Benin and Ghana, understanding the availability of inexpensive molecules (whether subsidized as here for ACTs or reimbursed through various insurance mechanisms), the distribution channels (formal or informal) used and how they are present in the country, is essential to build policies to combat diseases and assess their consequences on individual and public health as well as on the economy and society.

## Notes

1. Refer to Chapter 5 to understand the delay in WHO recommendations to introduce ACTs in Africa. See also Pourraz (2019).
2. See Ghana Demographic and Health Survey 2014, Chapter 12: https://dhsprogram.com/pubs/pdf/FR307/FR307.pdf and the 5th Demographic and Health Survey in the Republic of Benin, 2017–2018, p. 44–48: https://www.insae-bj.org/images/docs/insae-statistiques/sociales/Sante/Enqu%C3%AAte%20D%C3%A9mographique%20et%20de%20Sant%C3%A9%20au%20B%C3%A9nin%20%28EDSB%29%20de%202017-2018.pdf, accessed April 2020.
3. Recall that a country's pharmaceutical system is defined by all the processes for the supply and distribution of medicines available on its territory, whether public, private, or informal. See the Introduction of this book.
4. See the Introduction of this book for information on the data collection methodology.
5. In malaria, when parasitized red blood cells burst, they release pigments that color the urine and conjunctiva. In the Mono department, the color red is often used instead of yellow.

6. We can see from these examples that some common diseases are named after the causal element while others are named based on the symptomatology or treatment. People often specify that *hwecivio*, *hwecivoè*, *tanvio*, and *atikéssi* also mean *palu* (*malaria*) and/or also one of the other entities mentioned previously.
7. Severity here is associated with masculinity: *asì* in the Fon language means "wife, female" and *asú* means "husband, male." In the Mono department, people also spoke of red *atikéssi* and simple *atikéssi*.
8. We found the English term "malaria" and mosquitoes to be more routinely used in Ghana than in Benin. At first glance, especially when research starts first in Accra, Ghana may appear to be more strongly influenced than Benin by Western lifestyles and biomedical knowledge; however, this impression dissipates upon leaving the large city and its billboards, multiple road interchanges and its endless "go slow" (traffic jams).
9. The term *atridii* is another known term for popular *malaria*, but we found it only once in the interviews. It is used mostly in the Aburi area and the Eastern region.
10. First names used in the text are pseudonyms.
11. Chapter 10 of this book is devoted to healthcare treatments in Benin and Ghana, looking at self-medication and consultations with a specialist.
12. Until recently, ACTwatch conducted predominantly quantitative studies on the distribution and consumption of ACTs in 10 malaria-endemic countries, including Benin: www.actwatch.info (accessed February 2020).
13. See Chapter 3 in which the pharmaceutical systems of Benin and Ghana and the many actors at work there—public, private, and informal—are described in detail.
14. As part of the wave of reforms to Benin's pharmaceutical sector that has been underway since 2017, the CAME was dissolved in September 2020 and replaced with a new organization, the Société Béninoise pour l'Approvisionnement en Produits de Santé (Beninese Society for Health Product Supply or SoBAPS SA).
15. Chapter 9 is devoted to the issue of pharmaceutical promotion in Benin and Ghana.
16. The distribution of subsidized ACTs in the public and private sector in Ghana has been promoted by the AMFm (Affordable Medicines Facility-malaria) program, supported by the Global Fund. This was discussed in the previous chapter.
17. Depending on the fluctuating exchange rate, the euro is generally slightly higher than the dollar (1 euro ≈ USD 1.15). Specifying prices in euros for Benin and in dollars for Ghana, as is customary in these two countries, helps to highlight the influence of each of these financial and cultural contexts in Benin and Ghana, respectively.
18. We consider self-medication to be an individual's use of health products without the supervision of a professional they consider able to prescribe medicine, whether or not this person is actually authorized to do so. The issue of self-medication will be discussed at length in Chapter 10.
19. The mother of this "poor" family stood in sharp contrast to the other mothers of "poor" families. She had been educated up to year 9 in school and had previously lived in Parakou, the second largest city in the country. She was familiar with a large number of drugs and felt that she understood their effects.
20. Overall, public health facilities are more widely visited in the Mono department than in Cotonou, where a broader range of care is available. Private health centers do exist, but there are fewer of them than in Cotonou. The community outreach workers are village residents identified by the Ministry of Health and institutions that implement health projects locally to provide health advice and/or care, treatment, and vaccinations. In the case of malaria, they provide families with free ACTs for infected children under 5 years old.
21. Green-leaf CTAs were also widely distributed in Nigeria through the AMFm. That country is also a major supplier to Benin's informal markets (Baxerres & Le Hesran, 2011).

22. Chemoprophylaxis for malaria is no longer recommended by health authorities, except for pregnant women. We have shown previously that in Benin, popular perceptions of *malaria* lead people to engage in significant disease prevention behavior, using both plant concoctions and commercial products (Baxerres, 2013).
23. We decided not to describe the popular perceptions of ACTs in depth here since they do not represent the variations in ACT use in the two countries. In Benin, people are most familiar with the trade name "Coartem," because this brand was over-represented, if not the only available option, among subsidized ACTs for a long time. In both countries people describe the medicine as "the one taken four-four" or "the yellow ones." Unsubsidized ACTs were known by their trade names, with people using different names depending on their purchasing practices. In Ghana, some consumers know the term "ACT." There was a perception that ACTs were very efficient for treating *malaria* with few side effects, like temporary weakness. In Benin, ACTs were generally perceived as more effective than older antimalarial molecules, but this varied depending on the person's socioeconomic status and whether or not the products were subsidized. "Wealthy" and "middle-class" urban families perceived subsidized ACTs, distributed in public health centers, as less effective than unsubsidized ACTs. In these families, the side effects of (subsidized) ACTs could be described (too sweet, unpleasant smell, itching). In rural areas, subsidized ACTs were mostly associated with children.
24. This phenomenon also exists in Benin but is quantitatively much less significant. Only 3 of the 30 families surveyed using our qualitative methods had once used a standardized herbal medicine treatment for *palu*.
25. From the early 1960s to the early 1990s, chloroquine-based mass chemoprophylaxis was recommended in Africa by WHO for children (Sarrassat, 2009). This recommendation was later suspended and a policy of presumptive chloroquine treatment for uncomplicated malaria on the basis of a clinical diagnosis mainly focused on fever was recommended until the late 1990s, when malarial parasites developed chloroquine resistance (Souares, 2007). Other molecules were then recommended (mefloquine, SP), before the advent of ACTs.
26. Paracetamol is widely consumed in Benin and Ghana. It seems that in many countries there are specific perceptions of this molecule, and it is highly familiar to most people, some of whom no longer really consider it to be a drug, and thus potentially dangerous. In France, it is the only pharmaceutical product to escape the dichotomy of biochemical drugs between "natural" and "tainted" (David & Guienne, 2019).
27. It should be noted that people who use chloroquine may also report these side effects for quinine, and vice versa. There is thus a kind of differential appropriation of antimalarial drugs that depends on the individual. The personalization often attributed to commercial products—that a drug is suitable for one person's body but not for another's, even for the same health problem—has been described several times in the literature (Baxerres, 2013; Hardon, 1994).
28. At the time of our studies, quinine was still recommended for the treatment of severe malaria, either orally by prescription, as an injection or infusion, or as artesunate. Chloroquine was prohibited for malaria-related indications. It could be prescribed for the treatment of certain rare diseases, such as lupus erythematosus or rheumatoid arthritis. At the time of our study, people could only buy this compound through the informal drug market. We identified widely shared discourses and practices (most prevalent in the Mono department but also in Cotonou) that associate this molecule with the treatment of several other health issues: primarily stomach problems and constipation, but also for respiratory congestion, sleep problems, contraception, and unwanted pregnancies. As this chapter was being written, chloroquine was returning to the global limelight as a possible treatment for Covid-19. It has been the subject of vigorous scientific controversy, widely reported in the media and social networks.

29. We know that in the second half of the 20th century, chloroquine was more heavily promoted in French-speaking African countries, whereas SP was promoted in English-speaking countries. But these historical elements appear to be relatively insignificant compared to the pharmaceutical system currently operating in the country.
30. Two exciting fields of research can be used here: studies on consumption (Chessel, 2012; Trentmann, 2012) and on domestic culture (Miller, 2001; Pink, 2004).

## Reference list

Balkan, S., & Corty, J.-F. (2009). Paludisme: Les résistances traitées par une médiation sud-sud [Malaria: Resistances treated through South-South mediation]. In J.-H. Bradol, & C. Vidal (Eds.), *Innovations médicales en situations humanitaires. Le travail de Médecins sans Frontières [Medical innovations in humanitarian situations. The work of Médecins Sans Frontières]* (pp. 135–153). Paris, France: L'Harmattan.

Baxerres, C. (2013). *Du médicament informel au médicament libéralisé : Une anthropologie du médicament pharmaceutique au Bénin [From informal to liberalized drugs: An anthropology of pharmaceutical drugs in Benin]*. Paris, France: Les Éditions des Archives Contemporaines.

Baxerres, C., Anago, E., Hémadou, A. O., Kpatchavi, A. C., & Le Hesran, J.-Y. (2021). Le paludisme à l'ère de la santé globale, entre retour des velléités d'élimination et permanence des bricolages populaires. In A. Desclaux, A. Diarra, & S. Musso (Eds.), *Guérir en Afrique : Promesses et transformations* (pp. 275–294). Paris, France: L'Harmattan. Collection Anthropologies et Médecines.

Baxerres, C., Egrot, M., Houngnihin, R., & Le Hesran, J.-Y. (2015). Dualité de l'accès au médicament en Afrique de l'Ouest : Les ACT entre large distribution et consommation sous surveillance [Duality of drug access in West Africa: ACTs between wide distribution and consumption under surveillance]. In M. Badji, & A. Desclaux, (Eds.), *Nouveaux enjeux éthiques autour du médicament en Afrique. Analyses en anthropologie, droit et santé publique [New ethical issues around drugs in Africa. Analyses in anthropology, law, and public health]* (pp. 141–158). Dakar, Senegal: L'Harmattan.

Baxerres, C., & Le Hesran, J.-Y. (2011). Where do pharmaceuticals on the market originate? An analysis of the informal drug supply in Cotonou, Benin. *Social Science and Medicine*, *73*(8), 1249–1256.

Bonnet, D. (1986). *Représentations culturelles du paludisme chez les Moose du Burkina [Cultural representations of malaria among the Mossi of Burkina Faso]*. Ouagadougou, Burkina Faso: ORSTOM.

Brhlikova, P., Harper, I., Jeffery, R., Rawal, N., Subedi, M., & Santhosh, M. R. (2011). Trust and the regulation of pharmaceuticals: South Asia in a globalised world. *Globalization and Health*, *7*(10), 2–14.

Chessel, M.-E. (2012). *Histoire de la consommation [History of consumption]*. Paris, France: La Découverte.

Damien, B. G., Baxerres, C., Apetoh, E., & Le Hesran, J.-Y. (2020). Between traditional remedies and pharmaceutical drugs: Prevention and treatment of "Palu" in households in Benin, West Africa. *BMC Public Health*, *20*, 1425.

David, M., & Guienne, V. (2019). Savoirs expérientiels et normes collectives d'automédication [Experiential knowledge and collective self-medication standards]. *Anthropologie & Santé*, *18*, 1–13. http://journals.openedition.org/anthropologiesante/5089; DOI: https://doi.org/10.4000/anthropologiesante.5089.

Desclaux, A., & Egrot, M. (Eds.). (2015). *Anthropologie du médicament au Sud. La pharmaceuticalisation à ses marges [Anthropology of medicines in the South. Pharmaceuticalization at its margins]*. Paris, France: L'Harmattan.

Egrot, M. (2015). Produits frontières, légitimité, confiance et automédication : Interférences autour de quelques médicaments néotraditionnels circulant en Afrique de l'Ouest [Frontier products, legitimacy, trust and self-medication: Interference around some neotraditional drugs circulating in West Africa]. In *Les actes des rencontres Nord/Sud de l'automédication et de ses déterminants [Proceedings for North/South meetings on self-medication and its determinants]* (pp. 166–183). Cotonou, Benin: HAL.

Fainzang, S. (2001). *Médicaments et société [Medicines and society]*. Paris, France: Éditions PUF.

Faye, S. L. (2009). Du « *sumaan ndiig* » au paludisme infantile : La dynamique des représentations en milieu rural sereer Sinig (Sénégal) [From "*sumaan ndiig*" to child malaria: Trends in representations in rural Serer Sinig (Senegal)]. *Sciences Sociales et Santé*, *27*(4), 91–112.

Gregson, N. (2007). *Living with things: Ridding, accommodation, dwelling*. Wantage, UK: Sean Kingston Publishing.

Hamill, H., Hampshire, K., Mariwah, S., Amoako-Sakyi, D., Kyei, A., & Castelli, M. (2019). Managing uncertainty in medicine quality in Ghana: The cognitive and affective basis of trust in a high-risk, low-regulation context. *Social Science & Medicine*, *234*, 112369.

Hardon, A. (1994). People's understanding of efficacy for cough and cold medicines in Manila, the Philippines. In N. L. Etkin, & M. L. Tan (Eds.), *Medicines: Meanings and contexts* (pp. 47–67). Quezon City, the Philippines: Health Action Information Network.

Jaffré, Y., & Olivier de Sardan, J.-P. (1999). *La construction sociale des maladies: Les entités nosologiques populaires en Afrique de l'Ouest [The social construction of diseases: Popular nosological entities in West Africa]*. Paris, France: Éditions PUF.

Kamat, V. R., & Nyato D. J. (2010). Soft targets or partners in health? Retail pharmacies and their role in Tanzania's malaria control program. *Social Science & Medicine*, *71*(3), 626–633.

Kangwana, B. P., Kedenge, S. V., Noor, A. M., Alegana, V. A., Nyandigisi, A. J., Pandit, J., … Rogerson, S. J. (2011). The impact of retail-sector delivery of artemether–lumefantrine on malaria treatment of children under five in Kenya: A cluster randomized controlled trial. *PLoS Medicine*, 8(5), e1000437.

Kpatchavi, A. C. (2011). *Savoirs, maladie et thérapie en Afrique de l'ouest. Pour une anthropologie du paludisme chez les Fon et Waci du Bénin [Knowledge, disease, and therapy in West Africa. An anthropology of malaria among the Fon and Waci of Benin]*. Cotonou, Benin: Éditions Ablodè.

Miller, D. (2001). *Home possessions*. Oxford, UK: Berg.

Petryna, A., Lakoff, A., Kleinman, A. (Eds.). (2006). *Global pharmaceuticals, ethics, markets, practices*. London, UK: Duke University Press.

Pink, S. (2004). *Home truths: Gender, domestic objects and everyday life*. Oxford, UK: Berg.

Pourraz, J. (2019). *Réguler et produire les médicaments contre le paludisme au Ghana et au Bénin : Une affaire d'Etat ? Politiques pharmaceutiques, normes de qualité et marchés de médicaments [Regulating and producing malaria drugs in Ghana and Benin: A State affair? Pharmaceutical policies, quality standards, and drug markets]*. Doctoral dissertation. Ecole des Hautes Etudes en Sciences Sociales, Paris, France. Retrieved at http://www.theses.fr/2019EHES0014.

Sarrassat, S. (2009). *Mise en place des combinaisons thérapeutiques à base d'Artémisinine pour traiter le paludisme simple en Afrique Subsaharienne : De la théorie à la pratique [Establishment of artemisinin-based combinations to treat uncomplicated malaria in sub-Saharan Africa: From theory to practice]*. Unpublished doctoral dissertation. Université de Paris 6, Pierre-et-Marie-Curie, France.

Souares, A. (2007). *Mesure et déterminants de l'observance des prescriptions de combinaisons thérapeutiques dans le traitement de l'accès palustre simple chez l'enfant au Sénégal [Measurement and determinants of compliance with the prescriptions of therapeutic combinations in the treatment of uncomplicated malaria in children in Senegal]*. Doctoral dissertation. Université de Paris 6 Pierre-et-Marie-Curie, France. Retrieved at http://www.theses.fr/2007PA066056.

Trentmann, F. (Ed.). (2012). *The Oxford handbook of the history of consumption*. Oxford, UK: Oxford University Press.

Van der Geest, S., & Whyte, S. R. (Eds.). (1988). *The context of medicines in developing countries: Studies in pharmaceutical anthropology*. Dordrecht, The Netherlands: Kluwer Academic Publishers.

# 8 Standardized herbal medicines in Ghana

## The construction of a substantial share of the medicine market, especially for malaria

*Maxima Missodey and Daniel Kojo Arhinful*

### Introduction

The study of standardized phytotherapy medicines,[1] which some authors call "neo-traditional" (Simon & Egrot, 2012) and others "new traditional drugs" (Pordié, 2012), has been of increasing interest since the early 2000s in the social sciences. Mainly carried out in Asia (China, India, Indonesia, Sri Lanka), but also in Africa and Latin America, this research focuses on how States regulate these treatments, how their legal status changes when they circulate between countries (Hsu, 2009; Pordié & Hardon, 2015), their industrialization (Afdhal & Welsch, 1988; Bode, 2006; Pordié & Gaudillière, 2014), and their scientific experimentation (Micollier, 2011; Scheid, 2007). The international circulation networks of these medicines have also been studied (Hsu, 2009; Kouokam Magne, 2010).

In Africa, the emergence of these products must be considered in connection with the national initiatives to promote traditional medicines launched by the World Health Organization (WHO) beginning in the late 1970s in the context of the Primary Health Care policy. "The idea was that by using traditional therapies that were a priori more culturally acceptable, we could finally meet the challenge of equitable health development" (Baxerres & Simon, 2013, p. 8). In the context of postindependence Africa, when the new States sought to assert their national identity, standardized herbal medicines could also appear as strong identity symbols. In terms of health, "the hypothesis adopted was that the therapeutic indications of traditional healers could have real biological effectiveness, which remained to be evaluated and improved in order to obtain preparations usable in public health" (Baxerres & Simon, 2013, p. 9). It was then a question of "improving" the so-called traditional remedies by precisely identifying their botanical compounds, specifying dosages, and respecting hygienic rules for drying and storage, even if that meant bypassing the role of the therapist, still central in the medicine traditions from which these remedies come (Pordié, 2012). Sometimes under the impetus of the State, as we will see in Ghana, and more frequently via the increasing privatization of the health sector in African countries from the end of the 1980s, standardized phytotherapy medicines multiplied, although to different degrees depending on the country.[2] In the early 2000s, this trend was reinforced with the arrival of food supplements and phytotherapy products mainly from the United States and China (Simon, 2008).

These products have become increasingly marketed throughout various countries of Africa, even as they crystallize an intermingling of economic, technological, social, and health stakes.[3] This chapter will focus on how these stakes play out in the herbal medicine industry with a specific focus on malaria medicines, which feature prominently at the manufacturing phase, and medicines for sexual and reproductive health, which feature in the retail and consumption phase of the social life of the standardized herbal medicines.

Historically, herbal homemade remedies, popularly known as *abibiduro*,[4] have played a pivotal role in the health care and health-seeking behaviors of people in Ghana. As we will see, Ghana's first president, Kwame Nkrumah, made efforts toward standardizing traditional medicine and incorporating it into the health-care delivery system as part of his pan-Africanist agenda. Studies in Ghana on herbal medicines have focused on their increasing usage and their inclusion into the health-care delivery system (Amoah, Kakaney, Kwansa-Bentum, & Kusi, 2015; Aziato & Antwi, 2016; Osseo-Asare, 2014).

But from the early days of independence, these therapies have transitioned from homemade remedies to commercial products. As we will see in this chapter, their production has improved, both in terms of formulation—they are now available in dosage forms such as suspensions, tablets, and capsules (Bayor, Johnson, & Gbedema, 2011)—and in packaging (Senah, 1997). In the meantime, this transition moves herbal medicines from their therapeutic space to their commodified state. Pharmaceutical anthropologists have looked at medicines beyond their function as "materia medica" (Van der Geest & Hardon, 2006; Whyte, Van der Geest, & Hardon, 2002). Herbal medicines have taken on the unique characteristics of a commercial product in their development, i.e., manufacture, branding, and distribution, and in the final stage of their life, consumption. They develop both undeniably in a mimicry of pharmaceutical specialties (formulation, packaging, instructions) and a mistrust toward them (criticism of chemistry, enhancement of nature and tradition) (Hardon et al., 2008; Simon & Egrot, 2012). Thus, on the social and health level, they are the subject of discourse, perceptions, and variable practices that must be understood in relation to people's social, cultural, and economic characteristics. As with pharmaceuticals, not only dynamics of their popularity but also of the skepticism they arouse (Van Der Geest & Whyte, 2003) can be highlighted (Baxerres & Simon, 2013). In terms of individuals' health-seeking behaviors, therefore, herbal remedies may be used as a complement or as an alternative to commercial products; in either case, such use should be questioned and may prove to be variably beneficial or harmful, depending on the health problem being treated (Cohen & Rossi, 2011; Hardon et al., 2008). For malaria, a major health issue in Ghana especially for children under age 10, besides issues of history, regulation, industrialization, and commodification, it is important to understand the way standardized herbal medicines are used, as well as other "niches" developed in the manufactured herbal medicine industry.

## Policy for the development of standardized herbal medicines

Interest in the research and manufacture of herbal medicines is linked to the efforts of Oku Ampofo, who, with the support of another colleague, Albert Nii Tackie, founded the Centre for Scientific Research into Plant Medicine (CSRPM) in Mampong Akuapem, Ghana, renamed the Centre for Plant Medicine Research (CPMR) in 1975. Oku Ampofo's interest in plant medicine can be traced to many sources, including inheriting it from his father's cousin who used herbal medicines; his daughter's sickle cell anemia disease, which propelled him to research plant medicine as alternative to Western medicine; and finally the influence of pan-African ideologies and activities after studying medicine in Britain in the late colonial and early post-colonial period (Sutherland-Addy & Ansah, 2018). What sparked his interest was his medical practice upon his return to Mampong Akuapem, where most of those who visited his clinic were malaria cases (Osseo-Asare, 2014). Ampofo, one of the few Ghanaians to have received medical training in the United Kingdom at that time, worked on documenting plant-based recipes toward the end of the colonial period. He found that cryptolepis served as a useful herbal treatment for malaria. His personal attempt at bioprospecting medicinal plants was co-opted by the government for the creation of a national database of plants for the manufacture of medicines.

Several efforts have been made since the 1960s to develop herbal medicines in Ghana. Renowned bio- and phytochemists began to recognize the healing properties of herbs by incorporating science into herbal medicine production (Addae-Mensah, 1975). When the pharmaceutical division of the then Ghana Industrial Holding Company (GIHOC) was sold, Phyto-Riker, an American firm, bought it and began to produce generic pharmaceuticals. One, Phyto-Laria, was an herbal medicine produced from cryptolepis in 1999 as "a true herbal remedy" resulting from traditional knowledge (Osseo-Asare, 2014, p. 159).

Government efforts to standardize the practice of herbal medicine increased people's awareness of the use of these therapies as an additional or alternative form of treatment. In terms of research, the Centre for Scientific and Industrial Research (CSIR) was set up in 1975 to identify and document medicinal plants. In 1991, the government established the Traditional and Alternative Medicine Directorate, which began as a unit. The Food and Drugs Board was created in 1992, which later became the Food and Drugs Authority (FDA). The Ghana Federation for Traditional Medicine Practitioners (GHAFTRAM) was later formed in 1999 to be the mouthpiece for all the different practice groups, which included bonesetters,[5] traditional birth attendants, and faith healers, among others. The Traditional and Alternative Medicine Directorate of the Ministry of Health would make policy decisions in this field.

## Ghana's administrative and professional regulation of standardized herbal medicines

The regulation of standardized herbal medicines in Ghana constitutes a complexity of collaborative efforts among the existing regulatory bodies as well as contradictions and tensions. This situation stems from the different regulatory mechanisms put in place by governments. Prior to the establishment of the Food and Drugs Board in the 1990s, the control of drugs and the practice of pharmacy were under the 1961 Pharmacy and Drug Act (Act 64). The Provisional National Defence Council (PNDC), through the Narcotics Drugs Control, Enforcement and Sanction Law (PNDCL 236), established the Narcotics Control Board, which in 1992 separated the control of drugs other than narcotics from the practice of pharmacy.

The FDA was initially established as the Food and Drugs Board by PNDCL 302 in 1992, later amended in 1996 by the Food and Drugs Amendment Act 523 to become the FDA. Even though this entity was legally established in 1992, it was not until 1997 that the Board was actually inaugurated. It currently has an herbal medicine department that specifically oversees the registration of herbal medicinal products. The FDA is under the control and supervision of the Ministry of Health and is mandated by the Public Health Act (2012), Act 851: "There is hereby established a body corporate to be known as the Food and Drugs Authority. The object of the Authority is to provide and enforce standards for the sale of food, herbal medicinal products, cosmetics, drugs, medical devices and household chemical substances" (Ghana Public Health Act, 2012, pp. 80, 81).

Manufacturers are required to present an analysis report to the FDA from any of the testing facilities, usually the CPMR or Kwame Nkrumah University of Science and Technology (KNUST), along with the registration forms, which can be obtained from the FDA, a sample of the product, and the appropriate fees.[6] Some of the tests required for the product include a physicochemical test to ensure that the medicine is plant-based, and toxicology and microbial tests. The sample presented should not have pathogenic microbes like *Escherichia coli*, *Salmonella*, or *Staphylococcus*. A product sample with a trace of any of these will be rejected because they could cause conditions like diarrhea. For medicines for chronic conditions like diabetes or hypertension, further documentation beyond the physicochemical, toxicology, and microbial tests are required; therefore, it is not easy to register products for such conditions. The Head of the Herbal Medicine Department at KNUST at the time of this research indicated that most members brought their samples to KNUST upon the recommendation of the leaders of the Association. KNUST and GHAFTRAM have built a cordial relationship through the training workshops they have been jointly organizing since 2012.

Another act was also promulgated, the Traditional Medicine Practice Act, 575. The Act, gazetted in 2000, begins inter alia: "An Act to establish a Council to regulate the practice of traditional medicine, to register practitioners and license practices, to regulate the preparation and sale of herbal medicines and to provide for related purposes" (Ministry of Health, 2000, p. 5). It mandates the Traditional

Medicine Practice Council (TMPC) to regulate the practice as well as the practitioners of traditional medicines. The legal stipulation for the regulation of traditional medicine practice in Ghana ensures the registration of the premises, which include factories, clinics, herbal medicine shops, and vehicles as well as the practice of preparing the herbal medicines for clients.

The Traditional Medicine Practice Act for the registration of practitioners stipulates that: "No person shall operate or own any premises as a practitioner or produce herbal medicine for sale unless he is registered in accordance with this Act." The qualification for registration includes adequate proficiency in the practice of traditional medicine, endorsement of the application by either the district chairman of the Association; the traditional ruler of the community or the District Co-ordinating Director (Ministry of Health, 2000, p. 14).

The issuance of the TMPC license is dependent on the submission of an application form and payment, which covers the cost of training and issuing the TMPC operating license. This license is issued to a variety of practice groups, including herbalists (which includes manufacturers), traditional alternative medicine assistants, traditional faith healers, psychics, medical herbalists, and others.

According to manufacturers, a TMPC license is all that is required if the herbal medicines are prepared for use as extemporaneous mixtures for treatment. Manufacturers who decide to advertise and thus commercialize their herbal medicinal products are required to go to the FDA as mandated by the Public Health Act (2012), Act 851.

In addition to market authorization, Ghana also has regulations relating to advertisements of standardized herbal medicines, which forms an integral part of the herbal medicine business. Of the 14 manufacturers that participated in the research, 5 have been able to sustain continuous radio and television advertisements of their products,[7] which is reflected in the information obtained from the Advertisement section of the FDA that showed an increasing trend in advertisements of approved medicines.

The advertisements submitted to the FDA are reviewed on the basis of the content and approved if it does not violate their advertisement regulations (Table 8.1). An advertisement submitted for vetting per the FDA Guidelines is expected to be "accurate, complete, clear and designed to promote credibility and trust by the general public and health practitioners" (FDA, 2013, p. 4). Advertisements for over-the-counter (OTC) medicines, which include herbal treatments, are not supposed to overdramatize symptoms and signs.

*Table 8.1* Advertisement applications for standardized herbal medicines

| *Year* | *Applications received* | *Applications approved* |
|---|---|---|
| 2015 | 303 | 243 |
| 2016 | 293 | 201 |
| 2017 | 361 | 294 |

Source: Ghana Food and Drugs Administration, Authors.

The Public Health Act (Act 581) provides the regulatory requirement on advertisement of herbal medicines. "A person shall not advertise a drug, herbal medicinal product, cosmetic, medical device or household chemical substance to the general public as a treatment, preventive or cure for a disease, disorder or an abnormal physical state, unless the advertisement has been approved by the Authority" (Ghana Public Health Act, 2012, p. 114).

The Fifth Schedule of Act 585 outlines the diseases or cures for which herbal medicinal product advertisements are prohibited. These include sexually transmitted diseases, other forms of genitourinary diseases, acquired immune deficiency syndrome (AIDS), or other diseases connected with human reproductive functions, as well as diabetes, asthma, hypertension, obesity, and prostate cancer among others.

Herbal medicine advertisements come in various forms, but the most prominent are in electronic media; more recently social media advertisements have begun to feature prominently in this industry (Diabah, 2015). Although the restrictions on drug advertisements are clear, the same cannot be said for those on disease advertisements (Meixel, Yanchar, & Fugh-Berman, 2015). Various flexi banners advertising sexual and reproductive health conditions are one example of how businesses escape the regulatory clutches of the FDA. The daunting task of policing the media landscape by the FDA is managed through weekly and monthly schedules for monitoring the radio and television stations on which most of the advertisements for standardized herbal medicines are aired.

In spite of the seemingly different regulatory positions, the composition of the TMPC suggests a collaborative effort among the regulatory agencies to regulate herbal medicines. The membership of the TMPC includes:

- Five nominees from GHAFTRAM, at least one of whom shall be a woman;
- Two persons nominated by the Minister of Health, one of whom shall be the Director of the Traditional Medicine Services Division of the Ministry;
- Two representatives from universities and research institutions, one of whom shall be a pharmacist with an interest in traditional medicine and the other a person with an interest in biodiversity;
- The Director of the CSRPM;
- The chief executive of the FDA; and
- The Registrar appointed under Section 29 of Act 575 (Ministry of Health, 2000, pp. 8, 9).

In reality, the expectations of the FDA and TMPC in relation to the commercialization of herbal medicines seem to conflict with each other. Even though the TMPC license provides manufacturers with market authorization for their products per the FDA requirement, any product that is used externally or ingested should theoretically go through the registration process. Manufacturers, however, only emphasize the non-advertisement of the product, as confirmed by a manufacturer in an interview: "You have your membership card, you have your TMPC license, so you can sell. You can sell it in bits, but if you take it to the FDA, they would tell you not to sell the medicine until they are done with you [registration processes]" (interview with a manufacturer, Accra, March 23, 2017).

Since the standardization of the herbal medicine practice began at an organizational level before the regulatory authority was formed, GHAFTRAM mediates between the council and members on regulatory issues. Additionally, the application documents required for registration are expected to be endorsed by the District Chairman of the Association, where the Association in the Act refers to "an association or body of associations of Traditional Medicine Practitioners recognised by the Minister of Health" (Ministry of Health, 2000, p. 34).

Manufacturers also expressed how helpful GHAFTRAM has been in the process of seeking market authorization from the FDA. This was especially true for those who had recently begun commercializing their products and were now gaining ground in the business. The association became the entry point for some of these manufacturers. "What I realized is that, we have to run everything by the leaders [Ghana National Association of Traditional Healers]. I took it through one of the leaders, the organizer, and he indicated that for him he usually goes there (FDA) and the FDA is like home" (interview with a manufacturer, Accra, March 23, 2017).

Another aspect that exemplifies the collaborative efforts between the major stakeholders concerns training. The TMPC, FDA, Faculty of Pharmacy of KNUST,[8] and Department of Pharmacy of the University of Ghana organize periodic training programs for manufactures and practitioners. One of the TMPC's many functions is to "promote and support training in traditional medicine" (Ministry of Health, 2000, p. 7). The continuous training and education of herbal medicine practitioners is also related to regulation.

GHAFTRAM plays a pivotal role in these training sessions, especially in organizing member attendance and coordinating the workshops. Topics are based on member suggestions. For the stakeholders, these training sessions are not only regulatory requirements but are aimed at streamlining the activities of practitioners to protect public health. Practitioners concerned about how their practice was viewed by so-called elites see these training sessions as a means of carving out a professional niche for themselves. Their appreciation was expressed in their level of enthusiasm at these training sessions. "They [forefathers] did not go to school but had knowledge of the medicine, but now if you don't have an education, my sister… So there are things we go and learn. You should have a little education" (interview with a manufacturer, Accra, March 23, 2017).

The highlight of these training sessions for practitioners was the presentation of certificates. Photographers took advantage of the numbers to provide academic gowns (for a fee) to participants who were interested in taking pictures wearing them. The organizers did, however, advise participants against using the certificates and photos as portfolios for their practice, indicating an awareness of the realities surrounding the herbal medicine practice.

In the wake of standardization, attention is now increasingly being paid to professionalizing the practice in order to appeal to potential customers. Similar efforts toward professionalization have been seen elsewhere, such as in the

Tibetan neo-traditional medical system where some practices of the *amchi* (Tibetan neo-traditional healer) began to be modeled on biomedical practices. This was seen in the rationalization of their processes such as keeping treatment records and providing medical and prescription forms (Besch, 2006). As indicated by Janes (2002), these attempts by healers bring "with it economic returns of various kinds, along with various potential rewards, including influence, legitimacy, prestige authority and power" (p. 269).

In Ghana, some herbal medicine clinics or outlets attach the word "scientific" to their names. There is a conscious focus on the "science" of the practice in advertisements, which frequently use the terms *abaafo* (modern or scientific in the Akan language) and *nfidie* (machine). In the industrialization of herbal medicines, therefore, there is not only an attempt at a "reformulation regime" (Pordié & Gaudillière, 2014) of the medicines but the professionalization of the practitioners as well as the practice.

## The commodification and industrialization of standardized herbal medicines

Over the years, Ghana's pharmaceutical industry has transitioned from importation to manufacturing. This has been partly the result of WHO support to African governments toward local medicine production. Around the 2000s, Ghana's industrial policy led to the creation of drug manufacturing companies by Ghanaian pharmacists. These companies—such as Kinapharma, Danadams, and Ernest Chemists—began as import wholesalers for international companies (see Chapter 1). As of 2014, Ghana and Nigeria had the highest concentrations of registered manufacturers in the region, 36 and 120, respectively, out of a total of 166 (West African Health Organization, 2014).

Even though the State is responsible for medicine imports and manufacturing through the Ministry of Health (Senah, 1997), the private sector has become a dominant player in the manufacture and supply of pharmaceuticals. Herbal medicines are no exception in this transition and innovation in the pharmaceutical industry, as noted by Amoah et al.: "The recent revolution in the plant medicine industry has led to a large number of herbal products going through rebranding and packaging as well as rigorous national testing and licensing, resulting in herbal products with enhanced efficacy and reduced toxicity" (2015, p. 2).

Manufacturers identified packaging as a major transition in the herbal medicine industry. According to a manufacturer whose company was started by his grandfather, when they began making and selling the medicine, they did not have a label like they do now. It was packaged in Coca-Cola bottles, and the lids were secured with Sellotape to prevent leakage. The label was printed by hand on simple brown paper. He explained the arduous process of bottling manually and washing the bottled herbal medicines before they were labeled. Over time, they changed to a plastic bottle, which is what they currently use. The industry transitioned to the use of the plastic bottles to package herbal medicines in the late 1990s. It was around the same time that changes were made to the label.

Packaging innovation is of the utmost concern to the manufacturers, due to customers' interest in the "look" and "feel" of the medicine. Most of the effort put into the look of the product is focused on the consumer. Even though it is expensive to develop product packaging to an appreciable standard, manufacturers believe it is worth the goal of taking the medicine beyond the "local" level. "It is expensive. It is highly expensive bringing up the product to this level. But I always have a philosophy that, if it must be done, it must be done well irrespective of the cost. It has to be a product that upon seeing it, you would know it meets 'international' standards. And we are not doing it to meet local standards. We are doing it in such a way that, at the end of the day, it would cut across both the masses and the elites" (interview with manufacturer, Accra, August 30, 2017).

This packaging focus by manufacturers is also to capture the "elite" market. Historically, herbal medicines used to appeal only to rural or nonurban dwellers, so the product has to be "upgraded" to increase its attractiveness in other markets. While there exists some form of market hierarchy, as expressed in the quote earlier, potential customers with money are a target for production just as in any other business.

This emphasis has led to the development of an ancillary business for packaging. The next picture, taken during a KNUST workshop, shows a man displaying packages he had made for some herbal medicine manufacturers. He came to exhibit his wares so that others who might need his services could contact him.

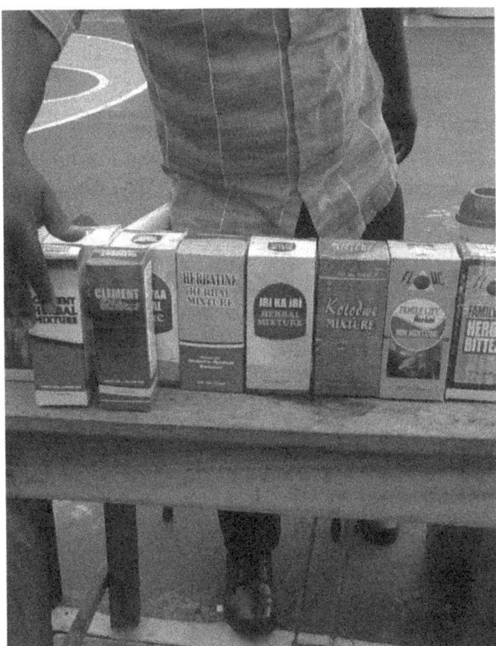


*Figure 8.1* Exhibition of herbal medicine packages.

Source: © IRD/Maxima Missodey, Kumasi, July 2017

He had his business card ready to give out to potential clients upon their interaction with him. Interestingly, he had packages of some known brands on the market that could serve as an added boost to his business.

The development of manufactured herbal medicines is characterized by tradition, the transmission of a heritage, and the hybridization of neo-tradition with industrial knowledge. Prior to commercialization, herbalists who held the belief that the knowledge of herbal medicinal preparations are divine gifts only received tokens willingly given to them by their clients. No fees were charged for the service offered. Among the Dagomba, one of the ethnic groups in Ghana, "money spoils medicines" (Bierlich, 1999, p. 321). Over time, herbal medicines have transitioned from their "sacred" position to becoming "profane" commodified products and so has the practice.

In terms of numbers, data show that an average of 500 registrations are filed annually for both new products and renewals. The regional distribution of herbalists shows that they are mostly in the populous regions of Greater Accra and Ashanti, as well as the Brong Ahafo, Central, Western, and Eastern regions, with a few from the Upper West region of Ghana (see Table 8.2 below).

As of January 2018, the FDA had registered a total of 151 herbal medicines for the Greater Accra region alone. There were different categories of manufacturers who had varied reasons for venturing into the business of herbal medicine production and who came from diverse backgrounds. Some were award-winning producers whose medicines were popular on the market, while others were only recently gaining ground in the business. Some had huge industrial manufacturing sites and others were involved in simple small-scale production using basic boiling machines. We categorized the 14 manufacturers we had selected on the basis of several factors: their production, distribution, and marketing; the visibility of their products on the market; and the size of their manufacturing companies. These companies can be broken down as follows:

- Seven who produced commercially for the markets. Their medicines are among the popular herbal medicine brands widely advertised in the herbal medicine space. They have manufacturing plants with employees for various segments of their production and marketing.

*Table 8.2* List of registered herbalists

| *Herbalists* | |
|---|---|
| *Year* | *Total number of registrations* |
| 2012 | 741 |
| 2013 | 1591 |
| 2015 | 833 |
| 2016 | 1027 |
| 2017 (January–August) | 1252 |

Source: TMPC Database (2017), Authors.

- Three who had clinics that produced medicines mainly to be used in their own facilities, with the remainder for the market.
- Four who were expanding into the business and therefore produced on a small scale.

Manufacturers assigned a hybridity of religious, utilitarian, and economic reasons for venturing into the business of herbal medicine. The categorization of herbal medicine manufacturers based on their motivation for venturing into the practice has not changed from what was described in the 1970s (Addae-Mensah, 1975), as we will see. A commonality among these manufacturers is the fact that at one point in time, the knowledge of how to prepare a particular medicine was handed down to them by a family relation or colleague. We find several modes of entry

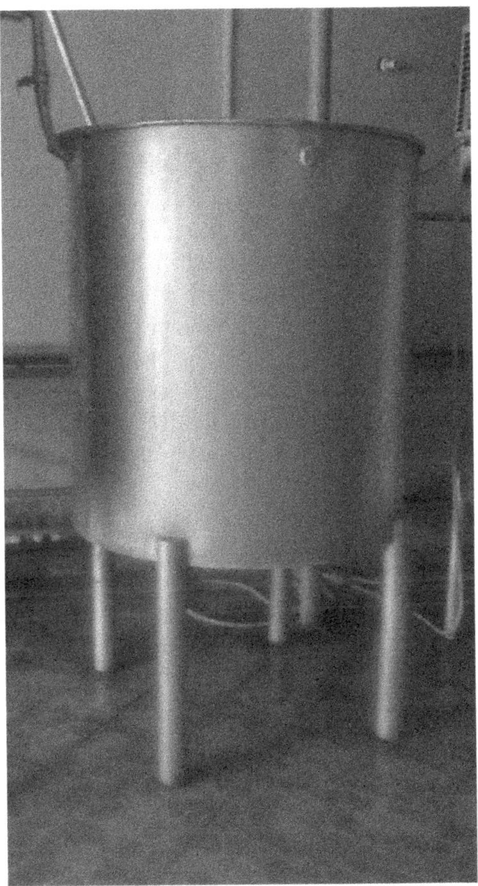

*Figure 8.2* Boiling machines for the production of standardized medicine for different manufacturers.

Source: © IRD/Maxima Missodey, Kumasi, August 2017

into the herbal medicine business: through heritage, going back for an old forgotten past, apprenticeship, divine revelation, and the pursuit of personal ambition. Three examples are given later.

### *Continuing a tradition*

Osmanu is the third generation to run the manufacturing company founded by his maternal grandfather, who by a writ transferred ownership to his daughter, Osmanu's mother. He has been involved in the business since childhood, when he would accompany his grandfather to the bush to collect medicinal plants and learned by observation. The business began in his grandfather's family house until he bought a piece of land for the manufacturing site. Osmanu studied science at the senior high school level but later transitioned to marketing before beginning his personal research into herbal medicines. He has since taken online courses in this field (interview with a manufacturer, Accra, August 11, 2017).

### *New entrants to the business*

Teye's passion for marketing and his assessment of the business potential of herbal medicines got him interested in manufacturing these products. He worked as a distributor for Nestlé Ghana before venturing into marketing the herbal medicines of a renowned herbal manufacturer. His marketing experience led him to realize the huge market potential of the herbal medicine business, so he decided to "retrace his steps to his roots" to start commercializing an old forgotten practice known as *sankofa*.[9] He went to his hometown and worked with his aunt to refresh his memory of the herbal remedies he had seen in his childhood (interview with manufacturer, Accra, January 12, 2017).

Another manufacturer, Wofa, who decided not to work in the public or civil service after secondary school, became involved in selling pharmaceuticals. He later decided to undertake an apprenticeship with an herbalist, having developed the interest from his aunt, who specialized in preparations for conditions like rheumatism, fertility issues, and complications with childbirth. Invoking the "grace of God," he mentioned that an herbalist whom he attends church with offered to teach him how to prepare some herbal medicines (interview with a manufacturer, Accra, August 28, 2017).

## The marketing of standardized herbal medicines

The kind of marketing strategy employed by the manufacturers depended on their capacity or resources. Their backgrounds also determined the geographic reach of their products: well-established businesses with popular brands supply the entire country and sometimes even outside Ghana's borders. This is driven mostly by the ability to advertise and market the products.

For small-scale manufacturers, the supply is dependent on recommendations from customers in certain locations. One of the marketing strategies these manufacturers employ is giving out samples of their medicines to customers for a trial. This is especially the case of manufacturers who do not have popular brands because they are not advertising, and those who are still working toward reaching wider markets. After the initial introduction of the product to the distributors, supply depends on request by the distributors.

Well-established manufacturers with popular brands supply their medicines across the country and beyond. They are able to reach their targeted markets because of their marketing capacity. Teye, for example, has four vans travelling to the Ashanti, Central, Eastern, Greater Accra, Northern, and Western regions of the country. These vans supply wholesalers and retailers in these locations. Additionally, his company exports to neighboring Nigeria, one of its leading countries for export.

Nii Kpakpo supplies his medicines across the country, but supply is also dependent on distributors' requests. He has mobile marketers who target the shops (herbal and OTC medicine shops). He uses the "sale or return approach" whereby he supplies the medicines after which he either gets his money when the products are sold or the products returned if not sold.

A feature of marketing or supplying that is common to both well-established and growing manufacturers is product requests based on consumer recommendations. Even for products made by well-established manufacturers, requests outside Ghana still depend on recommendations from satisfied customers. It must be noted that the phone numbers displayed on the packaging of these medicines also play a vital role in their coverage. Having direct access to the manufacturer establishes a connection between manufacturers and their consumers. Producers stay in touch with consumers and therefore are not alienated from either their products or their clients.

Manufacturers attribute various reasons to explain their sales outside the country; paramount among these are customer recommendations, supplies by self-appointed agents, and manufacturers' own efforts to target foreign markets. Teye, mentioned previously, attributed the penetration of the African and international market to his professional marketing background and his personal pan-African approach to marketing "our own locally manufactured products." "Why should we be trained and we are proud to be saying 'I am working with the Toyota company'? Why is it that we are not proud of our local things? What can we also take or how can we take something from our country and send it out there for them to also buy? I must take something that is specifically local to Ghana and also build it up; use my professional skills to build the product for it to also cross international borders" (interview with a manufacturer, Accra, January 12, 2017).

Another manufacturer whose medicines are found beyond the borders of Ghana is Wofa. He has customers come from Angola to buy his "Koo capsules." Wofa also mentioned that whenever he travels outside the country, he takes some of the medicines with him, especially to London and Canada. Krause (2008) reported the use of herbal medicines as one of the therapeutic options by Ghanaian migrants in London. This was facilitated by the networks of migrants who sent these medicines to them through "transnational therapy networks."

An inventory of herbal medicines stocked in the herbal medicine shop we studied revealed that some of the products had package information written in French. This could be one of the strategies for expanding beyond the Ghanaian or anglophone markets. The interweaving between English- and French-speaking markets in West Africa highlights the importance of these markets as one of the core elements in the reinvention of herbal medicine (Pordié & Gaudillière, 2014).

## Herbal medicines for malaria

Among the treatments used as first-line treatment by people questioned in our quantitative studies (see Introduction of this book) for what is popularly known as malaria (see Chapter 7), 14.29% had used exclusively standardized herbal medicines—and 17.86% had used exclusively homemade herbal medicines—which is quite significant. These data are for Accra, in the fairly heterogeneous district of Madina. Our research also found that 38% of all self-medication in Accra (Madina) and 37% in Breman Asikuma (Kuntenase) involves phytomedicines. Of these, 55% are standardized herbal medicines, and 45% are homemade medicines in Accra (Madina), while in Breman Asikuma, 33% are standardized and 67% are homemade.

It is interesting to note that all the people who use the standardized herbal medicines use them alone, without association with pharmaceuticals, which raises public health questions in the fight against malaria.

Generally, malaria mixtures[10] constituted a large proportion of the herbal medicinal products on the market (Komlaga et al., 2015). Ethnopharmacological surveys of herbal medicinal plants for malaria revealed they have a huge market and great economic value (Van Andel, Myren, & Van Onselen, 2012). Nine of the interviewed manufacturers produced malaria medicines either as their sole product or as additional products.

*Table* 8.3 Malaria medicines stocked in the studied herbal medicine shop

| *Name of medicine* | *Active ingredients* | *Indications* | *Price (GH C)* | *Price ($)* |
|---|---|---|---|---|
| Angel Herbal Mixture | *Cola gigantea*, *Solanum torvum*, *Spathodea campanulata*, *Bombax buonopozense*, *Vernonia amygdalina* | Menstrual pain, malaria, fever, loss of appetite, and body pains | 10.00 | 1.7 |
| Masada | *Cryptolepis sanguinolenta* | Malaria | 8.00 | 1.3 |
| Rooter Mixture | *Aloe schweinfurthii*, *Khaya senegalensis*, *Piliostigma thonningii*, *Cassia siamea*, flavor | Malaria, typhoid fever, and jaundice | 8.00 | 1.3 |
| Tinatett Malakare | *Carapa procera*, *Cryptolepis sanguinolenta* | Malaria fever, typhoid, tiredness, headache, stress, and body and joint pains | 13.00 | 2.22 |

Abranteɛ has been in business since 2008 and only sells a single product, in both a decoction and capsule form. This medicine is to treat malaria, and he explains his motivation for production thusly: "In Ghana, our main problem is malaria. Malaria kills us more than any other disease. It is not everybody who gets cancer or diabetes, stroke or whatever before they die. But you and I, we've experienced malaria before…." (interview with a manufacturer, Kumasi, August 2, 2017).

Nana, who also makes a malaria medicine, indicated a similar motivation. According to him, he had other products in line to be submitted to the FDA for approval but prefers to focus solely on the herbal mixture for malaria and maintain its quality until it does well on the market. In fact, it was during my observation in Breman Asikuma that I first discovered the product that Nana manufactured. It was very popular with customers.

Malaria remains a condition that manufacturers are cashing in on in spite of the several interventions and programs targeted at eradicating this disease. At the retail level in the herbal medicine shop and pharmacy we studied, our observations showed comparatively more sales of herbal remedies from the herbal medicine shop than in the pharmacy that also stocked these products. The location of the herbal medicine shop in the market could have been a contributory factor. Similarly, the purchase of "cosmopolitan medicines"[11] in the pharmacy was higher than the purchase of herbal medicines, at a ratio of 10:1. The pharmacist indicated that even though people bought herbal medicines, they did not do so in a consistent manner. Analgesics, antibiotics, anthelmintics, multivitamin syrup, and antimalarials were among the most frequently purchased medicines at the pharmacy. The herbal medicines mostly purchased during the observation period (May–July 2017) at the pharmacy in Accra included Rooter and Taabea Mixtures for malaria along with Adom Koo Capsules, which retailed at two capsules for GHC 1.00 and was purchased by people for piles (hemorrhoids), abdominal pain, and as a purgative. In the exit interviews, customers from the pharmacy stated

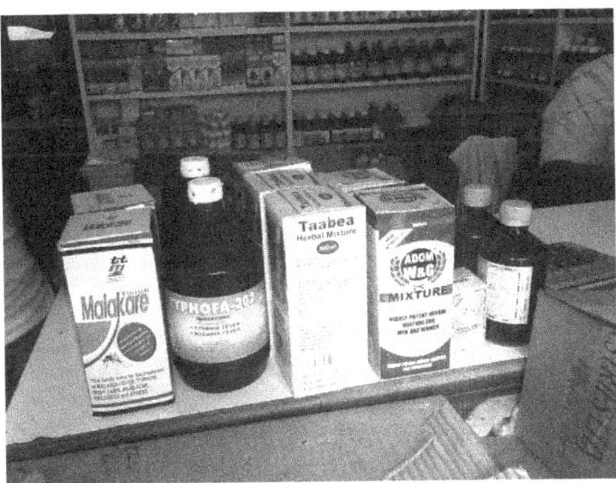


*Figure 8.3* Standardized herbal medicines for malaria in an herbal wholesale outlet at the Okaishie Market in Accra.

Source: © IRD/Carine Baxerres, Accra, September 2015

they had purchased standardized herbal medicines for malaria because of their efficacy.

In the rural area, the brands of herbal malaria medicine available in the OTC medicine shops in Breman Asikuma included Time Herbal Mixture, Mahay, Yaakson, Taabea, Enkaachi Malacure, Dwomoh, and Golden Herbal. With the exception of Enkaachi, Dwomoh, and Golden Herbal mixtures, all of the other brands were also found in urban Accra. This showed the extent to which manufacturers could market their products. The marketing of herbal medicines took various forms, including self-advertisement by small-scale manufacturers, distribution across the country by van, and advertisements on radio and television.

## Pharmaceuticalization of sexual and reproductive health

The next category of medicines to have flooded the herbal medicine market, after malaria and hemorrhoids, relates to sexual and reproductive health. While there are medicines for sexually transmitted infections for both men and women, there seem to be more herbal aphrodisiacs for men, commonly referred to in Akan as *mmarima eduro* ("medicine for men"), than *mmaa eduro* ("medicine for women"). This category of medicines reveals the extent of pharmaceuticalization associated with herbal aphrodisiacs.

Herbal medicines for sexual and reproductive health featured prominently in herbal medicine practice even before their commodification and proliferation on the market. The range of medicines in this category for women included medicines for infertility, while for men, there were medicines for sexual potency or male virility. Herbal aphrodisiacs as indicated by Lampiao, Miyango, and Simkoza (2017) generally have various functions among which are increasing libido or

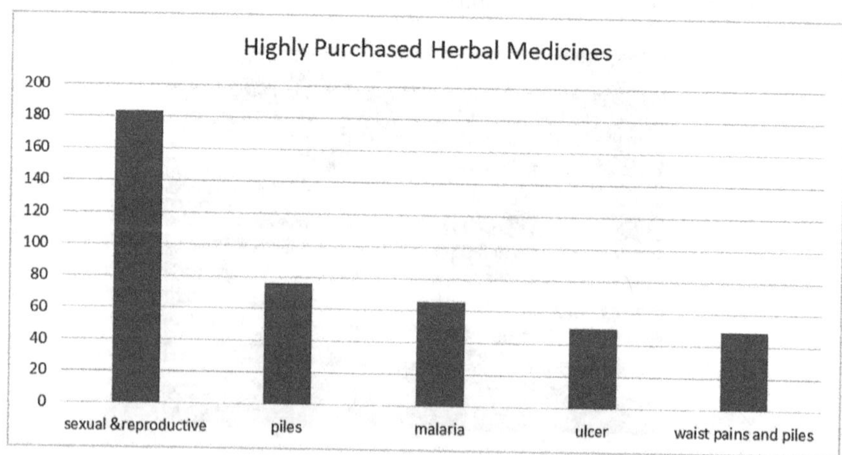


*Figure 8.4* Frequently purchased herbal medicines from studied herbal shop in Accra.

Source: Authors

sexual desire or arousal, increasing sexual potency, i.e., the effectiveness of erection, and increasing sexual pleasure.

Seven of the 14 manufacturers produced "man power" capsules. These represented the best-selling product for five of these seven companies and the only product for three of them. The "man power" capsules manufactured by the participants included nine different products with different names, two of which have their sexual connotations embedded in their names: Be4 Be4 and 230 instant capsules. The Be4 Be4 medicine, according to the manufacturer, is supposed to restore the sexually "weak" man to his previous days of "high performance," which was expressed in popular Ghanaian parlance as "before, before." The other product name expresses the dosage for the aphrodisiac: two capsules to be taken 30 minutes before sex. The manufacturers usually associate sexual weakness with abdominal pain, so the indication on these "man power" capsules apart from sexual weakness is abdominal pain.

The medicines in the sexual and reproductive health category for women were medicines to keep the vagina in a "healthy" state or one that will make sex more pleasurable for men. There were medicines for white [candidiasis] and a vagina "tightener." Two of the manufacturers interviewed had medicines for those conditions. Venecare can be taken by both sexes because of its use for sexually transmitted infections, but all of its other indications highlight conditions that affect women. These include candidiasis, vaginal itching, unpleasant discharges, painful intercourse and bleeding after sex, urinary tract infection, and menstrual pains. The manufacturer, Teye, endorsed his product by saying: "Venecare is the fastest selling product on the market. It's a wonderful product, scientifically tested" (interview with a manufacturer, Accra, January 12, 2017).

In Ghana, Enos (2001) noted that it was the unfounded fear and perception of vaginal enlargement after delivery that causes women to insert chemicals, herbs, and concoctions, a practice nicknamed "regular maintenance" to make the vagina tighter for the enjoyment of their male partners (p. 94).

## Conclusion

The industrialization of herbal medicines in Ghana began at the policy level with the efforts of Ghana's first president, Dr. Kwame Nkrumah, who sought to standardize the practice of herbal medicines as part of his pan-Africanist agenda. From those initial efforts to form an association, to streamlining the activities of herbal medicine practitioners, significant strides have been made toward regulating these products. From the 1970s through to the year 2000, numerous regulatory governmental agencies were established, such as the CPMR, CSIR, FDA, GHAFTRAM, and TMPC.

Although these agencies have a common purpose, their mandates often clash given the differences in their regulatory requirements. While the TMPC license offers manufacturers the opportunity to sell their herbal medicinal products, FDA requirements state that any product that is ingested or used must have FDA approval. There are, however, collaborative efforts involving training to bridge these gaps.

The standardization of the herbal medicine industry and the attempts at professionalization have culminated in the commodification of herbal remedies. Paralleling the pharmaceutical industry in general, the private sector has become a dominant player in the manufacture and supply of plant-based therapies. Both "heirs" and "new entrants" feature in the herbal medicine business landscape.

This heterogeneous business terrain is constituted by manufacturers who produce on a small scale to meet local demands as well as those with large-scale production capacity to meet regional and global markets using Ghanaian migrant networks. In terms of the kinds of products developed for the markets, manufacturers have developed niche markets for treating malaria and sexual and reproductive health issues. The consumption data on malaria indicate that herbal medicines are used alone for treatment without any other pharmaceuticals, often related to issues of efficacy after consumers do not get the desired expected results with "cosmopolitan" medicines.

The market for medicines to treat sexual and reproductive health issues is driven by demand as well as by the pharmaceuticalization of people's concerns in this domain. We find a proliferation of "man power" capsules for male virility, and medicines for women for keeping the vagina healthy and tight for sexual pleasure, highlighting the different sociocultural expectations for the sexes.

Herbal medicine has been industrialized in Ghana to the extent of products becoming commodified but cannot be compared to the level of Indian Ayurvedic medicines. Unlike those, where the "reformulation regime" has led to the mass production of medicines, which tends to "simplify and depersonalize the act of healing" (Pordié & Gaudillière, 2014, p. 63), Ghanaian standardized herbal medicine has retained certain traditional aspects despite the efforts toward rebranding. This could be a case of "alternative modernity," which must not be necessarily understood only as a "process of acculturation and local adaptation to the forms of knowledge, values and ways of acting that are originating in mostly a European modernity." "It involves a much complex dynamics resting on a dialectic constantly redefining and displacing the boundaries between the 'inside' and 'outside' and between what is accepted as 'modern' and promoted as 'tradition'" (Pordié & Gaudillière, 2014, pp. 4, 5).

## Notes

1. The term "standardized" here refers to the mass production of products using a specific model, with predefined characteristics.
2. In West Africa, the market for standardized herbal medicines is much more developed in English-speaking countries than in French-speaking countries.
3. Ideological (often the subject of controversy) and scientific (Pordié & Gaudillière, 2014) aspects of standardized herbal medicines are also very important, but we will not explore those aspects here.
4. *Abibiduro* is Akan, one of the most widely spoken languages in Ghana, and is the popular term for traditional medicine. Literally it means "African/Black medicine."

5. Bonesetters provide a kind of traditional orthopedic service. They are mostly located in the northern part of Ghana and are touted for their efficiency in their treatment of broken bones. They are often a preferred choice for patients with fractures.
6. According to the FDA fees schedule based on Legislative Instrument (L.I 2228), approved as Act 793 in 2009, the fees for the registration of a local herbal product for 3 years was GHC 360 (approximately USD 62) while the cost for foreign herbal products was for the cedi equivalent of USD 3600. The reanalysis fee per sample was GHC 50.00 (Ghana Public Health Act, 2012: Food and Drugs Authority Fees Schedule).
7. For more information on the methodology of this study, see the Introduction of this book.
8. With regard to training, the KNUST began offering a bachelor of science in herbal medicine degree in 2001.
9. Sankofa is an Akan philosophical concept that is symbolically depicted by a mythical bird that flies forward with its head turned backwards with an egg in its mouth (Quan-Baffour, 2012). It means "to go back to redeem," "return for it," "gazing back." It portrays the relevance of the past to the present and the future. The concept has mostly been used to foreground the relevance of the past indigenous knowledge to present development in herbal medicine.
10. Mixture is the commonly used term for herbal medicines that come in the form of decoctions.
11. "Cosmopolitan medicines" is used to refer to all other pharmaceuticals in general. This designation, as proposed by Frederick Dunn, was in recognition of the fact that what was commonly known as "Western" medicine has now become more "global and transcultural" (Tan, 1999, p. 10).

## Reference list

Addae-Mensah, I. (1975). Herbal medicine – Does it have a future in Ghana? *Universitas*, 5(1), 17–30.

Afdhal, A. F., & Welsch, R. L. (1988). The rise of the modern jamu industry in Indonesia: A preliminary overview. In S. Van der Geest, & S. R. Whyte (Eds.), *The context of medicines in developing countries* (pp. 149–172). Dordrecht, The Netherlands: Kluwer Academic Publishers.

Amoah, L. E., Kakaney, C., Kwansa-Bentum, B., & Kusi, K. A. (2015). Activity of herbal medicines on *Plasmodium falciparum* gametocytes: Implications for malaria transmission in Ghana. *PLOS ONE*, *10*(11), e0142587.

Aziato, L., & Antwi, H. O. (2016). Facilitators and barriers of herbal medicine use in Accra, Ghana: An inductive exploratory study. *BMC Complementary and Alternative Medicine*, *16*(1), 142.

Baxerres, C., & Simon, E. (2013). Les médicaments dans les Suds: Production, appropriation et circulation des savoirs et des marchandises [Medicines in the South: Production, appropriation, and circulation of knowledge and goods]. *Autrepart*, 63, 3–30.

Bayor, M. T., Johnson, R., & Gbedema, S. Y. (2011). The oral capsule-the most appropriate dosage form for croton membranaceus. *International Journal of Pharmaceutical Sciences and Research*, 2(1), 41.

Besch, N. F. (2006). *Tibetan medicine off the roads: Modernizing the work of the Amchi in Spiti*. Doctoral dissertation, Universität Heidelberg, Heidelberg. Retrieved from https://www.researchgate.net/publication/33429019_Tibetan_Medicine_Off_the_Roads_Modernizing_the_Work_of_the_Amchi_in_Spiti.

Bierlich, B. (1999). Sacrifice, plants, and western pharmaceuticals: Money and health care in northern Ghana. *Medical Anthropology Quarterly*, *13*(3), 316–337.

Bode, M. (2006). Taking traditional knowledge to the market: The commoditization of Indian medicine. *Anthropology & Medicine*, *13*(3), 225–236.

Cohen, P., & Rossi, I. (2011). Le pluralisme thérapeutique en mouvement. Introduction du numéro thématique «Anthropologie des soins non-conventionnels du cancer» [Therapeutic pluralism on the move. Introduction of the thematic issue *Anthropology of unconventional cancer care*]. *Anthropologie & Santé*, *2*, 1–8.

Diabah, G. (2015). From 'recharger' to 'gidi-power': The representation of male sexual power in Ghanaian radio commercials. *Critical Discourse Studies*, *12*(4), 377–397.

Enos, S. K. (2001). Badu Guan: A celebration of high fertility among the Akan people of Southern Ghana. In *Discovering normality in health and the reproductive body: Proceedings of a workshop* (pp. 91–101). Evanston, IL: Northwestern University.

FDA. (2013). *Guidelines for the advertisement of drugs, cosmetics, household chemicals and medical devices*. Accra, Ghana: FDA.

Ghana Public Health Act. (2012). *Ghana Public Health Act 851*. Accra, Ghana: Government Printer, Assembly Press. GPC/A753/350/11/2012.

Hardon, A., Desclaux, A., Egrot, M., Simon, E., Micollier, E., & Kyakuwa, M. (2008). Alternative medicines for AIDS in resource-poor settings: Insights from exploratory anthropological studies in Asia and Africa. *Journal of Ethnobiology and Ethnomedicine*, *4*(1), 16.

Hsu, E. (2009). Chinese propriety medicines: An "alternative modernity?" The case of the anti-malarial substance artemisinin in East Africa. *Medical Anthropology*, *28*(2), 111–140.

Janes, C. R. (2002). Buddhism, science, and market: The globalisation of Tibetan medicine. *Anthropology & Medicine*, *9*(3), 267–289.

Komlaga, G., Agyare, C., Dickson, R. A., Mensah, M. L. K., Annan, K., Loiseau, P. M., & Champy, P. (2015). Medicinal plants and finished marketed herbal products used in the treatment of malaria in the Ashanti region, Ghana. *Journal of Ethnopharmacology*, *172*, 333–346.

Kouokam Magne, E. (2010). Les médecines alternatives au Cameroun [Alternative medicines in Cameroon]. In L. Lado (Ed.), *Le pluralisme médical en Afrique [Medical pluralism in Africa]* (pp. 177–198). Conference proceedings. PUCAC-Karthala, Yaoundé, Cameroon-Paris, France.

Krause, K. (2008). Transnational therapy networks among Ghanaians in London. *Journal of Ethnic and Migration Studies*, *34*(2), 235–251.

Lampiao, F., Miyango, S., & Simkoza, H. (2017). Herbal aphrodisiac use among male adolescents and teenagers in a rural area of Blantyre district, Malawi. *International Journal of Reproduction, Contraception, Obstetrics and Gynecology*, *4*(3), 581–583.

Meixel, A., Yanchar, E., & Fugh-Berman, A. (2015). Hypoactive sexual desire disorder: Inventing a disease to sell low libido. *Journal of Medical Ethics*, *41*(10), 859–862.

Micollier, E. (2011). Un savoir thérapeutique hybride et mobile. Éclairage sur la recherche médicale en médecine chinoise en chine aujourd'hui [Hybrid and mobile therapeutic knowledge. Spotlight on Chinese medicine medical research in China today]. *Revue d'anthropologie des connaissances*, *5*, 41–70.

Ministry of Health. (2000). *Traditional Medicine Practice Act (Act 575)*. Accra, Ghana: Ministry of Health.

Osseo-Asare, A. D. (2014). *Bitter roots: The search for healing plants in Africa*. Chicago, IL: University of Chicago Press.

Pordié, L. (2012). Sortir de l'impasse épistémologique. Nouveaux médicaments et savoirs traditionnels [Getting out of the epistemological impasse. New medicines and traditional knowledge]. *Sciences Sociales et Santé*, *30*(2), 93–103.

Pordié, L., & Gaudillière, J. P. (2014). Introduction: Industrial Ayurveda: Drug discovery, reformulation and the market. *Asian Medicine*, *9*(1–2), 1–11.

Pordié, L., & Hardon, A. (2015). Drugs' stories and itineraries. On the making of Asian industrial medicines. *Anthropology & Medicine*, *22*(1), 1–6.

Quan-Baffour, K. P. (2012). Sankofa: 'Gazing back' to indigenous knowledge and skills for socio-economic development of Ghana. *Studies of Tribes and Tribals*, *10*(1), 1–5.

Scheid, V. (2007). Traditional Chinese medicine—What are we investigating?: The case of menopause. *Complementary Therapies in Medicine*, *15*(1), 54–68.

Senah, K. A. (1997). Money be man. *In The popularity of medicines in a rural Ghanaian community*. Amsterdam, The Netherlands: Het Spinhuis.

Simon, E. (2008). Importation of manufactured herbals in West Africa: The case of AIDS treatments in Benin. *Revue internationale sur le medicament*, *2*(1), 229–258.

Simon, E., & Egrot, M. (2012). « Médicaments néotraditionnels »: Une catégorie pertinente? ["Neotraditional Medicines": A relevant category?]. *Sciences Sociales et Santé*, *30*(2), 67–91.

Sutherland-Addy, E., & Ansah, M. A. (Eds.). (2018). *Building the nation: Seven notable Ghanaians*. Tema, Ghana: Digibooks Ghana Ltd.

Tan, M. L. (1999). *Good medicine: Pharmaceuticals and the construction of power and knowledge in the Philippines*. Amsterdam, The Netherlands: Het Spinhuis.

Van Andel, T., Myren, B., & Van Onselen, S. (2012). Ghana's herbal market. *Journal of Ethnopharmacology*, *140*(2), 368–378.

Van der Geest, S., & Hardon, A. (2006). Social and cultural efficacies of medicines: Complications for antiretroviral therapy. *Journal of Ethnobiology and Ethnomedicine*, *2*(1), 48.

Van Der Geest, S., & Whyte, S. R. (2003). Popularité et scepticisme: Opinions contrastées sur les médicaments [Popularity and scepticism: Constrasting opinions on medicines]. *Anthropologie et sociétés*, *27*(2), 97–117.

West African Health Organization. (2014). The Economic Community of West African States (ECOWAS) regional pharmaceutical plan. *WAHO essential medicines and vaccines programme*. Bobo-Dioulasso, Burkina Faso: West African Health Organization.

Whyte, S. R., Van der Geest, S., & Hardon, A. (2002). *Social lives of medicines*. New York, NY: Cambridge University Press.

Pordié, L. (2012). [illegible] Nouveaux médicaments et savoirs traditionnels [illegible]. New medicines and traditional knowledge [illegible] 91–110.

Pordié, L., & Gaudillière, J.-P. [illegible] Ayurveda [illegible] discovery [illegible] reformulation [illegible] and the market [illegible] 1–13.

Pordié, L., & Hardon, A. (2015). Drugs' stories and itineraries. On the making of Asian industrial medicines. Anthropology & Medicine, 22(1), 1–6.

[illegible] (2012). [illegible] Coming back to indigenous knowledge and skills for socio-economic development of Ghana. Studies of Tribes and Tribals, 10(1), [illegible]

[illegible] (2007). Traditional Chinese medicine—What are we investigating? The case of menopause. Complementary Therapies in Medicine [illegible]

[illegible] (1997). [illegible] The social use of [illegible] community. Amsterdam, the Netherlands: Het Spinhuis.

[illegible] (2008). [illegible] West Africa: The case of [illegible] treatment in Benin [illegible]

[illegible] (2013). [illegible] traditional [illegible]

[illegible]

# Part III

# Pharmaceuticalization: Medicines at the heart of health systems and societies

Moving beyond antimalarial drugs and returning to a broader perspective of the overall pharmaceutical supply in the countries considered, this third and last section of the book reports on the current dynamics generated by pharmaceutical markets in Global South societies, at both the health system and individual levels. Perfectly illustrating the concept of pharmaceuticalization, the activities of pharmaceutical companies' representatives target both prescribers and consumers, through the many distributors operating in health centers, wholesalers, pharmacies, over the counter (OTC) medicine shops, warehouses, and even informal vendors. Faced with this wide range of medicines, individuals develop knowledge that they mobilize to autonomously manage their own health. Nevertheless, they remain considerably limited by their financial situation, country, and place of residence (city or countryside), in these contexts where, since the Bamako Initiative of 1987, health-care expenses continue to largely be the responsibility of individuals. Thus, distanced from health professionals, they are vulnerable to the promotional assaults of economic actors and develop imaginaries around medicinal goods that mix colonial and postcolonial legacies, the new domination of Asian medicines, and the influence of Global Health. Pharmaceuticals generate multiple economic and social dynamics in the countries, extending beyond the firms themselves, for the many trades related to drug distribution and promotion. Unfortunately, however, although these trends have also stimulated health dynamics, this is not where they have had the greatest impact. The three following chapters discuss this phenomenon using anthropological and social epidemiological approaches.

# Part III

# Pharmaceuticalization: Medicines at the heart of health systems and societies

# 9 Pharmaceutical representative activities in Benin and Ghana

## Promoting firms while helping construct the pharmaceutical economy of African countries

*Carine Baxerres and Stéphanie Mahamé*

The sales representatives used by the pharmaceutical industry first appeared in the United States in the 1850s and in Europe shortly thereafter (Greffion, 2014). They emerged in the context of two distinct phenomena: one was the increasingly stiff competition between the nascent industry's "specialty" products and the compounded preparations made by community pharmacists (Bonah & Rasmussen, 2005); the other was the development of an internal sales department in industrial companies (Cochoy, 1999). These pharmaceutical companies achieved success through improved formulations and advertising, at a time when patents did not yet protect their pharmaceutical specialties (Chauveau, 1999; Greffion, 2014). In that era, pharmaceuticals were first advertised in the mainstream press and later in the medical press. Those industry representatives were called "detail men," "drug representatives," or "pharmaceutical sales representatives" in the United States (Dumit, 2012), while in France they were called "medical sales visitors" (since they visited doctors' offices), or "medical delegates" (Chauveau, 1999). This new sales tactic of the "medical visit" developed alongside press advertisements, and industry representatives became the predominant method of pharmaceutical firm promotion in Western countries around World War II.

In Africa, the pharmaceutical representatives' activities have gradually evolved in conjunction with the markets for medicines in the various countries since the introduction of manufactured industry products in the first half of the 20th century. This activity was initially performed by Western pharmaceutical firms that targeted exports of their products to countries under their influence: French firms to French colonies, English and American firms to the Commonwealth countries.[1] Sophie Chauveau (1999) notes that when Europe found itself in an economic crisis in the 1930s, the primary export market for France's pharmaceutical companies was their colonies. Even though these products were less expensive than those sold in Europe or in the United States (antiseptics, quinine-based treatments for tropical diseases, and other universal panaceas), they nonetheless represented one-third of the volume and one-quarter of the value of French drug exports. In the 1950s and 1960s, the subsidiaries and assembly plants that Western multinationals set up in certain countries, sometimes at the instigation of young African States, as in Ghana (see Chapter 1), also acted as their pharmaceutical reps. In West Africa, these were mainly Nigeria (May and Baker, Pfizer, and GlaxoSmithKline in the early 1950s; Ciba, Bayer, Wellcome, Boots, Hoechst, etc. in the 1960s), Ghana (Major & Company and Pharco Industry in the late 1950s; J.L. Morrison & Sons, Sterling Products, Kingsway Chemist, and Dumex Limited in the 1960s), and Senegal (Valdafrique Laboratoire Canonne—SA, established in 1942, Pfizer, Sanofi, and Institut Pasteur) (Peterson, 2014; Pourraz, 2019).[2] Starting in the 1970s, a period of massive upheaval in the global geography of the pharmaceutical industry (Abecassis & Coutinet, 2008; Cassier, 2019; Mulinari, 2016; Chapter 5 of this book), trade representatives from the emerging generic drug industry in Asian countries entered the fray. Their activities evolved over time as they penetrated the markets, first in English-speaking countries, then (in the late 2000s) in French-speaking countries (Baxerres, 2013; Singh, 2018). Some Indian firms and entrepreneurs also opened or bought out manufacturing companies in English-speaking countries during this period; examples from Ghana include Letap Pharmaceuticals, created in 1983, and M&G Pharmaceuticals, opened in 1989 (Pourraz, 2019). By the mid-1990s, local industry began developing in West Africa, especially in anglophone countries, through what has been described as the "Africanization" of pharmaceutical production (Mackintosh, Banda, Tibandebage, & Wamae, 2016; Pourraz, 2019). Local industry, too, uses pharmaceutical representatives.

In this chapter, we define pharmaceutical representatives as individuals whose job is to promote pharmaceutical companies' products to increase their prescription, sale, and consumption. We are using this basic definition because it allows us to account for the current dynamics in the contexts of the Global South that we study, in addition to those of the firms themselves. These contexts differ from those of the countries of the Global North, where similar studies have been conducted. This work highlights the stranglehold pharmaceutical firms have on doctors through their representatives, who in the vast majority of cases are direct employees of the firms (Greene, 2006; Greffion, 2014; Ravelli, 2015). We are of course interested in the facilities where the pharmaceutical representatives we observe in West Africa work, and we will describe them in detail. However, by starting with the actors closest to the field, the individuals themselves, we are able to study the actions they take in addition to promoting the firm's products; as we shall see, it is often these individuals who are the catalyst for the structures that subsequently develop. We use the term "representative" to reconcile the terms used in the analyses between Ghana, where it is the accepted term (in English), and Benin, where the usual term is "delegate" (from the French for "medical delegate"), which has an undertone of value that we would like to eliminate, as will be discussed later.

In this chapter, therefore, we are interested in the social dynamics generated by pharmaceutical representatives' activities in West Africa. This activity has evolved differently depending on the national contexts and the pharmaceutical legislation adopted within them. We will first analyze the differences and similarities in how this activity is structured in Benin and Ghana. Next we will examine the activities of pharmaceutical representatives in these two contexts to describe the logics used to monopolize markets by the various firms with a local presence, be they Western multinationals; Asian, European, or North African generic manufacturers; or local manufacturers from sub-Saharan Africa. Finally, we will highlight the effects of these representatives' activity, which extends beyond the companies, on the pharmaceutical economy of the two countries.[3]

## Benin and Ghana: Different operating modes of pharmaceutical representation

Pharmaceutical promotion is regulated differently by the laws of Benin and Ghana. In Benin, as in the other French-speaking countries of West Africa and in France, pharmaceutical promotion is legally completely decoupled from distribution. Wholesalers cannot legally promote medicines; only representatives of pharmaceutical companies can. In France, health authorities passed legislation in 1962—following the expansion of social security that began in 1945—in order to strictly regulate wholesaler activities, recognize the specific nature of the "wholesaler-distributor" profession, and prohibit them from pharmaceutical promotion (see Chapter 3). In Benin, the first wholesalers set up shop in the 1980s without any specific laws on their activities (see Chapter 2); legislation was adopted in the early 2000s.[4] Although there is no express provision for pharmaceutical promotion, this legislation is modeled on French law. Thus, in Benin as in France, the activity of pharmaceutical representatives is wholly linked to that of drug manufacturers. These francophone countries emphasize the medical, rather than the commercial, nature of this activity (Fournier, Lomba, & Muller, 2014). Pharmaceutical representatives constitute a professional group that has been and is being constructed "in contrast to the downgraded and downgrading categories of sales" (Greffion, 2014, p. 84).

In Ghana, where the authorities have expressly allowed considerable leeway for economic actors invested in medicines, pharmaceutical products can be promoted not just by the companies themselves, but by importers and wholesale companies as well (see Chapter 3). Numerous companies of different kinds are therefore involved. Legislation in that country has allowed companies to combine the activities of drug manufacturers, wholesalers, and representative-importers since 1957. "The purpose of this legal provision is to improve the viability of companies by allowing several trading and manufacturing activities to be combined, thus encouraging the establishment of economically viable firms" (Pourraz, 2019, p. 79). In Ghana, the term "sales representative" is used in the pharmaceutical sector just like it is in other business sectors.

In the next sections, we will see how these legislative differences in Benin and Ghana have affected the way pharmaceutical promotion is organized in the two countries.

***In Ghana, firm reps are active but eclipsed by importer reps***

There are two types of pharmaceutical representation in Ghana, based on the types of pharmaceutical companies and importer-distributors involved.

*Big Pharma's "ethical reps" and distributors*

European and North American multinationals use their own medical representatives (reps) for the scientific promotion of their products. These reps all have a pharmacy degree and are employed either directly by the company through a scientific office that it opens in Accra, or by one of its distributors on the company's behalf. This is the case for a dozen or so multinationals with a strong presence in Ghana: the British AstraZeneca and GlaxoSmithKline, the American Pfizer, the Swiss Novartis and Roche, the French Sanofi and Servier, the German Bayer and Denk, and the Danish Novo Nordisk.[5] Their products are distributed in the country through a few distributors—each company has three to six—who share the highly valued market for these drugs, which are considered to be very high quality. This explains the use of the adjective "ethical" that these representatives associate with the products and the promotion methods they claim to use, which we will come back to later. The scientific offices that these multinationals open in Accra, in the central and affluent districts of the city, generally include a country manager who is responsible for all operations, an accountant, sometimes several first-line managers who are focused on specific product lines, and several medical reps (between 10 and 60 depending on the company), who spend most of their time "in the field."

There are two types of importer-distributors for these "Big Pharma" products in Ghana: international groups and local wholesalers; these latter are among the largest such companies operating in the country. We encountered the two international groups invested in pharmaceutical distribution in Ghana: Gokals Laborex, the major shareholder of which is the French group Eurapharma that has been established in Ghana since 2008[6]; and World Wide Health Care Limited, a company that opened its doors in Ghana in 2011. This latter group had been created by, and at the time of our research belonged to, the Anglo-Indian Chanrai Summit Group based in Dubai, but was in the process of being acquired by a South African company, Imperial Logistics.[7] Some five or so Ghanaian wholesalers are invested in Big Pharma distribution, mainly Ernest Chemist, East Cantonment, and Oson's Chemist, which were established in the 1980–1990s.[8] These companies have either specialized in the import and distribution of these highly valued products, or are developing other strategies in parallel with products from other firms. These will be discussed later.

Each of these importer-distributors uses sales reps and medical reps for the Big Pharma products they represent. Distributors are carefully selected by pharmaceutical firms through calls for tenders and on the basis of criteria such as their financial capacity and the quality of their facilities. They are in direct competition with each other yet share the objective of maximizing the distribution of the

Big Pharma products they represent on the Ghanaian market.[9] They do not handle the administrative procedures for products' marketing authorization (MA) with the Food and Drugs Authority (FDA) of Ghana. They only conduct the necessary procedures for importing the products.

The medical reps responsible for promoting Big Pharma products work by product portfolio (most of those we met covered five or six products) and by territory (neighborhoods, cities, or regions). They are only responsible for scientific promotion and ordinarily do not get involved with sales, which are handled by the distributors' sales reps (discussed later). Since the 1990s, these medical reps have been under the umbrella of a professional association, the Association of Representatives of Ethical Pharmaceutical Industries or AREPI. The purpose of this association is to distinguish its members from other medical reps working for other pharmaceutical companies in Ghana, and to regulate the profession by publishing a code of ethics that, at the time of our research, they wanted to place under the aegis of Ghana's FDA. Their use of the term "ethical" skillfully combines the concepts that the products should be high-quality, innovative (not generic), prescription (not over the counter or OTC), and that the companies promoting them should have particularly ethical practices.[10]

### *Medical reps and sales reps of local wholesalers with a "monopoly" on Asian, European, and African firms*

Alongside the Big Pharma companies, the other pharmaceutical firms that put their products on the Ghanaian market, whether Asian, European, or African, all go through a locally operating wholesaler to whom they give the exclusive right to import and distribute their production. These wholesalers are said to have the "monopoly" on these firms' products. Some wholesalers, who are generally quite robust financially, also engage in contract manufacturing with one or more firms, mainly Asian but also European, which manufacture products for them under their own brand name.[11] Most local Ghanaian firms combine distribution with their production activities and therefore also have wholesaler status (Pourraz, 2019). In addition to the promotion and distribution of their products, firms leave the administrative procedures for MA to these various wholesalers as well.

These wholesalers hire medical reps and even greater numbers of sales reps to promote the different products; their numbers vary depending on the size of the company and the number of products they have to promote. Tobinco, one of the largest, promotes about 200 products from 8 different pharmaceutical firms (5 based in India, 1 in the United Kingdom, 1 in China, and 1 in Indonesia) and employs 80 sales reps and 20 medical reps for this purpose. In comparison, Biotic Pharmacy, which distributes around 20 products from 2 companies (1 Pakistani and 1 German), employs 6 sales reps and 4 medical reps. In one instance, the director of a small company that recently started importing a single product from a foreign firm promotes that product alone, filling both the sales rep and the medical rep roles.

In theory, these two types of representatives perform very different functions. Medical reps interact with prescribers in hospitals, clinics, and health centers and scientifically promote the products. Sales reps are responsible for the actual sales activities. "It's a two-way affair, the sales rep is basically a business person, his interest is in the business, and then the medical rep is an expert. All the medical reps are pharmacists, registered pharmacists, so it's more about trying to draw attention of the medical doctor to what products are available, what new compositions are there, what the advantage is... so they are more the people who generate the business, generate the orders, and then the sales reps come in to look at those orders and handle the transaction. So they pick the order, do the order, process the order, do the delivery, follow up on payment" (interview with the brand manager at a Ghanaian wholesaler, Accra, February 2015).

Of course, the type of representative who is sent to the field will be different depending on whether the products being promoted are prescription or OTC, innovative or generic. Innovative prescription products, regardless of how innovative they actually are, will require many medical reps, while generics, even prescription generics, and especially OTC products will mainly require sales reps. For this reason, and unlike the promotion of Big Pharma products by medical reps presented earlier, sales reps play the essential role for the products of Asian, smaller European, and African firms.[12] They are organized by territory (by neighborhoods in major cities or by regions of the country) and by type of customer (hospitals and clinics, wholesalers, and retailers).

## *A shifting landscape of pharmaceutical representation in Benin*

There are currently three kinds of pharmaceutical representatives in Benin, organized around the type of structure that employs them. We will describe the respective importance of each and how it has changed as this area of activity has evolved in the country.

### *Direct-labos: Professionals employed by the firms themselves*

An emblematic figure of pharmaceutical representation, *direct-labos* are employees of the firm they represent. They are responsible for visiting prescribers and pharmacists, tracking MA applications with the pharmacy directorate (Directorate of Pharmacies, Medicines, and Diagnostic Investigations [DPMED] at the time of our research),[13] and gathering sales statistics from wholesalers. Being a *direct-labo* in a multinational company is the dream of all young people entering the profession. It is the most highly valued and coveted position in pharmaceutical representation in Benin, and the origin of the profession in the country.

The late 1960s saw the disappearance of small- and medium-sized pharmaceutical companies around the globe and the concentration of companies into what would later be called Big Pharma (Greffion, 2014). These large companies went on to create their own sales departments, and it was at this point in time that the figure of the *direct-labo* representative, as seen in Benin, was born. Initially these were primarily European expatriates or others assigned temporarily in the countries. In the 1980s and 1990s, firms began to hire young college graduates in the French-speaking countries of Africa to fill these positions. The presence of subsidiaries of the major pharmaceutical companies in Senegal and Côte d'Ivoire was a contributing factor, due to the availability of young people newly trained at those countries' polytechnic institutes, for example. At that time in Benin, *direct-labos* were a kind of all-powerful representative, with high salaries and company cars at their disposal; some were even envied by doctors.

The position of *direct-labo* remains idealized to this day, feeding the imaginary that surrounds the pharmaceutical representative profession in Benin as well as in Côte d'Ivoire, where we also conducted research. But the trend in the pharmaceutical industry, as described in the literature (Greffion, 2014) and as we observed in Benin, is to outsource certain activities, such as research and development, and marketing. As a result, very few of these representatives remain in Benin. At the time we collected our data, only the Servier company was still employing *direct-labos*. In Ghana, however, we noted an apparently recent trend in the opposite direction in which Big Pharma companies contract their representatives directly.

### *International agencies: Stakeholders in the large and still often French groups*

In the early 1990s, the sales figures for these large pharmaceutical firms decreased, and they began to make extensive use of service providers to promote their products (Greffion, 2014). "When the generic companies first entered the system, their profits [Big Pharma] started to go down a bit, so they invested less, and most of these laboratories began entrusting the majority of their products to representation agencies. So that's how the agencies started to take shape" (interview with the head of a representation agency, Abidjan, September 2019).

The international promotion agencies that operate today on the African continent were established gradually during this period. They are cheaper for firms than *direct-labos*, and are more flexible, more efficient, and allow for better organization of the labor market. In fact, they position themselves as a specialized system for managing the human resources of pharmaceutical representatives. Their major selling point is that they have a detailed knowledge of various laws and practices of the francophone countries of West Africa. They can thus ease the burden for the Big Pharma firms, who no longer have to focus on the specific laws of each country, manage relations with each of the national administrations, or deal with the potential hassles of every field agent. Some of these companies were founded by former *direct-labo* employees of Big Pharma, as evidenced in this interview excerpt: "At a certain point, the African market, especially with the arrival of generics companies, well, the African market no longer interested them. So, they entrusted the products they had to former civil servants.[14] That's how Pharmaco[15] was born; Pharmaco was created by a Swiss man (…), who worked in Africa for a long time for Roche. So Pharmaco was managing Roche's products and now has many other products" (interview with the first-line manager of an international agency, Cotonou, January 2019).

The international agencies each employ an average of 20–50 people in Benin to promote products and, depending on the terms of their contracts with the firms, manage regulatory affairs. Until recently, most of these agencies were French or Franco-Ivorian companies with the legal status of export wholesalers in France. Companies from other countries are gradually getting involved in this activity. The largest of them are part of complex economic groups (holding companies) that include companies involved in the entire drug chain (manufacturing, distribution, logistics, promotion). Some examples with regard to promotion include Eurotech, part of the French group Tridem that was purchased in 2017 by the Chinese company FoSun; Planetpharma Promotion, a Franco-Ivorian company belonging to the Ubipharm group; and Ethica, also Franco-Ivorian, bought by the French group Eurapharma discussed earlier in the Ghana section.[16] These three agencies share the representation contracts for all the Big Pharma companies. The relatively large Asian generics companies, which are positioned in subsidized markets (see Chapters 5 and 6) and present in several French-speaking African countries, do not have the energy or resources to address various laws and customary ways of doing things specific to each country and face a significant language barrier, so they also entrust the representation of their products to these agencies.

Some international agencies set up offices in what they consider to be the "major" countries (Cameroon, Côte d'Ivoire, and Senegal) and subcontract to local agencies or hire field agents who are considered *direct-labos* but who would more accurately be called "direct-agencies." Others choose to set up offices in each country, or one common office for two countries, under the responsibility of a country manager and supervisors.

### *Local agencies: Emerging Beninese players*

Local agencies emerged in the early 2000s in Benin and more broadly in francophone West African countries, during a period in which the patents for several drugs were expiring, pharmaceutical markets in these countries were becoming more liberal,[17] and these markets were being taken over by Asian firms (Abecassis & Coutinet, 2008; Baxerres, 2013; Singh, 2018). One of the representatives we met in Côte d'Ivoire expressed it in these terms: "Today, people understand that it was a job different from sales, and then more and more agencies were created because at the time, to be honest it was only European laboratories… European ones, I mean for the most part. Now, with globalization, there are Indian laboratories here. There are Chinese laboratories, there are Pakistani ones (…) and as they couldn't come here directly, they started by having pharmaceutical representation agencies. And here we are today (…) there are so many now, there are so many…" (interview with the regulatory affairs officer of a European firm, Abidjan, September 2019).

In Benin, local agencies are more numerous (about 50) than the other types described but do not have the highest sales or largest market presence. These agencies were created by former *direct-labos* or employees of international agencies, and their staff size ranges between 1 and 50 employees. They sign contracts with pharmaceutical companies, either directly with firms, or with distributors or international agencies that subcontract activities to them. Local agencies can be divided into two subcategories based on their economic significance and the types of pharmaceutical companies with which they contract.

One subcategory consists of medium-sized local agencies that contract with international agencies or with European, Asian, or North African generics companies. These agencies operate on a relatively structured basis, with fully equipped offices and administrative staff (accountant, secretary, sales manager, etc.) in addition to their "field" representatives. Some of these medium-sized local agencies are also present in Côte d'Ivoire and Togo, and some even compete with the international agencies and the firms they represent in terms of prestige and image. Some have websites, and employees wear uniforms that highlight the agency rather than the client company. Candidates for employment in these agencies must have a car. Representatives have employment or service contracts, receive bonuses, and even get paid time off.

The other subcategory consists of small local agencies that partner with one or more small Asian firm(s), primarily Indian and Pakistani but occasionally Chinese. These agencies have very limited resources and their representatives often travel by motorcycle. Most of the reps are quite young, and their level of formal preparation is often limited to a baccalaureate plus 6 months of training in private schools.[18] For the most part, they work without a written contract, have low salaries—as low as CFA 50,000 (EUR 76) per month—and are not paid on a regular schedule. These agencies' operations are less structured, with no dedicated office for business activities and no administrative staff.

Asian firms that contract with these small local agencies periodically send a country manager to monitor their interests within the agency. The country manager accompanies representatives on their "field" visits and assists the agency head with DPMED administrative procedures. This practice is extremely controversial, including in agencies that host such country managers, who claim to have no choice in the matter. They have very poor relations with other types of representatives, who accuse them of all sorts of dubious practices, including corruption and the practice of paying health-care professionals to prescribe their products. Even so, these country managers play a central role in how small Asian firms construct markets: by carefully studying the markets, products, and practices of their competitors.

Now that we have described the structure of pharmaceutical representation activities in the two countries—changing in Benin, more established in Ghana—let us see how these differences affect the way pharmaceutical companies invest locally.

## Market-capture strategies: Contrasts and similarities in Benin and Ghana

Benin and Ghana have legislated different legal statuses for medicines, which help us understand the strategies used by pharmaceutical firms. In Ghana, there are three different classes of medicines: "prescription-only medicines" that require a doctor's prescription; "pharmacy-only medicines" that pharmacists can recommend themselves because of their expertise; and "OTC medicines."[19] Although Benin does have a list of drugs sold only on medical prescription and a list of "products on recommendation," the texts do not distinguish by class or table other than for narcotic drugs and psychotropic substances.[20]

Another difference between the two countries that impacts representatives' activity is the legal status of retail distribution actors (strong pharmacist monopoly in Benin, two distribution licenses in Ghana)[21] and how they are located throughout the national territory. OTC medicines sellers are commonly found throughout Ghana—numbering 10,424 in 2015—particularly in the working-class districts of cities and rural areas. Legally, they are only required to distribute a limited list of products including OTCs and medicines included in public health programs (antimalarials, contraceptives, and so forth). In contrast, pharmacies in Ghana are exclusively found in major cities. They distribute all of the classes of drugs provided for by legislation.

In Benin, the main actors in formal private retail distribution are pharmacies. These are found in major urban centers, though in recent years, the increasing number of trained pharmacists in the country has expanded their range to more rural areas. Pharmacies reach rural areas through pharmaceutical depots, which they supervise remotely, but nationwide there are relatively few such depots (165 in 2018). The informal drug sales sector, which previously played a key role in pharmaceutical distribution and access to medicines (Baxerres, 2013; Chapters 3, 7, and 10), had been heavily suppressed by the authorities as we began collecting data about representatives in Benin. We were therefore no longer able to study whether reps had specific strategies for this sector.[22]

### *A trend toward market segmentation in Ghana and competition in a more homogeneous market in Benin*

#### *Ghanaian segmentations by therapeutic class, legal status, and territory*

Most of the economic actors in the pharmaceutical sector in Ghana, whether manufacturers or importer-distributors, are highly specialized in terms of medicines' legal status (prescription-only medicines, pharmacy-only medicines, or OTCs) and therapeutic classes (medicines to treat chronic diseases, or acute diseases and common symptoms). These elements determine the investment pharmaceutical reps make with different clients.

Some representatives specifically target health facilities and prescription products. These include Big Pharma's "ethical reps" and their distributors' medical and sales reps. One example are representatives for one of the multinationals with a local presence, which specializes in Ghana in the treatment of chronic diseases (hypertension, diabetes, cancer, dermatological disorders). But this category also includes the medical and sales reps for the local wholesalers who represent some large Asian generics manufacturers, such as a wholesaler that specializes in prescription products from India (drugs to treat diabetes, hypertension, liver and kidney diseases, etc.). This segment of the pharmaceutical market has the advantage of generating very large orders, via the country's entire public sector through various levels of its health pyramid, but also via private clinics and mission hospitals.[23] The establishment of the National Health Insurance Scheme (NHIS) in Ghana in 2003 provides pharmaceutical companies with a major client, and cornering this market is a major economic issue.[24] However, according to the testimonies of several of the actors we interviewed, the NHIS is experiencing significant difficulties that have resulted in it paying its bills several months late. "The national health insurance, they don't pay… they just don't pay… their reinvestment is very slow… the last reinvestment national health gave to the hospital was April last year (…), so how do you stay in business if after eight months the person still owes you? It doesn't make sense" (interview with the director of operations for an international distributor, Accra, February 2015).

Many firms and wholesalers have therefore decided to focus on the private retail market (pharmacies and/or OTC medicine shops), in which pharmacy-only and OTC medicines represent the large market of self-medication without any medical consultation. The director of a wholesaler-importer explained it this way: "Prescription-only medicine is really hurting me really badly because I don't get my money cycle in good shape. You supply and it takes you between six and eight months to get your money back. It stifles business. Now we want to do OTCs where we can concentrate on the private-sector market, where we can really make payment within a month to get your money" (interview with the manager of a Ghanaian wholesaler-importer, Accra, March 2016).[25] For example, one wholesaler-importer in Ghana, who imports only seven products from an Indian firm (an antimalarial, a deworming agent, three painkillers, a decongestant, and a cough suppressant), only targets private wholesalers as clients.

Drug reps in Ghana—backed by the companies they represent—always decide how aggressively they will focus on the wealthy or poor districts in the capital, other major cities, or rural regions based on their target clients (health facilities, pharmacies, OTC medicine sellers). However, they also consider how extensively they are located around the country and the relative financial status of the end users.

For example, a wholesaler-importer who has signed contract manufacturing agreements with a small German company, two Chinese companies, and one Indian company, and has the "monopoly" on an American company that has generics manufactured in India, owns two wholesale stores in Accra, one in Kumasi (the second-largest city located in the center of the country), as well as an office with warehouses, one medical rep, one sales rep, and one minibus and one driver in each of Ghana's ten regions. This wholesaler-importer thus ensures that the products it represents are well distributed throughout the country. In comparison, Big Pharma's two international distributors do not have much presence outside Accra. Gokals Laborex has no depots outside Accra and mainly targets public hospitals and private clinics along with all wholesalers. It generally does not directly target retailers, but when it does these are only "high-level pharmacies" in Accra and certainly not OTC medicine shops. The pharmacist superintendent of World Wide Health Care Limited stated in our interview that he prefers to focus on a few large clients, such as the Korle Bu National Reference University Hospital in Accra, rather than spreading out across numerous small clients. So Big Pharma's "ethical reps" are primarily found in Accra and with prescribers in major public hospitals and large private clinics. In contrast, wholesalers who specialize in OTC products manufactured in Asia will send their sales reps primarily to nonimporting wholesalers, pharmacies, and OTC medicine sellers; they take care to have a significant presence throughout the country specifically for these latter clients.

Some of the largest local wholesaler-importers are of course playing on all fields, both in terms of end users' socioeconomic status and coverage of the entire country. A brand manager with Ernest Chemist, a company with 15 wholesale stores in 7 of the 10 regions of Ghana, explains: "We represent different companies and each of the companies has different target markets, so we have companies that we represent that target the top end, the high-class market. We represent other companies that also look at the middle, and then we have locally produced products that look at the middle to lower class. So we look at all the classes involved and we have different products, different prices to cover everybody" (Accra, February 2015). Tobinco, mentioned earlier, which specializes in products made in Asia for acute and common health problems (antimalarials, painkillers, deworming agents, antibiotics), also sends its medical reps but especially its sales reps to both health facilities and nonimporting wholesalers and retailers. It also has a nationwide presence. The extent of their activities and the capital accumulated since their creation means these two major Ghanaian companies have also been investing in pharmaceutical production for several years.

Some Big Pharma companies also do not limit themselves to prescription products and chronic diseases, or to the city of Accra, but are positioning themselves on the OTC market throughout the country. The portfolio of a Sanofi medical rep we met consists solely of OTC products (antacids, vitamins, cough medicines). She works exclusively with wholesalers and pharmacy salespeople and, at the time of our interview, was thinking about how to best position herself with OTC medicine sellers. Only 9 of the 60 medical reps working for this firm are based in Accra; the other 51 are posted across the country. Similarly, Novartis' scientific office in Accra has two first-line managers, one of whom specializes in cardiovascular products, the other in painkillers and antimalarial drugs. They each manage several medical reps, although this latter manager explained that when talking about painkillers and antimalarials we should really refer to these representatives as "pharmacy reps" since that is where the market for these products is found.

### *Activities in Benin are concentrated yet distributed throughout the hierarchy of health facilities and formal retailers*

As we saw earlier, there are fewer legal categories for medicines in Benin than in Ghana. Because OTC medicines are not recognized, pharmaceutical companies tend to all target the same therapeutic markets.[26] Formal retailers are also mainly located in Benin's cities. These two elements show that the activities of drug reps are overall much more concentrated therapeutically and geographically in Benin than in Ghana. Even so, here too we find that end users with different financial means are targeted within the hierarchy of the health facilities and formal retailers that are available.

The representatives of the Big Pharma firms and their generics branches mainly focus on large private clinics and public university hospitals. Their second choice of clients are medium-sized private clinics and so-called zone public hospitals, which are also reference centers, where they mainly target well-known professors and doctors, as well as hospital pharmacists who place orders for the products used internally. But university and zone hospitals are also a true competitive arena between Big Pharma and the large generics companies, as this excerpt from an interview with a former employee of the American firm Pfizer illustrates: "I had an account at the CNHU [national university hospital center], I had an account in dialysis. And the CNHU ordered about 1000 boxes of Almor[27] per year. Then those guys came [Macleods, a major Indian generics company] to take that client away from me. No, but I did everything I could. I used all my connections, because the person who places that order is a pharmacist, a dean… who was the hospital pharmacist. When I heard about the problem, I made an appointment with him and I went to see him and I said, 'Dean, I'm your little brother, I'm a pharmacist like you. You can't take this account away from me and give it to the Indians. Come on, you're a health professional', and I tried to convince him. I kept the account there until I left the company. They couldn't change" (interview, Cotonou, June 2019).

We can see that the large generics firms are competing with multinationals in university and zone hospitals. If they are unable to win over the well-established doctors, who are in the habit of prescribing Big Pharma products, the generics representatives mainly target interns, doctors studying to be specialists (DES)[28] and midwives who write a significant number of prescriptions. "There are others who really only prescribe European products. The older doctors for example, with new products, you can go see them 10,000 times, they will never prescribe them. Those guys are very attached to the old products" (interview with the representative of a European generics manufacturer, Cotonou, June 2019). These generics manufacturers—from every continent—have the largest market shares and are present throughout the prescription chain, from reference hospitals to small health centers. In each prescribing site, representatives observe, learn, listen to prescribers and adjust their visit schedule based on the end client's purchasing power. As the rep quoted earlier expressed it, "There is all this information that we are trying to find out, and then they [the prescribers] themselves tell us, and at the nearest pharmacies too, we conduct surveys to find out their prescribing habits (…) so when you go to see him [the prescriber], he'll tell you straight out, 'I don't prescribe expensive things because here, the population here, people can't afford them' (…). My products are even a bit expensive. In the range of CFA 3500 to 21,000 [EUR 5.5–32]."

Representatives working for small Asian firms position themselves mainly in district public health centers and small private practices run mostly by midwives and nurses. These practices, located in working-class neighborhoods, attract a clientele with meager means. This same representative expressed it this way: "Some prescribers, it depends on the area where they are. They don't like expensive products so they have to prescribe Indian products. So if they are in an area where there are only people with low purchasing power, they have to make do with Indian products."

Various firms construct markets around pharmacies as well as health centers. Some agencies have representatives who exclusively solicit pharmacies. In a pharmaceutical market that mainly comprises generics and where the law on substituting originator drugs with generics by retailers dates back to 1999, a significant part of the market construction strategy involves working with pharmacies. Pharmacies are also the main category of authorized retailers. For some firms, particularly the smaller ones, salespeople in pharmacies may be more important than prescribers. The representative of a Franco-Ivorian generics company we shadowed rarely visits health centers. "We then went to a health center, a small clinic in Godomey [a suburb of Cotonou]. I told him I thought he only did pharmacies. He told me that they are his main target, but that he also goes to health centers where clients have low purchasing power. For example, it wouldn't do him any good to go to upmarket health centers where people use insurance most of the time. His products will not be prescribed there" (field notebook, Cotonou, August 2018).

Note that 169 of the 276 pharmacies (61%) in Benin are located in either the city of Cotonou (97) or its surroundings (43 in Abomey-Calavi, 29 in Porto-Novo).[29] Representatives therefore logically concentrate their activities in this geographic area. They generally target their clients first by type of health center and second by type of prescriber. If the main client targets appear insufficient to meet the monthly or quarterly goal, they broaden their actions to encompass less lucrative and hard-to-reach areas. "The delegate told me that he also goes to completely remote centers like Zinvié [a lakeside village on the outskirts of Cotonou] to round off the ends of the month" (field notebook, Cotonou, July 2018).

Once a month, representatives visit the secondary cities located within a radius of 100–300 km of Cotonou. For cities located beyond this perimeter, the largest agencies use the services of "multi-card" representatives (who represent several firms simultaneously) who are based in those areas. In addition to the informal sector, the formal market in rural areas is composed of a few private pharmaceutical depots and, more recently, a few pharmacies. Public health centers distribute essential generic drugs, sold under international nonproprietary names (INNs), which are prescribed by a health-care professional. These products are not promoted by company representatives but are subject to other market rules, such as calls for tender (see Chapter 2). This excerpt from an interview with a physician sums up the situation in remote areas: "In my four years of working in Segbana [a small commune in northwestern Benin], I have never seen a single delegate. So in order to stay informed about the products, I ask the Kandi pharmacy to regularly send me the catalog of available products. Otherwise, I work a lot with the CAME [Central Purchasing Office for Essential Medicines and Medical Consumables] products that are available in the center. (…). The pharmacy is really the last resort" (March 2019).

### *Strategies in both countries: Scientific but primarily commercial and relational*

#### *Scientific promotion*

Traditionally, pharmaceutical representatives primarily focus their activities on prescribers and the scientific promotion of products (Greene, 2006; Greffion, 2014; Ravelli, 2015; Scheffer, 2017). That is the raison d'être for Big Pharma's "ethical reps" in Ghana as well as all pharmaceutical representatives in Benin, at least in theory. This activity can take place at a variety of venues: a scientific symposium organized when a product is launched; smaller group meetings,

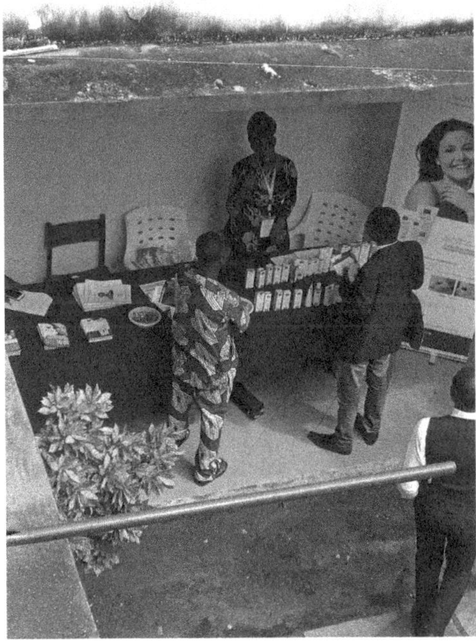

*Figure 9.1* Promotional stand at a scientific event in Cotonou.

Source: © IRD/Stéphanie Mahamé, Cotonou, February 2019

frequently organized to train various prescribers (doctors, nurses, midwives) on a specific health issue; over a working lunch; at a training session at the beach; and of course during the well-known "medical visit," which remains the key tactic.

Each one requires specific strategies. Kristin Peterson's studies in Nigeria (2014, ch. 6) illustrate how, when a pharmaceutical innovation is introduced (regardless of the actual degree of innovation), marketers must first approach specialist physicians—recognized opinion leaders in the therapeutic field concerned—who will be able to introduce the product and thus influence their colleagues, especially those who are younger and less experienced. Clinical meetings are then key to promoting the product. They often report on the clinical trials that companies have conducted on their products and that will help representatives convince their clients of these products' usefulness (Dumit, 2012; Ravelli, 2015).

One ethical rep explained his approach during visits: "So you interact with the physicians and try to understand their practice. If it is an antihypertensive I am supposed to sell that day, [that] I want him to prescribe that day, I ask him questions about hypertension, his practice. What he looks out for in the medicine before he prescribes. So as I listen to him, I find the loopholes where my product comes in, with the advantages. (…). Yes he may know of it but I will just draw his attention to those benefits he is looking for in the product. (…). Some of them will tell you (…) they prefer other drugs they want to use. They give you their reasons (…), so you just end the call then make plans for how to tackle their objections. Whatever reasons why he decided to choose another product, you go back, then find reasons why when you meet him again he should now consider your product" (interview, Accra, December 2015).

In Benin, these various scientific promotion activities are grouped under the term "public relations." Although the relationship between representatives and prescribers is described in the Global North as being increasingly difficult,[30] in the contexts we studied medical visits always seem to produce significant results with prescribers. This is why reps try to stop by often to keep their products "front of mind" and prevent competitors from supplanting them in the minds of prescribers they previously won over, as these observation notes show: "The delegate says to them 'I heard that you are prescribing my competitors'. One of the two midwives replied 'we don't see you anymore, your competitors are here every day, we can't remember everything, you have to come by and remind us of the products'" (field notebook, Cotonou, April 2019). A maximum of four products are presented at each visit to avoid overloading the client with too much information at one time. Several elements are used to leave the prescriber with a strong memory of the visit and particularly of the products presented. For example, references to WHO prequalification are often made in relation to artemisinin-based combination therapies (ACTs) against malaria.

### *Social activities related to the sale itself*

In Ghana today, however, these traditional scientific activities of pharmaceutical representation no longer occupy anything close to the bulk of representatives' working time. An Indian expatriate explains why, based on his experience in both Indian and Ghanaian markets: "Initially, around 10 to 15 years back, when we were all working as medical representatives, (...) meeting with a qualified doctor and talking about our products, our promotion, was enough to get the business and recommendation from them. Now, that is not the case. It has been totally changed. (...). Because of the Internet and electronic media, if a doctor wants to have any information about any molecule, it's easily available. (...). So they are easily getting the information which was earlier being imparted by the medical representatives, so their role has been minimized" (interview, Accra, May 2015). In the Ghanaian context, sales-centric activities are considerable: checking that stocks are moving properly, collecting checks once the payment period is due, offering customers the opportunity to reorder, negotiating payment methods (cash, credit, granting varying lengths of credit), and so forth. These sales activities are supposed to be carried out exclusively by sales reps, which explains some testimonials stating that sales reps are ultimately more important than medical reps. However, medical reps also engage in these activities. One ethical rep described himself to us as a "medical sales representative."

In Benin, there is a certain hierarchy in promotional activities. While representatives, most of whom are fairly young, are responsible for medical visits and maintaining social relations with doctors, sales-related activities are more the responsibility of supervisors, sales managers, or agency heads. They go "out in the field" to maintain social relations with pharmacists involved in retail and wholesale distribution, monitor stocks with wholesalers, and record sales statistics. Representatives also work on some sales-related activities. They cultivate social relations with counter salespeople, frequently check the availability of "their" products in pharmacies, and try to place their products in pharmacies and health centers that do not yet sell them. Although in Benin they do not make direct sales, companies set monthly, quarterly, and annual sales targets for them. They call this "making their numbers," which amounts to what they refer to as "indirect" sales.

These sales-centered activities (direct in Ghana or indirect in Benin) require reps to invest in very significant social engagement. In Ghana, these are referred to as business relations. Sales reps for wholesaler-importers spend a great deal of time "in the field" greeting customers, maintaining contacts, expressing birthday and anniversary congratulations, and attending ceremonies for both happy events (marriage, birth) and unhappy ones (funerals), all the while conducting various sales-related activities. The brand manager of a Ghanaian wholesaler-importer quite convincingly explains it this way: "You look at customer service quality, and then customer reception. Those are the things that are competitive now, and then customer care in general, how much we know about our customers, what is the relationship, how do we nurture the relationship between the two: yourself and the customer, so that it does not become like once in a while when they need something then they walk in. But then it's a constant friendship, what I call 'a professional marriage that does not end'. Whether you need something from me or not, we have a relationship, and we would continue to nurture and grow it, and automatically, any day or anytime, I will be the first one on your mind" (Accra, February 2015). Our data thus strongly demonstrate the social construction of the market and the relational dimension of competition, as described by sociology and economic anthropology (Steiner, 2005).

Logically, these activities do not primarily target prescribers but rather vendors, those behind the counters of retail and wholesale stores in Ghana and behind pharmacy counters and in wholesaler-distributor offices in Benin. A Big Pharma representative in Ghana explains: "The other side [of our work] basically has to do with talking to the pharmacies, number one, why they shouldn't do substitution; number two, how to keep the products to ensure that we can maintain that efficacy throughout the lifespan of a product. (…). And we do a little bit of the marketing aspect, how to display your goods at the pharmacy to make sure that when customers walk in they can see what they want so that at least, they can also say 'ok, I want this; I've used this before, this is what I prefer'" (interview, Accra, March 2016). Work sessions, training sessions, and product launches are organized specifically for these front desk sellers, as they are known. The people in charge of placing orders for hospitals, clinics, and wholesale companies, and the accountants working in these various facilities are also "targets" that should not be overlooked.[31]

In Benin, representatives do not hesitate to use their relationships with doctors practicing in a specific area to influence the people in charge of pharmacy orders, as we were able to observe during several shadowing sessions with a doctor in a mission health center: "While we were there, a pharmacy called him to ask for advice on product placement, to which he responded warmly. He said that he had no problem with it, but that he did not know what the other doctors preferred. (…) The delegate who was in the pharmacy for the placement of a product and had asked the pharmacy to call the doctor came by after leaving the pharmacy. He came to thank him for helping him to convince the pharmacy" (field notebook, Cotonou, August 2018).

### *Gifts and special attention to boost sales*

Commercial strategies, described previously in the literature (Fugh-Berman & Ahari, 2015), help to maintain these social relations: offering promotional items (pens, jackets, mugs, caps, T-shirts, hand sanitizer,[32] umbrellas, calendars, bags, cell phone covers, etc.), remembering birthdays (cakes) or holidays (chocolates and flowers for Valentine's Day), invitations to luncheons, and providing free samples, which an "ethical rep" in Ghana told us was the main promotional tool for the firm he represents.

Larger gifts may also be offered to good clients, such as televisions, air conditioners, refrigerators, water fountains, microwaves, or "scientific" trips abroad for conferences or pharmaceutical fairs. Discounts may be given for large purchases; good clients may even receive extended credit periods or credits for "fast moving products," which is not the usual practice.

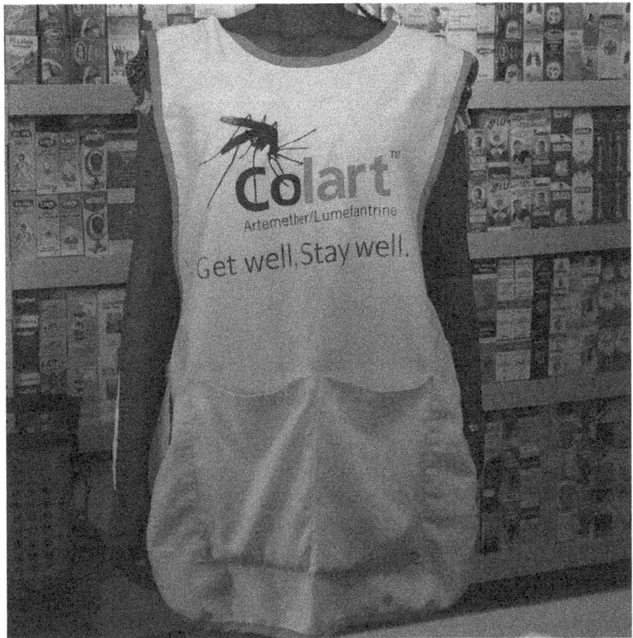


*Figure 9.2* Pharmacy seller's white shirt in Accra.

Source: © IRD/Carine Baxerres, Accra, September 2015

In Benin, since sales are decoupled from promotion, these commercial strategies are an extension of the public relations mentioned earlier and are therefore mainly focused on prescribers personally ("scientific" trip abroad), but also on medical societies (pediatrics, ophthalmology, surgery, etc.), hospitals, and health centers (support pledges for various activities). "On the way out of the midwives' on-call room, we stopped in front of a classroom where the DES students and the professor had just finished a meeting. We greeted them and they all responded, smiling. The delegate had told me on the way there that they had provided a large digital screen and a computer for their classes. Now they can run course content or any presentation right from a smartphone. The prof asked his DES students 'do you prescribe their products? Because we should return people's favors'. They hastened to answer yes, yes, yes" (field notebook, Cotonou, January 2018).

All representatives in Benin and Ghana engage in such sales and promotional activities for the market segments or types of end users targeted by the firms they represent. Big Pharma reps say they do not engage in "unethical" promotional practices and seek the proper balance between incentives and legality. "We are a multinational company; we are listed on the stock exchange, not in Ghana, so we are bound by all those corruption laws and all of those things. (…). So we try and weigh, we are not giving gifts above 20 dollars, those kinds of things (…), to our disadvantage because our competitors can easily give ACs and fridges and all that but we can't" (interview, Accra, February 2015).

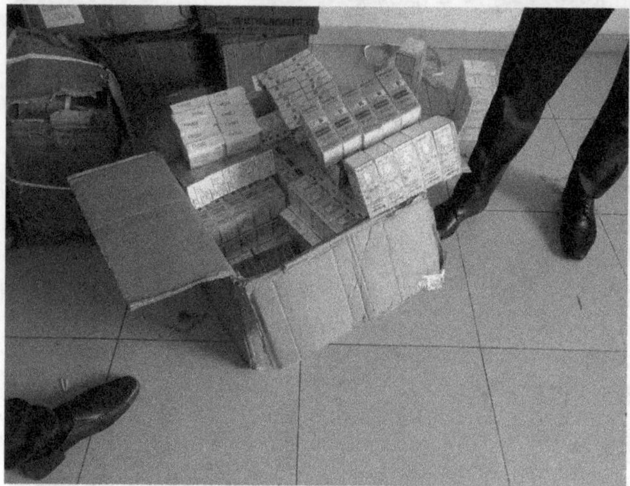

*Figure 9.3* Samples for medical visit in Benin.

Source: © IRD/Stéphanie Mahamé, Cotonou, September 2018

## Conclusion

In Europe and North America, there is talk of the "medical visit crisis" (Ravelli, 2015, p. 70). Due to the global decline in pharmaceutical companies' capacity for innovation, increased international competition linked to the growing numbers of generic manufacturers, the decline in public spending, and the deterioration of the industry's image with prescribers, since the mid-2000s companies have tended to employ fewer and fewer pharmaceutical representatives.[33] In West Africa, however, pharmaceutical representation activity is far from on the decline. The fact that it is not only focused on scientific promotion but also more broadly on sales, whether direct or indirect, undoubtedly has something to do with this. Also contrary to what is described in the Global North, this activity is aimed at a broad range of actors that goes well beyond just physicians: nurses, midwives, nurses' aides, salespeople in pharmacies and OTC medicine shops, accountants and order managers in health facilities, wholesalers, and so forth. Finally, in the Global North when products move into the public domain and their prices drop drastically, promoting them is no longer profitable (Ravelli, 2015). In West Africa, where the pharmaceutical market is even more dominated by generics than in the Global North, this is not a major consideration, especially since the labor costs of representatives are much lower.

More established in Ghana, changing in Benin, tied to national pharmaceutical regulations, different economic actors in both countries are the keystone of this pharmaceutical representation: wholesaler-importers in Ghana and promotion agencies in Benin. Beyond the very significant issue of the international economic actors invested in pharmaceutical promotion and distribution, many of whom are still French in this region of the world where that country's influence is undeniable,[34] it is striking to note that in both countries, the key economic players in pharmaceutical promotion are largely national players with national capital. The importance of the definition of "pharmaceutical representative" adopted in the Introduction is now quite clear. Our work highlights that, although in different proportions in Ghana and Benin, these field professionals themselves generate definite and endogenous pharmaceutical dynamics in their country, independently of the firms they represent.

In Ghana, our research shows that the pharmacy field has been built through the activity of sales reps, who, as one pharmacist dismissively stated, do "trading... trading, anybody can buy and sell" (interview, Accra, March 2016). The most important economic players today, many of whom are now involved in pharmaceutical manufacturing, started out as sales reps (Baxerres, 2018).[35] The promotion of medicines, whatever the products or companies involved, from whatever corner of the world, has led to the construction of Ghana's pharmaceutical economy, strengthening and advancing local actors. The Tobinco company discussed in this chapter has grown by promoting the products of a small Indian firm that a pharmacist told us "is not known in India... when I say it's not known, it hasn't got a name; in fact it's not a big company... it's a very small company" (interview, Accra, October 2014).

In Benin, the dynamics of pharmaceutical representation are still emerging and the pharmacy field is currently so disrupted that it is difficult to imagine its future. Moreover, the government regulation in place up to this point has tended to limit economic actors' room to maneuver (see Chapter 3). Despite this, representatives are playing an increasingly important role in local pharmaceutical dynamics, which are no longer dominated by wholesaler-distributors alone. The rise of representative agencies is certain. Paid between 10% and 18% of the firms' sales figures, agencies achieve a financial power that allows them to diversify. Some local agencies have obtained approval to import and sell medical equipment (beds, gynecological tables, electric respirators, surgical equipment, etc.), and others have founded training schools in the fields of pharmaceutical promotion and pharmacy sales.[36]

Through their representatives, pharmaceutical companies from different regions of the world are setting up local operations in Africa and gaining market shares in a highly competitive context.[37] While still based on governmental regulation and the country's pharmaceutical distribution structure (whether or not the ubiquitous OTC medicine shops are formally included), the firms develop territorial and therapeutic strategies: segmentation in Ghana, concentration in Benin. But beyond these differences, in these contexts where health care is still mainly the responsibility of end users,[38] similar underlying strategies appear in how these users are targeted based on their financial situation. Product pricing and brand reputation determine how aggressively firms in both Benin and Ghana target health facilities and retail distributers, and whether these are centrally located or in rural districts, high-end or low. Through the intermediary of their representatives, they even intervene in people's private lives to recommend medications.

This intermediary is skillfully constructed not only through prescribers and the many actors involved in distribution and health care that representatives so carefully cultivate, but also through those actors' friends, neighbors, colleagues, and families.[39]

## Notes

1. As colonization was ending, the main sources of medicines for Ghana were the United Kingdom, West Germany, Italy, Switzerland, the Netherlands, and the United States (Pourraz, 2019). In Dahomey, medicines at that time came primarily from France, but also arrived from Senegal and Morocco, where some companies had established manufacturing sites (Baxerres, 2013).
2. These companies could also engage in representation activities for other pharmaceutical companies for whom they import and distribute medicines in African countries; this was the case of Major & Company and J.L. Morrison & Sons in Ghana (Pourraz, 2019).
3. See the Introduction of this book for more information on the data collection methodology.
4. See Decree 2000-450 of September 11, 2000 regarding the application of Law 97-020 of June 11, 1997 regarding the conditions for practicing the medical and paramedical professions with private clients and relating to the opening of wholesaler-distributor companies in the Republic of Benin.
5. The opening of scientific offices seems to be a fairly recent trend among multinational drug companies in Ghana. For example, Novartis opened its scientific office in 2014, and Denk did so after 2010.
6. Eurapharma was discussed in Chapters 1 and 2 and appears below in the discussion of Benin. The policy of this pharmaceutical company, long a fixture in the French-speaking countries of Africa, is to associate itself with an existing local company and purchase more than half of its shares. In Ghana, Laborex—a name often used by Eurapharma subsidiaries in various countries—has joined forces with Gokals Limited, a Ghanaian company founded in 1998 by a Ghanaian entrepreneur of Indian origin. A section of Gokals Limited that specialized in generics was not affected by this takeover and has continued on its own path. It continues to operate today under the name Gokals Limited.
7. For more on these two international companies, see https://www.chanraisummitgroup.com/home.html and https://www.imperiallogistics.com/overview.php, accessed in July 2020.
8. Other companies may be mobilized for specific actions, such as programs related to Global Health, like the AMFm (Affordable Medicine Facility-malaria) discussed in Chapter 6.
9. For example, they may distribute products at the lower end of the price range set by the Big Pharma companies. Some explain that in order to keep these firms as clients, they may agree to pay for their medical reps to promote products that are at the end of their life cycle or no longer sell well, or OTC products that do not necessarily need scientific promotion. Competition is fierce between importer-distributors in Ghana, and the local actors who were there first take a very dim view of the competition from international wholesalers, which they consider unfair.
10. This is objectively not always the case. The Big Pharma products that they promote are not all innovative and not all prescription, far from it. The quality and promotion of these products will be discussed in the next section of this chapter as well as in Chapter 11. Here again, as with the term "specialty," which we discussed previously in French-speaking contexts (Baxerres, 2013), there is some linguistic ambiguity (or abuse of language) adroitly used for commercial purposes in the pharmacy world.

11. These issues of "monopoly" and "contract manufacturing" are discussed in Chapter 6.
12. Sometimes agents who act as medical reps for these firms do not have a pharmacy degree or training in medicine or pharmacy.
13. The DPMED was reorganized in early 2020 and renamed the Beninese Agency for Pharmaceutical Regulation (ABRP: https://www.abrp.bj/organisation.php). For more on this subject, see Chapter 1.
14. In Benin, the term "civil servant" covers both public and private sector employees who have open-ended contracts and are firmly established in their place of work.
15. Pharmaco is an international agency based in South Africa that operates in several countries in sub-Saharan Africa. See their website: https://pharmaco.co.za, accessed September 2020.
16. See the websites of Tridem Pharma (https://www.tridem-pharma.com/), Ubipharm (http://www.ubipharm.com/fr), and Eurapharma (http://www.eurapharma.com/fr/), accessed in September 2020.
17. In the early 1990s, several countries, such as Benin, Burkina Faso, Mali, and Niger, transitioned to a more democratic political regime, which resulted in the opening of their markets. On the pharmaceutical front, the State ceded its monopoly on supply, which allowed private initiatives to develop, such as the establishment of private wholesale companies and representation agencies.
18. Since the mid-2000s, Benin has witnessed an explosion of "pharmaceutical delegation" training schools, a trend that originated in Côte d'Ivoire and quickly spread to Benin. These schools are usually founded by people who have no ties to the world of medicine but who think it will be a profitable niche. In fact, beginning in the 1990s, private initiatives in the health and education sector have spiraled out of control in Benin as in other French-speaking African countries (Baxerres, 2013).
19. The list of medicines included in each of these three classes can be found here: https://fdaghana.gov.gh/wp-content/uploads/2017/06/NEW-DRUG-CLASSIFICATION-LIST.pdf, accessed March 2019.
20. See Law 97-025 of July 18, 1997 on the Control of Drugs and Precursors.
21. These aspects are extensively developed and analyzed in Chapter 3, where the various actors involved in retail distribution in Ghana and Benin are described in detail.
22. In their work on the construction of the antidepressant market in India, Stefan Ecks and Soumita Basu describe how reps behave toward rural practitioners who are not licensed to prescribe these drugs. In that context, informal markets are not a barrier to the reps' activity (Ecks & Basu, 2014).
23. The types of care facilities available in Ghana and Benin are presented in detail in the following chapter.
24. Note that the prices of products reimbursed by the NHIS are set by the NHIS, unlike other products in Ghana whose prices are set by free market forces. Competition between economic actors is therefore not a factor in this specific market segment on prices.
25. Interviewees stated that repayment times have been long from the very inception of the NHIS, and that they have gradually worsened since 2003. This was not the case when the policy at health facilities was "cash and carry" (cost recovery).
26. However, we have seen a tendency for Big Pharma reps to focus more on promoting molecules for the treatment of chronic diseases and mental health and to somewhat neglect the promotion of their older products, which have garnered strong reputations but are now largely generics.
27. Amlor® is the originator product of amlodipine, an antihypertensive patented by Pfizer.
28. Interns are students in their 6th year of medical school while DES [*diplôme d'études spécialisées*] are doctors who have obtained their general practitioner degree and are studying in a specialty field.

29. Source: list of authorized pharmacies in the Republic of Benin, DPMED, January 2018.
30. In Western countries, although firms know just how much they can push to be available without being invasive, the various industry scandals make relations between pharmaceutical representatives and doctors increasingly difficult (Greffion, 2014; Greffion & Breda, 2015).
31. The pharmacist superintendent of a wholesaler-importer in Ghana explained how, to solidify his relationships with health facility administrators, he volunteers his own time to help them prepare bids.
32. Some of our research took place during the Ebola outbreak in West Africa.
33. Jérôme Greffion (2014) explains that there have been three phases of expansion followed by decline in the number of pharmaceutical representatives since 1945. However, the decrease seen from 2005 onward is the largest of these.
34. This observation may perhaps also be explained by French pharmaceutical regulation of wholesale distribution and by the specificity of the "wholesaler-distributor" profession it regulates (see Chapter 3). It should be still noted that these two activities are performed jointly in the large French international groups discussed in this chapter, including in Benin where promotion and distribution must be separated and where companies with a local presence perform one or the other exclusively.
35. An upcoming book by Carine Baxerres focusing on the Ghanaian history and contexts will be dedicated to these dynamics, both pharmaceutical and economic.
36. These dynamics are the subject of the thesis that Stéphanie Mahamé is writing about pharmaceutical representatives and their activities in Benin. It will be defended in 2021 and is jointly supervised by the Abomey-Calavi University of Benin and the EHESS of Paris in France.
37. In a Latin American context, Cory Hayden illustrates the confrontation between representatives of multinational pharmaceutical companies and those of the "similar medicines" industry in Mexican markets (Hayden, 2015).
38. As we have seen, including in Ghana where the NHIS is one of the most successful in Africa, it faces many challenges. These will also be discussed in the next chapter.
39. Quentin Ravelli (2015, p. 36) writes on this subject of the "values of informal use" of drugs, "in particular those of doctors whose scientific authority will then act in domino fashion on the uses of their patients, and subsequently their relatives." In the contexts that we study, the "informal use values" that influence large sections of society are those of all the actors involved to some degree in health care presented in this chapter, in addition to physicians.

## Reference list


Abecassis, P., & Coutinet, N. (2008). Caractéristiques du marché des médicaments et stratégies des firmes pharmaceutiques [Characteristics of drug markets and pharmaceutical firms' strategies]. *Horizons stratégiques*, *7*, 111–139.

Baxerres, C. (2013). *Du médicament informel au médicament libéralisé : une anthropologie du médicament pharmaceutique au Bénin [From informal to liberalized drugs: An anthropology of pharmaceutical drugs in Benin]*. Paris, France: Les Éditions des Archives Contemporaines.

Baxerres, C. (2018). D'intermédiaire informel, devenir détaillant, grossiste puis producteur pharmaceutique : Les trajectoires « vertueuses » des hommes d'affaires du médicament au Ghana [From informal intermediary to becoming a retailer, wholesaler, and then pharmaceutical producer: The "virtuous" trajectories of drug businessmen in Ghana]. In C. Baxerres, & C. Marquis (Eds.), *Regulations, markets, health: Questioning current stakes of pharmaceuticals in Africa* (pp. 30–40). (Conference proceedings). HAL, Ouidah, Benin. https://hal.archives-ouvertes.fr/hal-01988227.

Bonah, C., & Rasmussen, A. (Eds.). (2005). *Histoire et médicament aux 19ème et 20ème siècles [History and medication in the 19th and 20th centuries]*. Paris, France: Éditions Glyphe.

Cassier, M. (2019). La fin du partage artagecapitalismes de la copie face au capitalisme de la rentre globale : Une nouvelle géographie des industries de santé [The end of sharing? Copying capitalism in the face of global income capitalism: A new geography of health industries]. *Mouvements les idées et des luttes*, 98, 108–119.

Chauveau, S. (1999). *L'invention pharmaceutique: La pharmacie française entre l'état et la société au XXe siècle [Pharmaceutical invention: French pharmacy between the State and society in the XXth century]*. Paris, France: Inst. d'Édition Sanofi-Synthelabo.

Cochoy, F. (1999). *Une histoire du marketing: Discipliner l'économie de marché [A history of marketing: Disciplining the market economy]*. Paris, France: La Découverte.

Dumit, J. (2012). *Drugs for life. How pharmaceutical companies define our health*. London, UK: Duke University Press.

Ecks, S., & Basu, S. (2014). "We always live in fear": Antidepressant prescriptions by unlicensed doctors in India. *Culture, Medicine and Psychiatry*, 38(2), 197–216.

Fournier, P., Lomba, C., & Muller, S. (Eds.). (2014). *Les travailleurs du médicament. L'industrie pharmaceutique sous observation [Drug workers. The pharmaceutical industry under observation]*. Toulouse, France: ERES.

Fugh-Berman, A., & Ahari, S. (2015). Following the script: How drug reps make friends and influence doctors. In S. Sismondo, & J. A. Greene (Eds.), *The pharmaceutical studies reader* (pp. 123–132). Chichester, UK: Wiley Blackwell.

Greene, J. A. (2006). *Prescribing by numbers: Drugs and the definition of disease*. Baltimore, MD: Johns Hopkins University Press.

Greffion, J. (2014). *Faire passer la pilule. Visiteurs médicaux et entreprises pharmaceutiques face aux médecins : Une relation socio-économique sous tensions privées et publiques (1905–2014) [Pass the pill. Medical visitors and pharmaceutical companies confronting doctors: A socio-economic relationship under private and public tensions (1905–2014)]*. Doctoral dissertation, Ecole des Hautes Etudes en Sciences Sociales/ENS, Paris, France. Retrieved from http://www.theses.fr/2014EHES0133.

Greffion, J., & Breda, T. (2015). Façonner la prescription, influencer les médecins. Les effets difficilement saisissables du cœur de métier des grandes entreprises pharmaceutiques [Shaping prescriptions, influencing doctors. The hard-to-grasp effects at the heart of large pharmaceutical companies' professions]. *Revue de la régulation. Capitalisme, institutions, pouvoirs*, *17*, 1–26.

Hayden, C. (2015). Generic medicines and the question of the similar. In S. Sismondo, & J. A. Greene (Eds.), *The pharmaceutical studies reader* (pp. 261–267). Chichester, UK: Wiley Blackwell.

Mackintosh, M., Banda, G., Tibandebage, P., & Wamae, W. (Eds.). (2016). *Making medicines in Africa: The political economy of industrializing for local health*. London, UK: Palgrave Macmillan.

Mulinari, S. (2016). Regulating pharmaceutical industry marketing: Development, enforcement, and outcome of marketing rules. *Sociology Compass*, *1*(10), 74–86.

Peterson, K. (2014). *Speculative markets: Drug circuits and derivative life in Nigeria*. London, UK: Duke University Press Books.

Pourraz, J. (2019). *Réguler et produire les médicaments contre le paludisme au Ghana et au Bénin : Une affaire d'Etat ? Politiques pharmaceutiques, normes de qualité et marchés de médicaments [Regulating and producing malaria drugs in Ghana and Benin: A State affair? Pharmaceutical policies, quality standards, and drug markets]*. Doctoral dissertation, Ecole des Hautes Etudes en Sciences Sociales, Paris, France. Retrieved from http://www.theses.fr/2019EHES0014.

Ravelli, Q. (2015). *La stratégie de la bactérie. Une enquête au coeur de l'industrie pharmaceutique [The bacteria strategy. An investigation at the heart of the pharmaceutical industry].* Paris, France: Seuil.

Scheffer, P. (2017). *Quelle formation à l'indépendance est-elle possible pour les étudiants en médecine, par rapport à l'influence de l'industrie pharmaceutique ? [What training is possible for medical students' independence, in light of the pharmaceutical industry's influence?].* Doctoral dissertation, University of Paris 8, France. Retrieved from https://formindep.fr/wp-content/uploads/2017/08/th%c3%a8se-Paul-9-mars-2017.pdf.

Singh, S. (2018). *Entry and operation strategies of Indian pharmaceutical firms in Africa under the dynamics of markets and institutions.* Doctoral dissertation, Aix-Marseille University, France. Retrieved from http://www.theses.fr/2018AIXM0238.

Steiner, P. (2005). Le marché selon la sociologie économique [The market based on economic sociology]. *Revue européenne des sciences sociales*, 43(132), 31–64.

# 10 Self-medication versus consultation

## Individual autonomy and dependence in health decisions

*Carine Baxerres, Kelley Sams, Roch Appolinaire Houngnihin, Daniel Kojo Arhinful, Jean-Yves Le Hesran*

### Introduction

Individuals can address their health problems in one of two ways: on their own, in their home or close social environment; or with the help of specialists, which as a rule involves payment. Medications play an important role in both the intimate sphere of the home and the professional sphere outside, regardless of where the drugs lie on the spectrum, from biochemical molecules to standardized or nonstandardized herbal treatments. Both therapeutic and commercial, they are used by individuals to treat their own health and by professionals who write prescriptions based on their diagnoses. A focus on medications allows us to analyze the ways in which people manage their health and to understand the choices they make to do so. What interests us as anthropologists, epidemiologists, and public health specialists in the context of our research in Benin and Ghana is understanding the mechanisms that explain why people either treat themselves at home or seek out a biomedical professional and the temporalities and logics they use to move from one to the other.[1]

The literature in the social sciences, social epidemiology, and public health on health-care-seeking behavior is vast, in contexts in both the Global South (Fournier & Haddad, 1995; Mahendradhata, Souares, Phalkey, & Sauerborn, 2014; Ridde et al., 2018; Sams, 2017) and the Global North (Chaix, Navaie-Waliser, Viboud, Parizot, & Chauvin, 2006; Goldberg, Melchior, Leclerc, & Lert, 2002; Jacquet et al., 2018; Vallée & Chauvin, 2012), to name but a few. A whole series of context-specific social, economic, and structural factors have been proposed to explain behaviors. The premise of a recent study in France, based on the work of Robert Castel (2009), was that health-care practices can be understood as being shaped positively by individuals' own choices or negatively by the constraints to which they are subject, depending on their characteristics (Brutus, Fleuret, & Guienne, 2017). In his study of undocumented migrants in the United States, Nolan Kline describes how the political context of immigration influences health-care utilization and leads to the development of informal structures and alternative practices (Kline, 2017). In countries of the Global South, the emphasis is generally on economic, structural, and even "cultural" constraints, favoring a "single story" rather than alternative accounts that go against this dominant narrative (Mkhwanazi, 2016).

For the purposes of this chapter and to answer our question, we will examine three important concepts. The first is the *social determinants* that shape individuals' objective conditions (social class, income, education level, family situation, etc.).[2] The health-related institutional and social supports that individuals can mobilize must be taken into account as well, i.e., insurance mechanisms, characteristics of health-care offerings and medication availability, and belonging to social networks (Castel, 2009).

The second is the concept of *autonomy*, a basic definition that highlights "the capacity to think, decide, and act on the basis of such thought and decision freely and independently and without let or hindrance" (Gillon, 1985, p. 1806). Here again, institutional and social supports must be incorporated when analyzing autonomy with regard to health issues. The concept of autonomy and medication use has been researched extensively in relation to the issue of self-medication, the subject of several studies in France in recent years (cited throughout in this chapter), a country with its pharmaceutical monopoly under pressure from the European economic community (see Chapter 3). Self-medication may be defined narrowly (the use without a prescription of commercial specialty products to treat a health issue) or broadly (the use of any existing health products, or even health-care practices, including "prescriptions" written by other actors—from social circles or distribution or care facilities that are not legally authorized to do so—as well as "disguised self-medication," when the patient asks his or her doctor to include specific products on the prescription) (Brutus et al., 2017; Bureau-Point, Baxerres, & Chheang, 2020; Fainzang, 2012; Moloney, 2017). We consider self-medication by individuals to be the use of health products without the supervision of a professional who individuals recognize as being able to "prescribe," whether or not that person is actually authorized to do so.

The third concept of *popular knowledge* will be useful for us to understand what guides individual practices. Raymond Massé defines popular knowledge as "sociocultural constructs that reflect the vision that populations have of the world of health and illness." It is authentic knowledge, collected in a true "cultural system of common sense." "Constructed from a set of basic elements (beliefs, attitudes, values, etc.)," this cultural system "allows the individual to interpret the illness" and "to build models that explain the causes, progression, and treatment of his or her illness" (Massé, 1995, pp. 14 and 236).[3] While not particularly novel, these three concepts will be important in our discussion here of public health.

In this chapter, we will show how, in the Beninese and Ghanaian contexts we studied, medication is an indicator both of individuals' autonomous and positive management of their health, and of inequalities in their personal health and utilization of health services by socioeconomic status, urban or rural context, and country of residence. We will see that, depending on the health services and medication available to them and the health issues they face, people make different trade-offs in varying temporalities between several forms of self-medication and consulting a professional. These trade-offs may reveal individuals' *autonomy* with regard to health or their *dependence* on the health-care system[4] in relation to their *social determinants*. These determinants also highlight that autonomy and dependence are not contradictory but instead are extensively interrelated. Although the overall logic of health-seeking behavior appears to be relatively universal for people in both Benin and Ghana, we will see that structural and especially economic constraints affect some more than others. To understand these, we must first set the scene and describe the health-care services and medicines available in the two countries.

## Differing health-care services and medication options in Benin and Ghana

The Ghanaian biomedical health-care system took root during colonial times led by the British (UK colonization: 1874–1957). In 1923, the Gold Coast Hospital, Korle Bu, was built, and for many years considered the most advanced facility in Africa (Arhinful, 2003). The biomedical health-care system in Benin was also launched during the colonial period (French colonization: 1894–1960) but a bit later than in Ghana, at the beginning of the 1930s (Baxerres, 2013). While these two countries share a similar geographic location, and have been confronted with similar Global Health actors and policies (Baxerres & Eboko, 2019), several national differences seem important in the types of health-care services and pharmaceuticals that are available in both countries.

Until the Bamako Initiative was implemented in this country in 1988, Benin provided free biomedical health services for its population, whereas Ghana charged people for health care from the late 1960s/early 1970s and in 1985 reintroduced full user fees and cost recovery for medication.[5] The privatization of health care can be seen in Benin beginning in 1986 based on World Bank and International Monetary Fund recommendations. From that time, the national government limited the number of public servants in the health sector (Savina & Boidin, 1996). Young medical professionals were compelled to find new job prospects, which most frequently meant setting up their own practices or working in an already existent private health center. This led to an increase in small private health facilities in Cotonou and in Southern Benin from the late 1980s. These small private health centers often function in ways that are at odds with the legislation that defines them. Yet, it is not easy to categorize them into two groups of formal and informal health centers (Baxerres, 2013).[6]

Since 2003, Ghana has implemented the National Health Insurance Scheme (NHIS), which is still today one of the most advanced public health insurance systems in sub-Saharan Africa (Antwi, 2019). In Benin, it was not until 2017 that the Insurance for Building Human Capital (ARCH) was launched, but things do not seem to be happening quickly (Deville, Fecher, & Poncelet, 2018; Gbénahou, 2019).[7] While these policy-level factors are not the only influences of how health-care services are used by people, they are very important in determining what

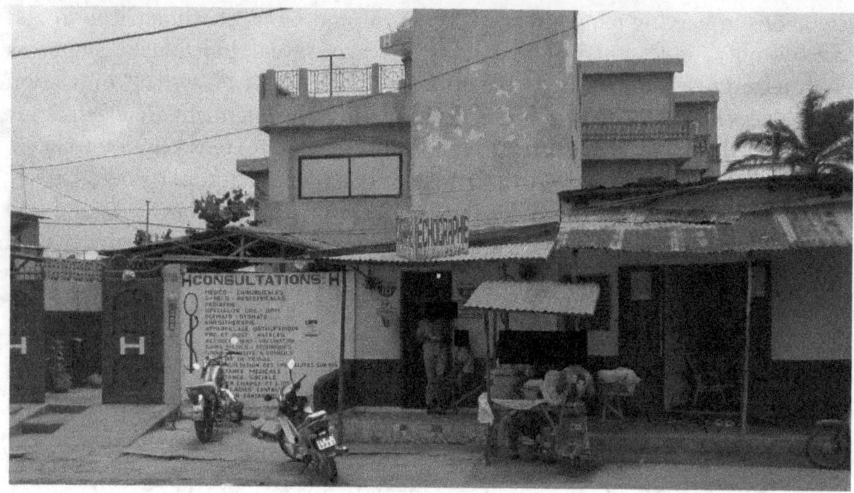


*Figure 10.1* Small private health center in Cotonou.

Source: © IRD/Aubierge Kpatinvoh, September 2015

types of facilities are available and at what costs. The multiplicity of biomedical care, offered by different types of institutions (public, private for-profit, private not-for-profit, informal), has developed differently between Benin and Ghana and between urban and rural contexts.[8]

The city of Cotonou has a large variety of health-care services, including all levels of the public health system (national reference hospital, district hospital, neighborhood health center, city health center, and even independent maternity ward), several mission hospitals, large private clinics, and many small private health centers (Figure 10.1). The availability of health-care services, the involvement of professionals, and specializations vary according to the facility. Loosely following the public health pyramid's recommendation of services that should be offered at each level, the private sector is very heterogeneous in the services offered, as well as in the relationship between the prices charged and the services received. Accra also had a great diversity of biomedical health-care facilities, larger than that of Cotonou due to a large wealthy population. The different levels of the public health pyramid are present in the city as well as private hospitals and clinics of different sizes but with few mission hospitals. However, in Accra, the same type of small private health centers seen in Cotonou do not exist.

The available types of biomedical services were very different between the rural research sites of the two countries. For example, in Benin, the types of services offered in semirural settings in the Mono department were distributed similarly to Cotonou, but on a much smaller scale. The public health centers followed the public health pyramid for this area; there were also mission health centers, some small private health centers, and a few larger private facilities. In Comé, a city in Mono with a population of 80,000, there were over 15 private health centers.

In the small city of Lobogo, population 17,000, there were at least 6. However, this was very different in rural Ghana; in Breman Asikuma and the surrounding areas, only one private health center was found: a maternity home that also offered general health-care services. Most of these facilities were different levels of public facilities (district hospital, health center, community-based health planning, and services [CHPS] compound), or occasionally a mission facility such as the one found in the district capital, Breman Asikuma, where the public district hospital is a mission hospital (see Figure 10.2 below).

Unlike in Benin, there were no small, informal private health facilities in rural Ghana. The "injection doctors" described in the past (Senah, 1997) did not seem to be continuing their activity in the research sites during the time of data collection. While the Government of Benin favored a policy of community health workers to share health advice and products with people, as promoted by many Global Health actors (WHO, USAID, Global Fund, etc.), in Ghana, rural populations were mainly reached through CHPS compounds (nurses, health assistants), that, when possible, sometimes conducted outreach visits to remote villages and hamlets.

Examining the pharmaceutical medications that are available at these health facilities in both countries is interesting. Officially, in Benin, medication can only be distributed by public or mission facilities. Private health centers can only prescribe medications for patients who go on to purchase from private retailers. In Ghana, private and public outlets of pharmaceutical distribution were intertwined and all facilities that offered health care were also authorized to sell pharmaceuticals. Apart from these different actors in health-care services, pharmaceuticals are also (and primarily) available to the population from private retailers: private

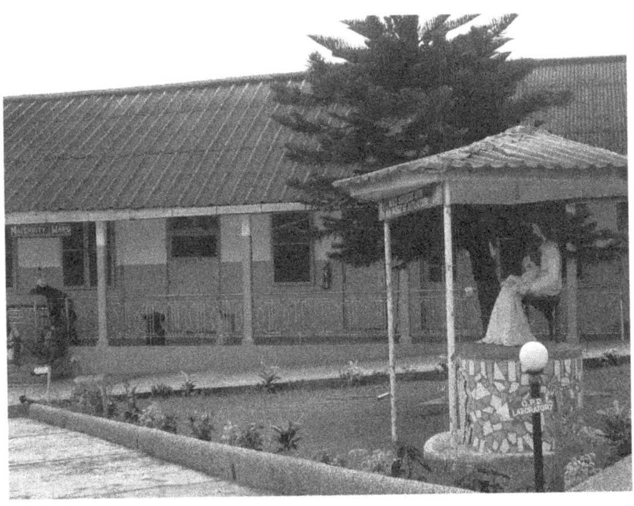

*Figure 10.2* Public district mission hospital of Breman Asikuma in Ghana.

Source: © IRD/Carine Baxerres, November 2015

pharmacies, mainly in cities (exclusively in the case of Ghana); over-the-counter (OTC) medicine shops in rural areas and in working-class neighborhoods in cities in Ghana; pharmaceutical depots in rural areas in Benin; and informal sellers in urban and rural areas in Benin.[9]

We will now analyze how people navigate these biomedical health-care services and drugs to manage their own health and that of their family. What logics emerge and which actors play a significant role in the two countries and in the urban and rural contexts we investigated?

## Understanding "essential" management of family health events

The population survey we conducted among approximately 600 families in each of the different contexts—urban and rural in Benin and Ghana—allowed us to quantify families' needs for health care, health management practices, and the realities of health-care-seeking behavior.[10]

These surveys indicate that in the various study areas, 70–90% of the ailments adults encounter on a daily basis are treated at home without requiring any biomedical consultation.[11] This rate is significantly higher in rural areas in both countries—90 versus 78% in Benin, 77 versus 70% in Ghana—likely due to a lower availability of health care and perhaps also to the lower availability of quickly accessed cash that is associated with agricultural and livestock activities (Baxerres & Le Hesran, 2010).

It is interesting to note that in all four of the contexts studied, the people we spoke to mentioned very similar day-to-day health problems. Our survey covered "health events" experienced in the previous 7 days.[12] People mostly reported very general symptoms: headache (12–30%), aches and pains (15–30%), fatigue (2.5–11%), and stomachache (4–9%). Symptoms indicative of infectious diseases (runny nose, cough, fever) (5–11%) were also reported. Popular nosological entities associated with malaria, known as *palu* in Benin and *malaria* in Ghana (see Chapter 7), also ranked high on the list of the most frequently encountered ailments (15–26%). Underscoring once again the discrepancy between "biomedical" and "popular" disease entities, this was true regardless of the local malaria epidemiological facies, despite higher parasite transmission in rural areas and more limited transmission in urban areas, due to pollution and a less favorable environment for mosquitoes. The chronic disease most often mentioned by the families surveyed was hypertension, commonly known as *tension* in Benin and *pressure* or *BP* in Ghana. It is significantly more prevalent in the city of Cotonou (6%) than in the other sites surveyed (between 1 and 3%), where it nevertheless represents a major health concern (reports are made on a weekly basis).[13] When we ask people about the origin of the health events, the causes evoked may differ between urban and rural environments and relate to people's living conditions: city dwellers more often associate their symptoms with pollution, noise, and stress (physical and mental fatigue) while rural inhabitants attribute them to harsh working conditions (heat, sun, physical fatigue). There also seem to be different ways of talking about symptoms in Benin and Ghana: "Fatigue" was more often mentioned in Benin, and "headaches" and "pain" in Ghana.

For these very common daily ailments, the same therapeutic classes of drugs were generally used by families that did not first consult a biomedical professional in the four contexts studied: analgesics (20–30%), antimalarial drugs (10–16%), anti-inflammatory and antirheumatic drugs (5–10%), vitamins and tonics (6–10%), and antibiotics (4–6%). Several particular molecules from these therapeutic classes are mainly used: paracetamol (analgesic), ibuprofen (anti-inflammatory), quinine and artemisinin-based combination therapies (antimalarial drugs),[14] and amoxicillin and metronidazole (antibiotics). These six molecules or combinations account for more than 50% of the drugs consumed by people in all of the areas.

Why do so many treatments involve these specific drugs? Because they are on the list of essential medicines defined by the health authorities of both countries. They have a long history as effective compounds and are available in generic form. They are also the drugs most frequently prescribed by health professionals. These molecules have very broad indications (fever, pain, broad-spectrum antibiotics) and are effective against numerous health problems. They therefore constitute an "essential" pharmacopoeia, one that is minimal and safe for families and can be used to treat most common ailments, similar to what health centers offer, and in many people's minds just as effective. A study we conducted in Cotonou of nearly 14,000 medical visits in three public health centers clearly shows that people consult providers primarily for infectious or parasitic problems such as acute respiratory infections (13.1%), malaria (21.8%), and infectious syndromes (30%). The notation of "infectious syndrome" on health center records indicates that the origin of the infection is unknown. This is a "catch-all" diagnosis that shows how difficult it is for providers to make an accurate diagnosis in the absence of additional tests (such as blood cultures). We will come back to this point in the conclusion.

Returning to families' use of pharmaceuticals and what individuals consider to be self-medication, we conducted exhaustive data collection during our participatory observations in urban and rural pharmaceutical distribution sites in Ghana and Benin. Standing at the counter alongside the vendors, we observed that, depending on the distribution site—pharmacies or OTC medicine shops in Ghana; pharmacies, pharmaceutical depots, or informal vendors in Benin—between 62 and 82.5% of drug purchases followed a spontaneous request from customers: either oral, showing an empty drug container (box, blister pack, tube), or presenting a piece of paper with the name of the product(s) (see table 10.1).[15]

Our quantitative and qualitative studies thus clearly show that, regardless of the differences in regulations, pharmaceutical distribution methods, and healthcare services, self-medication is by far the most common modality for purchasing medications in both countries. Let us now examine how qualitative studies can help us understand these findings and flesh them out with regard to social determinants and living situation.

*Table 10.1* Medication purchase modalities in various distribution sites

| Purchase modality | Benin | | | Ghana | | |
|---|---|---|---|---|---|---|
| | Urban pharmacies (n = 972) | Rural pharmacies (n = 1123) | Rural informal vendors (n = 521) | Urban pharmacies (n = 370) | Urban OTC shops (n = 703) | Rural OTC shops (n = 1040) |
| Spontaneous request (%) | 73 | 65 | 70 | 62 | 82.5 | 78 |
| Prescription (%) | 20 | 30 | 0 | 21.5 | 0 | 1.5 |
| Request for advice (%) | 7 | 5 | 30 | 16.5 | 17.5 | 20.5 |

Source: Authors.

## When people feel in control of their health problems

### *Self-medication as explained by the importance of popular knowledge*

Through the in-depth interviews we conducted with families in various contexts studied in Benin and Ghana, it became clear that, whatever their socioeconomic status, people initially managed their health problems or ailments either on their own or with help from their family and friends. People have extensive knowledge about health and medicines that they logically mobilize when confronted with a health issue. The interviews that we conducted are interspersed with statements like "I took batrim [for Bactrim® or cotrimoxazole], three tablets in the morning for three days, to soothe my stomach ache" (father of a "poor" family, Mono department, Benin, January 2015); or "when I develop boils or have joint pain, I just go to the drugstore to buy medicine like quick action efpac" (grandfather, "middle class" family, Breman Asikuma, Ghana, March 2016); or "because I get hypoglycemia quickly, when time goes by and maybe I haven't eaten, when I start shaking, I take vitamin C… UPSA-C, that's what I take. So, if I take that and I still don't feel better, I take calcium or magnesium in addition" (mother of a "wealthy" family, Cotonou, December 2014). Depending on the families and places of residence, this knowledge includes both pharmaceuticals and herbal remedies, which are taken as an alternative or simultaneously.

Thus, rather than just for mild symptoms or health problems, as have often been reported in the literature, this frequent self-medication is primarily used to treat health issues that people have under control or believe they have under control. This excerpt from an interview with a mother of a "poor" family living in Cotonou talking about her 14-year-old daughter illustrates this point: "Adèle does not get sick very often, the only time she has been sick is with jaundice (*ictère*)[16] (…), she had that last year, (…) it was really serious, if we hadn't taken good care of her, she would have passed. Her father had to buy the medicines that help the blood, and I sought out coconut and kinkeliba tree roots that I prepared.

That's what I gave her first and it got better" (December 2014). Another example is a mother from an upper class household in Accra who explained how she treated her son's recent illness, and also treated her other children as well: "He was coughing persistently, it was not going, it goes it comes, it goes it comes, it goes it comes, so I just decided to buy the flemex. It wasn't going. I mean after a week, so I bought the antibiotics to add and gave them piriton… because all three [children] have allergies" (March 2015). This observation has also been made in other contexts, including in France and in relation to chronic diseases (Brutus et al., 2017; Fainzang, 2012). "The criterion is that of known rather than benign disorders, as this experiential knowledge may relate to serious disorders, but ones the patient knows and, above all, recognizes" (Brutus et al., 2017, p. 9). Thus, when people are familiar with the health problem, they logically do not turn to a health professional. In some families, initial at-home management even seems like a necessary step, proving that the parents (often the mother) take good care of their children. During a bimonthly follow-up with a "wealthy" family in Cotonou, the mother explained that "she cannot go to the hospital for an ailment for which she knows the treatment; if the child cannot get warm, coughs, or catches a cold she's not going to run to the hospital" (July 2015).

As Brutus et al. (2017) show in French contexts, self-medication is not merely a linear practice, a step in an individual's health-care path before turning to professionals. Yet again indicating the importance of the popular knowledge individuals mobilize for their health, in several situations we studied, individuals decided to combine practices from the domestic sphere with a biomedical consultation. A mother from a "poor" family living in the Mono department in Benin explained that she had given "home" medicines (referring to informal vendors) to her 18-year-old son for "worm problems," then went to the hospital, and upon returning home she gave him more "home" medicines, which was when the problem ended (bi-monthly monitoring, April 2015). In Ghana, we found a similar situation, with a mother in an Accra "middle-class" household who explained, "I remember, there was a time I sent my daughter to the hospital…the [medicines] which were given to me, I came home and gave them to the child but still, at the end of it all, I went with her again to the pharmacy to buy [medicine] for her before she got better" (January, 2015). In both countries as well, we found mothers or fathers who would give herbals in addition to medicines prescribed by health centers.

The knowledge that people mobilize for health and medicines in the different contexts we have studied is built through a syncretism between practices transmitted from generation to generation and biomedicine (Baxerres, 2013). As Laurent Brutus et al. noted in French contexts, the relationship with biomedical professionals is also important in Benin and Ghana. "Self-medication is not so much characterized by the absence of medical advice, but by how it is transformed, and the use the patient makes of it" (2017, p. 9). Thus, in Benin and Ghana, people acquire knowledge when they go for a consultation in a biomedical health facility. They then follow that same advice again in the future for symptoms they consider to be similar. They also learn from the biomedical professionals in their social environment who have a broad range of skills (from the specialist physician to the nurse, midwife, nursing assistant, and even the pharmacy salesperson, medical representative, or hospital administrator). People also learn from and are influenced by their entire social environment: neighbors, colleagues, and immediate and extended family, as previously described in the literature (Jansen, 1995; Quintero & Nichter, 2011). Marion David and Véronique Guienne talk about "collective prescriptions for behavior or consumption" (2019, p. 3). The Internet and social networks, particularly WhatsApp, are now increasingly used in Benin and Ghana to convey information about health, illness, and treatments. Finally, the media (radio, television, newspapers) are another significant vector of information, through public health awareness messages, information about health development projects, and even advertisements for different kinds of health products.[17]

Similar to what recent research conducted in France has demonstrated, we find in the context of our research that self-medication also occurs through experimentation or testing that people perform on themselves when they experience symptoms. "If you want to use leaves, use them to clearly see how they work. In the same way, you're going to focus on a single drug for a while and see how it works… that gives you a clear idea of what really cured the disease" (father of a "middle-class" family, Mono department, January 2015). Laurent Brutus et al. talk about a "daily experimentation on one's own that is primarily based on experience," which is to be understood both in the sense of "having the experience of," as we saw above with regard to consultation experiences, and in the sense of "experimenting" (2017, p. 10). Sylvie Fainzang (2014) evokes a true "experience-based-medicine." People perform these tests by self-medicating, which if effective, enables them to avoid consulting specialists. A mother in a semirural Breman Asikuma "middle-class" household explained, "when [my husband] notices that any of the children is sick then he tells us to use herbal medicine for a while to see if there would be a good result. If there's anything more to do then we would take them to the hospital…most times he wants to see the result first. And most of the time too it doesn't get to that, to take them to the hospital" (interview, November 2014). The concept of "experiential knowledge" may be interesting to consider here. Without wanting to mobilize a "fashionable" notion, used outside its usual health domain (chronic diseases, disability), it seems to us that by evoking this idea for frequent daily drug consumption rather than to treat acute symptoms, we are able to demonstrate how individual "testing" of the body is important in these situations and that it results in collectively constructed knowledge that is transmitted to the individual.[18]

### *Products and purchase sites conditioned by social determinants*

Self-medication is widespread in Benin and Ghana, regardless of socioeconomic status, context, and place of residence. However, the products and pharmaceutical distribution sites utilized differ depending on the families and their country (Benin or Ghana) and context (urban or rural) of residence.

"Wealthy" families in Cotonou and Accra are more likely to go to pharmacies, while "poor" families in these two capital cities are more likely to go to OTC medicine sellers (in Ghana) or informal vendors (in Benin). The medicines used for self-medication in rural areas are commonly purchased from OTC medicine sellers in Ghana and informal vendors in Benin, regardless of socioeconomic status. Our quantitative data show that in rural Benin these sources account for 70% of the pharmaceuticals used to self-medicate versus 30% in the city of Cotonou.

In Benin, the drugs used for self-medication are sometimes purchased from health centers, more often in rural areas than in cities, without a prior consultation. The percentage of sales following a "spontaneous request" for drugs by the "patient," who then becomes simply a "client," can be as high as 15–20% of total sales in the pharmacy of certain health centers (a public neighborhood health center and a small mission health center that we observed, for example). Indicative of the phenomenon of drug commodification in health centers in Benin (Baxerres, 2013), these centers—whether private or public, urban, or rural—are never utilized for the purposes of practicing self-medication in Ghana.[19]

We also observed a kind of gradation in the self-medication practices of families that may involve a succession of different types of products, purchased in different places. Some people start self-medicating with plants before using pharmaceuticals (or vice versa) and then may return to other herbal remedies later. Others start with one type of pharmaceuticals (e.g., analgesics) before turning to others (e.g., antimalarials) later when the fever, in this example, does not go down. Some people start self-medicating with leftovers from previous prescriptions before going to buy other products if the problem persists. Others in Benin start by using drugs purchased from informal vendors before using those purchased at the pharmacy, at times interspersing these with drugs purchased in a health center (without prior consultation).[20] "Poor" families are generally the most likely to self-medicate multiple times before consulting a professional.

Herbal treatments are an important object that warrants some attention. Our quantitative studies show very different realities on this subject in Benin and Ghana. In Cotonou, households self-medicated with herbal treatments in response to the "health events" in the previous 7 days 4% of the time, compared to 94% for pharmaceuticals (2% combined both types of remedies). In the rural area of Lobogo, 14.8% of the treatments used were herbal, versus 66% for pharmaceuticals and 8.6% combining the two. In contrast in Ghana, herbal treatments were much more widely used in Accra, in nearly 30% of cases, compared to 15% in rural areas. Phytotherapy was more frequently used alone (not in combination with pharmaceuticals) in Ghana, where a nonnegligible percentage of herbal medicines are standardized (see Chapter 8). In Benin, the phytotherapy used was mainly prepared at home (concocted with ingredients bought at the market or collected from the surrounding environment). Offering standardized phytotherapy products thus seems to modify the public's understanding and exclusive use of them vis-à-vis pharmaceuticals.

## When individuals feel the need for outside professional advice

### *Comparable logics but inequalities in temporality and options*

A similar logic for when to seek help from biomedical professionals was used in both countries and regardless of socioeconomic status. Individuals will consult a professional when the health problem does not go away, returns, or worsens after one or more self-medication practice(s). A father of a "poor" family living in the Mono department of Benin explains: "after three days, if it doesn't get better, it isn't working, you have to know that it's beyond the pills you buy, then you have to go to the hospital" (interview, January 2015). A mother from an upper class semirural family in Ghana used a similar logic to explain seeking help: "After I heard the child cough…I thought maybe it is just a small unexpected cough. Later the cough persisted so I went to a drugstore nearby…he gave [me] cough medicine for the child. After I gave the medicine to the child, he started vomiting phlegm… later we took the child to the hospital, and there we heard it was asthma" (interview, November 2014). Similar logics were expressed in Cotonou and Accra, irrespective of socioeconomic status. A mother from an Accra upper class household explained, "when someone is not feeling well, you have to know a particular place. If for example it is headache, you go to the pharmacy… The first aid is a painkiller to calm it down. If it is not working, you go to hospital" (interview, February 2015).

The fact that the health problem is considered serious at this point (the symptoms are multiplying and/or prolonged, the patient appears to be quite unwell) and that it is a cause for concern justifies going to see a doctor in all the contexts studied. Therefore, in some situations, when the problem appears to be severe from the outset or when people cannot explain it or do not understand it, the self-medication stage may be skipped or considerably shortened. Patients may also consult a professional early on when they are seeking a specific biomedical technique, whether they believe they understand the health problem (when they request an injection) or not (when they request a medical examination).

Although these logics of health management are broadly similar across families, it is when individuals seek help from the external sphere that social and residence-based inequalities are most clearly expressed. In the various contexts studied, we found that when the problem was not solved through self-medication, the more precarious the person's socioeconomic status, the longer it took to see a professional. Our bimonthly monitoring visits with the various families show that this most often ranges from a few hours to 1 day for "wealthy" families to possibly several days (more than 1 or 2 weeks) for "poor" families. The anxiety that leads to the consultation often appears to be more pronounced in "poor" families than in "wealthy" ones. A mother from a "poor" family living in Cotonou explains, "I don't go to the hospital like this myself; before going, I have to know that it is really out of my league. If an illness arrives and I treat it at home myself without any improvement, I take it to the hospital. That's how it is, but that doesn't happen very often" (interview, February 2015).

Thus, the connection families develop with health facilities, which we observed for about a year, often appears characteristic of their socioeconomic status in both urban and rural areas. In Benin, for example, Myriam's family—consisting of herself, her husband, and their three children—is "poor" and lives on the outskirts of Cotonou. She explained in an interview that they had not been to the hospital for a very long time. During the bimonthly follow-up, Myriam was the only one to have had a consultation; she was supposed to go back for a checkup, but since she had no money, she prepared herbal tea instead. When her youngest (3-year-old) son had "measles," she gave him herbal tea and went to a small private health center to buy medicine without a consultation. Her 10-year-old daughter had a health problem that worried them considerably, but they did not go to the hospital; instead they gave her a variety of pharmaceuticals and herbal teas. In comparison, Aubierge's family, which is "wealthy," resides in the Mono department and consists of both parents and their five children, ranging in age from 17 years to a few months, regularly visit the health center. During the bimonthly monitoring period they had gone in a total of seven times. Two of the children (ages 4 and 14) were brought directly to the clinic when they had a fever. In Ghana as well, lower class households visited health facilities less than upper class households. Discourse about care-seeking was very different between the socioeconomic categories, with upper class families insisting on the importance of a biomedical approach. For example, one mother from an Accra lower class household stated, "as for me in particular, I have never been to the hospital. I don't know if I was taken when I was young but as far as I can remember, anytime I am sick, I either go to the pharmacy or the drugstore; then I buy what I need to buy and go, but when I realize that the medicines from those places are not working, then I get my herbs and cook it and drink it" (interview, January 2016). In contrast, a mother from an upper class Accra household stated, "The adults, I will be honest with you, we like to self-medicate, but when it comes to the kids, we don't take chances. We go [to the clinic]…I take them" (interview, March 2015). Generally in both countries, "wealthy" families more frequently (or quickly) bypass the self-medication stage.

A family's socioeconomic status also influences the type of health centers they use. However, the urban or rural context and the country of residence also have a strong impact on this point. In both Accra and Cotonou, for example, "wealthy" families are more likely to go to expensive private clinics or to the major public national reference hospitals to consult specialist physicians. "Poor" families are more likely to go to public health centers where they see nurses, or, in Cotonou, to small, inexpensive (often partly informal) private health centers. By contrast in rural areas, as we have seen, families do not have as many health-care options. Regardless of their socioeconomic status, all the families we studied in Breman Asikuma in Ghana go to public health centers for consultations or to the local mission facility.[21] This is also predominantly the case for the families studied in Benin's Mono department, even though they also have a few private health centers at their disposal.

The range of health-care options in a specific context may, as with self-medication practices, lead to a kind of gradated reliance on biomedical professionals. A mother from an urban upper class household in Accra described how she sought care from a private hospital for illnesses that seemed serious or unfamiliar, otherwise she would go to a public hospital or self-medicate. Families in Benin may first go to a small private health center close to home before seeking care at one or more other health facilities seen as having a higher level of competence, if necessary. We were told several stories of families navigating grueling obstacle courses to obtain health care. For example, a father from a "poor" family in Cotonou told us about his 11-month-old child, who had a fever he thought could be *palu*. He gave the boy paracetamol and ibuprofen, followed by moringa tea made from leaves he had taken from a tree near his home. When the fever did not go away, the next day he took the child to a small private health center nearby where he received several injections morning and evening for 3 days. But there was still no improvement so they went to a second small private health center where the child received another injection, but since he was really sick at this point, the father was advised to go to the nearest public district hospital.

Deciding which type of health center to visit is also heavily dependent on whether or not the family has health insurance, and the agreements this insurance has with specific health facilities. Contrary to expectations, the NHIS in Ghana did not have a strong impact on health-care utilization at the time of our studies. People are much more likely to have insurance coverage in Ghana than in Benin (our quantitative surveys show that nearly 70% of Ghanaians have insurance, mainly through its NHIS, compared to 10% of people living in Benin's capital and less than 4% in its rural areas).[22] However, many appear to be behind in their payments (only 44.24% of the families in Accra in the quantitative survey had renewed their annual membership). But even among those who have insurance, the fact that their expenses may be covered does not necessarily mean that they consult a biomedical professional more quickly or more often, particularly for the acute health issues on which our surveys were more specifically focused. Indeed almost half of the people with health insurance who we surveyed in Accra declared they had not used it during their last health problem. This may be due to the fact that not all health expenses are covered by insurance. Furthermore, seeking help from a biomedical professional for frequent health issues that are perceived as not being (too) serious did not appear to represent a sufficient advantage, but in fact may be seen as a waste of time (indirect costs) compared to visiting a pharmaceutical retailer (pharmacy, OTC medicine shop). "When we do lab tests, for that you have to pay money…At times when you go there [to the hospital], they say 'this medication is not covered by the Health Insurance' or 'that medication is out of stock'. And the medicines they will give you are those that cost 3 and 4 cedis [USD 0.5–0.7] but for the expensive ones, there is no way you're going to get it. (…). So if I have the money and I can [go to] the pharmacy, it's better than me going to waste much time over there. At times, maybe you'll come [from the hospital] and you wouldn't have that money to go buy medicine at the pharmacy for the child…which means that, the hospital you visited, what was the use?…So I feel that the pharmacy is where I should go and show them the children for medication to be given to them. It is better for me" (interview with a mother from an urban Accra "middle-class" household, January 2015). Despite very strong political will for the NHIS in Ghana, one of the most advanced insurance programs in Africa, the program appears to have stagnated in growth while raising concerns of equity and sustainability (Antwi, 2019).

### *Distribution actors involved in health-care service provision*

In both countries, certain actors in the pharmaceutical distribution sector have significant influence on how families use outside professionals. As illustrated in the table 10.1, OTC medicine sellers in both rural and urban areas of Ghana, and informal vendors in rural Benin, offer advice in a relatively high number of cases (17–20% of cases in Ghana and 30% in rural Benin).

Because they are able to offer treatments for common health problems without the downside of a consultation in a health center—especially a public facility, with its long waiting times, direct and indirect costs, poor reception, and tense relations between providers and patients (see Bogart et al., 2013; Jaffré & Olivier de Sardan, 2003)—some consider these distribution actors to be professionals people can turn to when home remedies have failed to solve the problem. Individuals therefore view this as consultation and not as a form of self-medication. These pharmaceutical retailers' broad accessibility, both geographic (they are numerous) and financial (their products are generally less expensive than those of pharmacies), surely explains their popularity. In Accra, OTC medicine sellers are especially important for "poor" families.[23] However, in rural areas in both countries, where they are often the only outlets for medications (there are no pharmacies in rural Ghana; informal vendors are the most common retailers and often the only ones found in rural Benin), OTC medicine sellers in Ghana and informal vendors in Benin influence the health-care practices of the vast majority of families, whether they are "poor," "middle-class," or "wealthy."

In Benin, we did not conduct systematic observations of informal vendors in Cotonou as part of the Globalmed research program. However, our previous study in this city (Baxerres, 2013) found that they only play a minor role as health advisors, likely due to the greater connections that people have with health professionals in Cotonou than in rural areas and the greater media influence in that city.[24] This was confirmed by the family interviews conducted as part of this study. Of the 15 families we worked with in Cotonou, only two, both "poor," showed signs that their health-care practices were influenced by informal vendors. In rural areas, on the other hand, interviews found this influence to be significant. The mothers and fathers of families living in the Mono department, regardless of their socioeconomic status, often told us that they had learned about a particular drug they were taking through the informal vendors. "It was a night that I was so cold[25]… I bought para [paracetamol] that I took for two or three days but it didn't

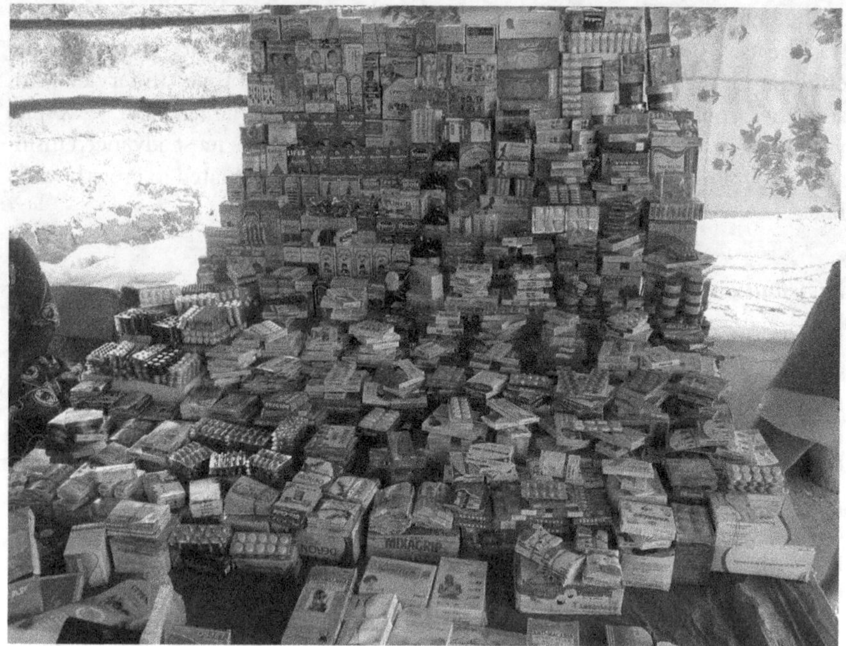


*Figure 10.3* Stand of an informal saleswoman in Benin rural area.

Source: © IRD/Carine Baxerres, April 2014

work, so one day I went to see a lady who sells at a sidewalk pharmacy. I told her about it, and she recommended that I take para C. Later that evening, the cold came back and I was shivering, then I drank that tablet and 15 minutes later I started sweating and the cold stopped... I was so happy, if I had had any money I would have gone and given it to the lady... that's when I started taking this tablet" (interview, "middle-class" father, December 2015).

The prescribing or even consultation role that the saleswomen play is evident in this statement by a "poor" father: "If you go over there and say 'sell me pills for body pain', she'll sell you this. They are the ones who know the names... if you only have pain in a particular area, tell them the part where it hurts, and they will sell you their medicine... even when you go to the doctor, they will ask, 'where does it hurt?'" (interview, December 2015).

In Ghana, many owners of OTC medicine shops have a very positive reputation and are seen in their neighborhood as preferred advisors regarding health. Some families indicated that they have a lot more confidence in attendants of OTC medicine shops than doctors. "I remember, there was a time I sent Princess [her daughter] to the hospital, I gave her the medicines which were given me, but still, she did not feel better... at the end of it all, I went with her again to the drugstore[26] to buy medicine for her before she got better, so I don't depend on hospitals most of the time... he [the owner of OTC medicine shop] is really knowledgeable about medicines" (interview with a "middle-class" mother, Accra, January 2015).

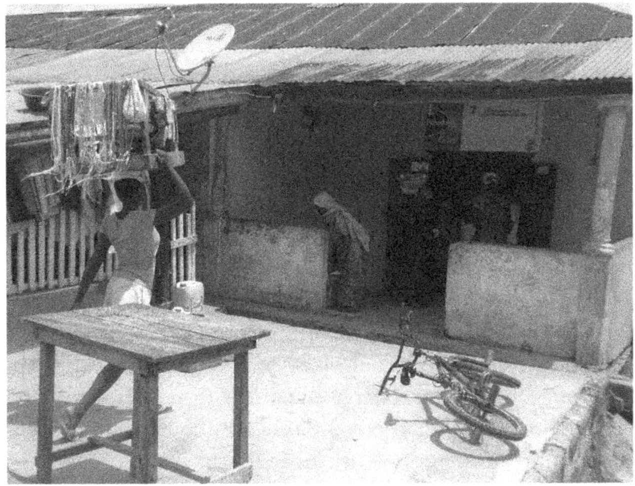

*Figure 10.4* A very popular OTC medicine shop in rural Ghana.

Source: © IRD/Eunice Ayimbila, May 2016

OTC medicine sellers play an even more important role in health care than informal medicine sellers in Benin. Indeed not all attendants have health backgrounds (few of them were retired midwives or nurses, for example), but some effectively combined their activity of selling medications with medical care such as giving infusions and injections, in spite of these practices not being officially permitted. At one OTC medicine shop in Accra, the owner had a small room behind the store where injections were given. There were beds where patients could be detained for a while. The owner compared the quality of health care to that received at the hospital. "Because of the treatment here, having time for you, talking to you, and doing all these things for you. People come from far. It is just like you have gone to the hospital but they don't pay for consultation..." (interview, OTC medicine seller, Accra, November 2015). Most OTC medicine sellers said they maintained excellent customer relationships and offered the best of care to their clients. Perceived expertise of the OTC medicine sellers then also contributed to the use of these shops as a primary resource. The mother of an Accra lower class household described a women medicine seller who she liked purchasing medications from, "She usually comes in the evening. She is very good. She gives a lot of advice before she gives the medicines. If it is too much for her too, she would tell you that you should go to the hospital" (interview, January 2016).

## Conclusion

In this chapter, we first discussed the dialectic of peoples' health-related autonomy/dependence or empowerment/vulnerability in the Global South contexts in which we worked. Studies in recent years in France illustrate both the normative context of contemporary individualism, which promotes autonomy, and the fact that modern-day patients take responsibility for their own health, thus freeing them from the yoke of "medical paternalism" and "the mirage of autonomy." They highlight the fact that autonomy is often manipulated by governments for economic purposes in a desire to control health-care spending, and that it therefore remains relative, particularly in the irrevocable link between patients and biomedical professionals (Brutus et al., 2017; Fainzang, 2012).

The situations we described in Benin and Ghana, in contexts where health expenditures are only infrequently covered by an insurance system, underline different realities. Here, self-medication reflects a form of positive autonomy, regardless of socioeconomic status or life contexts. Mobilizing their extensive "experiential knowledge," individuals draw on a wide range of health products at their disposal: pharmaceuticals offered in various distribution outlets, and herbal remedies either purchased or gathered from nearby courtyards, gardens, or bushes. Without dismissing the potential risk inherent to some of these practices (for example, overconsumption of anti-inflammatory drugs to treat aches and pains as we noted),[27] our data show some actual room for individuals to maneuver in how they manage their health. We believe this is not highlighted enough in the Global South.[28] However, it should be recognized, following first Anne-Marie Mol, then Emmanuelle Simon, Arborio, Halloy, and Hejoaka (2019), that this autonomy is essentially built collectively, as we have seen in Benin and Ghana, which may seem contradictory. These authors prefer to speak of "the logic of care" and "associated knowledge."

However, when people do not or no longer feel able to manage their health problems either on their own or in their social environment, this autonomy is largely constrained by their social determinants and place of residence. Socioeconomic inequalities in health are very clearly expressed in the contexts we studied, including in Ghana with its NHIS. We indicate the issue of the delay in seeking care: in both countries, the poorest people sometimes find themselves in significant distress that can lead to human tragedy, as evidenced by the high malaria mortality rate among children under 5 years of age in Africa.

Our comparative study in two countries that are close geographically but far apart in terms of health-care services and medicine availability allows us to make original observations about territorial inequalities in health. We have seen that the inhabitants of the capital cities and the semirural and rural areas we surveyed do not have the same options for health care. In these latter geographical contexts, we do not see socioeconomic inequalities in the choice of which pharmaceutical retailers or health professionals to consult, as available services are largely the same regardless of socioeconomic status. This is especially true in Ghana, where people only have access to OTC medicine shops and public health centers or mission hospitals. However, we do find inequalities in how promptly families seek professional treatment. Privatization of health care, very visible throughout Accra and Cotonou, and less evident in semirural Benin, is virtually non-existent in the research site that we studied in semirural Ghana. Heath facilities that are present in Breman Asikuma appear to be considerably "nationalized" since it is almost exclusively public.

This leads us to one final discussion: the place of providers. As we have seen in Benin, all kinds of health centers sometimes sold medications to individuals who had not been examined by staff at the center. The sale of pharmaceuticals appears to have gained a position there in the provision of care. In Ghana, health facilities were not visited solely to purchase medication, which was done at OTC medicine shops, or pharmacies. Unlike in Benin, there were no small private informal health facilities in rural Ghana. From another point of view, OTC medicine sellers are key actors in the distribution of pharmaceuticals but also in basic health-care services (injections, IVs). Then, it appears that, much more than in Benin, the distribution of pharmaceuticals in Ghana gained importance as a type of care. The presence of the numerous OTC medicine shops seemed to thwart the drive for the small private informal health-care centers that were found in Benin. This means that most providers do not even have access to basic clinical training (nurses, health-care aides).

One might legitimately question the place and role of biomedical professionals in the contexts we studied, where pharmaceutical retailers have a substantial presence, whether formal as in Ghana or informal as in Benin. According to a "disempowerment of the doctor" dynamic described in Western contexts, such as occurred between the two World Wars when American antibiotic manufacturers favored broad-spectrum molecules, thus encouraging less specific diagnosis (Podolsky & Kveim Lie, 2016), or when, more generally, the pharmaceutical industry relies on direct-to-consumer advertising campaigns (Dumit, 2012), one wonders whether the extensive and omnipresent pharmaceutical distribution in the Global South contexts we studied is a factor in devaluing the status of biomedical expertise. Given the current disenchantment with health services (our quantitative survey in public health centers in Cotonou found there were often fewer than 20 consults per day), cursory clinical examinations, and stereotypical prescriptions limited to a few essential drugs, it is important that health authorities reverse this trend by increasing what biomedical professionals can offer so that their clinical diagnoses are seen as providing true added value to patients beyond what they can do for themselves in their social environment or in their homes.

## Notes

1. The health-care professionals we have chosen to focus on in this chapter are biomedical and pharmaceutical practitioners. Although other types of professionals may be consulted in the contexts we studied (e.g., traditional healers, practitioners of Chinese medicine, and religious healers), this is relatively rare. Traditional healers are more often consulted about family, relationship, or professional problems, while herbal medicine in the domestic sphere is frequent. The use of herbal remedies will be discussed. It should also be pointed out that people make extensive use of health products to prevent future illnesses or to maintain their good health (Baxerres, 2013). These practices are more highly developed in Benin than in Ghana. However, they will not be described in this chapter, as we wanted to focus on how individuals manage current health problems.

2. Although "social determinants of health" is becoming increasingly important in public health, some scholars such as Gregory Simon have noted that this term does not take in account the role of resilience and hope. Simon advocates for the term social "influencers" rather than "determinants." See: https://medium.com/@KPWaResearch/whats-wrong-with-the-term-social-determinants-of-health-8e69684ec442, accessed September 2020.
3. The concepts of "popular" or "local" knowledge in health are more frequently used in Global South contexts, while "lay knowledge" is used more often in the Global North and is considered in the provider-patient relationship. The two are essentially equivalent.
4. As Sylvie Fainzang (2012) reminds us, "dependence" is used as an antonym of "autonomy" in the field of disability, when, following an accident or illness, a person becomes dependent on outside help for their daily activities. We find it relevant to our argument here, to emphasize that people's health care practices may be largely dependent on external factors and that their ability to decide and make free choices is thus biased.
5. In 1992, the "cash and carry" system was introduced. Health facilities were required to pay for drugs that they collected from medical stores, and patients were required to pay for services before being treated, all as a way of efficiently managing the drugs at a sub district level (Arhinful, 2003).
6. Indeed, whether or not a center has been authorized to operate does not strictly depend on the quality of care, the apparent cleanliness of the facility, or the status of its director (doctor, nurse, or midwife) and his or her actual presence in the health center. Many small health centers have obtained authorization through improper means: the reported director is not the one who actually runs the facility, authorizations are granted to nursing care facilities or childbirth clinics even though they offer a wider range of services and prescriptions. Some hospitalize patients without being authorized to do so; others perform deliveries without midwives on staff.
7. In 2008, before the ARCH, the Beninese authorities had established the Universal Health Insurance Scheme (RAMU), but implementation was quickly aborted. At this time only formal sector workers and their dependents are covered by Benin's National Pension Fund (FNRB) or private insurance companies. They still represent less than 10% of the country's population (Gbénahou, 2019).
8. Note that our data were collected between 2014 and 2017. However, there have been significant changes in Benin since 2017, related to reforms by the administration of President Patrice Tallon, such as the current ban on performing biomedical functions in both the public and private health sectors and the closure of many private health centers. These reforms undoubtedly impact the biomedical services currently available in that country.
9. See Chapter 3 for more information on these different actors in pharmaceutical distribution. In Ghana, OTC medicine shops are managed by non-pharmacists with a minimum academic level who must attend mandatory post-registration training sessions on a regular basis and are authorized to sell only OTC medicines and some public health program products such as antimalarials or contraceptives. They were numerous in the country (10,424 at the time of our study). Private pharmaceutical warehouses in rural Benin are also managed by people who do not have a degree in pharmacy. Owners are authorized to sell essential medicines from a limited list and are under a pharmacist's supervision. They shut down if a pharmacy opens within a 10-km radius. Linked to this strict legislation, their number is very few in rural Benin (165 in 2018). In Benin, the large number of informal vendors distribute medicines outside the formal channels imposed by the State: in markets, shops, stalls, on the side of busy roads, door-to-door, at home, on public transport, etc.
10. See the Introduction of this book for more information on the methodology used, quantitative and a combination of qualitative and quantitative here, and qualitative next.

11. We are discussing adults here so that we can analyze the numerous quantitative data points we have for the four different sites (two per country). This is not to suggest that these practices are very different for children (self-medication rates are between 70 and 84% for children in the four contexts), but that we have chosen to focus here on adults.
12. We created this "health notion" in social epidemiology for the purposes of this study. The idea was to ask families about broader issues than just the "health problems" defined by biomedicine. By using the term "health event," we can include all the reasons why people use medication.
13. However, hypertension can be hard to gauge. If the disease is treated properly, it does not cause acute symptoms. If not, its symptoms are nonspecific (headache, shortness of breath, swelling in the legs). This suggests that popular perceptions of *tension* or *pressure/BP* and treatment practices and the use of preventive medicines to prevent this disease are particularly fruitful to study regarding the issue of (non)-diagnosis and (non)-biomedical monitoring.
14. Quinine is used mainly in Benin (see Chapter 7).
15. These pieces of paper show that this was either an order placed by a third party with the person, advice from a relative, or a prescription from a health professional by telephone or without a prescription pad. In the latter cases, which were few, the person is not self-medicating. Since we were unable to distinguish between these situations, we counted them as "spontaneous requests," so this category may be slightly overestimated.
16. The French term was used in this interview conducted in the Fon language.
17. In a French context, Sylvie Fainzang discusses the multiple sources for gaining knowledge that people mobilize when they self-medicate, of a "baroque, composite, and recomposed knowledge." She also discusses a specific form of "circular knowledge" between patients and their physicians, in which the latter are able to reappropriate the testimonies of the former regarding the effectiveness and effects of treatments and use them during subsequent consultations (Fainzang, 2012).
18. The first use of the concept of experiential knowledge in health dates back to the 1970s, but it has increasingly been the subject of scientific production since the 2000s (Simon, Arborio, Halloy, & Hejoaka, 2019). Such knowledge "is developed through collective and sustained sharing among peers and is the result of a personal reflective process and work. Experiential knowledge automatically emerges in an interactional configuration between the patient and other patients within various mediation spaces such as peer groups, support groups, or the Internet and social networks" (p. 59). Emmanuelle Simon et al. note that there is no gap between experiential and scientific knowledge, as health-care professionals also develop experiential knowledge. Simon et al. also emphasize that experiencing the illness is not enough to develop experiential knowledge. Like us, Marion David and Véronique Guienne (2019) also utilize this notion in relation to self-medication.
19. However, unused prescribed drugs are commonly later taken for self-medication in both countries, as described in other contexts (Brutus et al., 2017; Fainzang, 2012).
20. Chapter 11 discusses the concept of a drug's "subjective quality," which in Benin partly explains these gradations of use by the various distribution points.
21. Although Breman Asikuma had limited health services, families in the study did not report traveling to seek care. One husband from a rural upper class family described seeking care and buying medication in Accra, but he was already in the city for other reasons. He did not travel there specifically for treatment.
22. In rural areas, however, 46.55% of respondents were affiliated with a *tontine*, a local savings system.
23. Note that pharmacy vendors in Accra also play a significant advisory role (16.5%), just behind OTC medicine sellers, which is not the case in Benin in Cotonou or even in the Mono department, where pharmacy vendors recommend products to

their clients in only 5–7% of cases. Regulation of pharmaceutical distribution combined with the health care services offered in both countries seem to allow formal retailers in Ghana greater free rein in offering advice than in Benin.

24. Data collected from a retailer in one Cotonou neighborhood showed that out of 205 customers, 82% had approached the retailer with a direct request for the drug they wanted. In the pharmaceutical sector of Cotonou's central market, this was true of 94% of the 260 "lay customers" (non-professionals) observed.
25. *Avivo* in the Mina language, which means "cold" or "shivering."
26. The term "drugstore" was used by respondents to refer to both pharmacies and OTC medicine shops, and many respondents described not knowing the difference between these two categories. In this case, the mother was referring to an OTC medicine shop.
27. These risks appear relatively minimal in French contexts (Brutus et al., 2017), unlike in North American where they are seen more broadly, such as in the opiate crisis.
28. Our research in Cambodia revealed very different realities. Linked to the country's political history, particularly the Khmer Rouge regime, people have developed much less room for maneuvering in terms of health care and a heavy dependence on pharmaceutical retailers (Bureau-Point et al., 2020). The inclusion of herbal medicine in the analysis might have demonstrated a form of autonomy restricted to that type of health product.

## Reference list


Antwi, A. A. (2019). *The pathway of achieving the universal health coverage in Ghana: The role of social determinants of health and "health in all policies."* Doctoral dissertation, University of Lille, France. Retrieved from http://www.theses.fr/2019LIL1A002.

Arhinful, D. K. (2003). *The solidarity of self-interest. Social and cultural feasibility of rural health insurance in Ghana.* Doctoral dissertation, African Studies Centre, Leiden University, The Netherlands. Retrieved from https://openaccess.leidenuniv.nl/handle/1887/12919.

Baxerres, C. (2013). *Du médicament informel au médicament libéralisé : Une anthropologie du médicament pharmaceutique au Bénin [From informal to liberalized drugs: An anthropology of pharmaceutical drugs in Benin].* Paris, France: Les Éditions des Archives Contemporaines.

Baxerres, C., & Eboko, F. (Eds.). (2019). Global health: Et la santé ? [Global health: And health?]. *Politique Africaine*, 4, 156.

Baxerres, C., & Le Hesran, J.-Y. (2010). Quelles ressources familiales financent la santé des enfants ? Les difficultés du recours aux soins pour traiter le paludisme en milieu rural sénégalais [What family resources pay for children's health? Challenges in seeking care to treat malaria in rural Senegal]. *Tiers Monde*, *202*, 149–165.

Bogart, L. M., Chetty, S., Giddy, J., Sypek, A., Sticklor, L., Walensky, R. P., … Bassett, I. V. (2013). Barriers to care among people living with HIV in South Africa: Contrasts between patient and healthcare provider perspectives. *AIDS Care*, *25*(7), 843–853.

Brutus, L., Fleuret, S., & Guienne, V. (2017). Se soigner par soi-même. *Recherche interdisciplinaire sur l'automédication [Taking care of yourself. Interdisciplinary research on self-medication].* Paris, France: CNRS éditions.

Bureau-Point, E., Baxerres, C., & Chheang, S. (2020). Self-medication and the pharmaceutical system in Cambodia. *Medical Anthropology*, p. 765–781. https://doi.org/10.1080/01459740.2020.1753726.

Castel, R. (2009). *La montée des incertitudes. Travail, protections, statut de l'individu [The rise of uncertainties. Labor, protections, and individual status].* Paris, France: Seuil.

Chaix, B., Navaie-Waliser, M., Viboud, C., Parizot, I., & Chauvin, P. (2006). Lower utilization of primary, specialty and preventive care services by individuals residing with persons in poor health. *European Journal of Public Health*, *16*(2), 209–216.

David, M., & Guienne, V. (2019). Savoirs expérientiels et normes collectives d'automédication [Experiential knowledge and collective self-medication standards]. *Anthropologie & Santé, 18, 1–13. http://journals.openedition.org/anthropologiesante/5089; DOI: https://doi.org/10.4000/anthropologiesante.5089.*

Deville, C., Fecher, F., & Poncelet, M. (2018). L'assurance pour le renforcement du capital humain (ARCH) au Bénin : Processus d'élaboration et défis de mise en œuvre [Insurance for building human capital (ARCH) in Benin: Development process and implementation challenges]. *Revue française des affaires sociales*, *1*, 107–123. https://doi.org/10.3917/rfas.181.0107.

Dumit, J. (2012). *Drugs for life. How pharmaceutical companies define our health*. London, UK: Duke University Press.

Fainzang, S. (2012). *L'automédication ou les mirages de l'autonomie [Self-medication or mirages of autonomy]*. Paris, France: Éditions PUF.

Fainzang, S. (2014). Managing medicinal risks in self-medication. *Drug Safety*, *37*, 333–342.

Fournier, P., & Haddad, S. (1995). Les facteurs associés à l'utilisation des services de santé dans les pays en développement [Factors associated with the use of health services in developing countries]. In H. Gérard, & V. Piché (Eds.), *Sociologie des populations [Sociology of populations]* (pp. 289–325). Montreal, Canada: Presses de l'Université de Montréal.

Gbénahou, H. B. M. (2019). Comprendre les faibles taux d'adhésion et de cotisation aux mutuelles de santé : Exploration dans quatre communes du Bénin [Understanding low membership and mutual health insurance contribution rates: Survey conducted in four municipalities in Benin]. *Anthropologie & Santé*, *18*, 1–19. http://journals.openedition.org/anthropologiesante/4847; https://doi.org/10.4000/anthropologiesante.4847.

Gillon, R. (1985). Autonomy and the principle of respect for autonomy. *British Medical Journal*, *290*, 1806–1808.

Goldberg, M., Melchior, M., Leclerc, A., & Lert, F. (2002). Les déterminants sociaux de la santé : Apports récents de l'épidémiologie sociale et des sciences sociales de la santé [Social determinants of health: Recent contributions from social epidemiology and the social sciences of health]. *Sciences Sociales et Santé*, *20*(4), 75–128.

Jacquet, E., Robert, S., Chauvin, P., Menvielle, G., Melchior, M., & Ibanez, G. (2018). Social inequalities in health and mental health in France. The results of a 2010 population-based survey in Paris metropolitan area. *PLOS ONE*, *13*(9), e0203676.

Jaffré Y., & Olivier de Sardan, J.-P. (Eds.). (2003). *Une médecine inhospitalière: Les difficiles relations entre soignants et soignés dans cinq capitales d'Afrique de l'Ouest [Inhospitable medicine: The difficult relationships between caregivers and patients in five capitals in West Africa]*. Paris, France: Karthala.

Jansen, J. M. (1995). *La quête de la thérapie au Bas-Zaïre [The quest for therapy in Lower Zaire]*. Paris, France: Karthala.

Kline, N. (2017). Pathogenic policy: Immigrant policing, fear, and parallel medical systems in the US South. *Medical Anthropology*, *36*(4), 396–410.

Mahendradhata, Y., Souares, A., Phalkey, R., & Sauerborn, R. (2014). Optimizing patient-centeredness in the transitions of healthcare systems in low- and middle-income countries. *BMC Health Services Research*, *14*, 386. https://doi.org/10.1186/1472-6963-14-386.

Massé, R. (1995). *Culture et santé publique. Les contributions de l'anthropologie à la prévention et à la promotion de la santé [Culture and public health. Contributions of anthropology to prevention and health promotion]*. Montreal, Canada: Gaëtan Morin.

Mkhwanazi, N. (2016). Medical anthropology in Africa: The trouble with a single story. *Medical Anthropology*, 35(2), 193–202.

Moloney, M. E. (2017). "Sometimes, it's easier to write the prescription": Physician and patient accounts of the reluctant medicalisation of sleeplessness. *Sociology of Health & Illness*, 39(3), 333–348.

Podolsky, S. H., & Kveim Lie, A. (2016). Futures and their uses: Antibiotics and therapeutic revolutions. In J. A. Greene, F. Condrau, & E. Siegel Watkins (Eds.), *Therapeutic revolutions. Pharmaceuticals and social change in the twentieth century* (pp. 18–42). Chicago, IL: The University of Chicago Press.

Quintero, G., & Nichter, M. (2011). Generation RX: Anthropological research on pharmaceutical enhancement, lifestyle regulation, self-medication, and recreational drug use. In M. Singer, & P. I. Erickson (Eds.), *A companion to medical anthropology* (pp. 339–350). Hoboken, NJ: Wiley Blackwell.

Ridde, V., Asomaning Antwi, A., Boidin, B., Chemouni, B., Hane, F., & Touré, L. (2018). Time to abandon amateurism and volunteerism: Addressing tensions between the Alma-Ata principle of community participation and the effectiveness of community-based health insurance in Africa. *BMJ Global Health*, 3(3), e001056.

Sams, K. (2017). Engaging conceptions of identity in a context of medical pluralism: Explaining treatment choices for everyday illness in Niger. *Sociology of Health & Illness*, 39(7), 1100–1116.

Savina, M. D., & Boidin, B. (1996). Privatisation des services sociaux et redéfinition du rôle de l'Etat : Les prestations éducatives et sanitaires au Bénin [Privatization of social services and redefinition of the role of the State: Educational and health services in Benin]. *Tiers Monde*, 37(148), 853–874.

Senah, K. A. (1997). *Money be man. The popularity of medicines in a rural Ghanaian community*. Unpublished doctoral dissertation, University of Amsterdam, The Netherlands.

Simon, E., Arborio, S., Halloy, A., & Hejoaka, F. (Eds.). (2019). *Les savoirs expérientiels en santé : Fondements épistémologiques et enjeux identitaires [Experiential knowledge in health: Epistemological foundations and identity issues]*. Nancy, France: Presses universitaires de Nancy.

Vallée, J., & Chauvin, P. (2012). Investigating the effects of medical density on health-seeking behaviours using a multiscale approach to residential and activity spaces: Results from a prospective cohort study in the Paris metropolitan area, France. *International Journal of Health Geographics*, 11, 54.

# 11 When subjective quality shapes the whole economy of pharmaceutical distribution and production

*Carine Baxerres, Adolphe Codjo Kpatchavi, Daniel Kojo Arhinful*

Since its emergence in the 1980s, the anthropology of pharmaceuticals has focused both on how products are used and the ways they are distributed (Van der Geest & Whyte, 1988), yet these two questions are not always explored simultaneously. How pharmaceutical companies influence prescriptions and consumption has been highlighted, especially in the context of rich countries (Collin & Otero, 2015; Dumit, 2012; Greffion & Breda, 2015; Moynihan, Heath, & Henry, 2002; Vega, 2011). Speculation logics of the multinational pharmaceutical industry as well as legislation on intellectual property and their impact on the economy of "emerging" countries, such as India, Nigeria, and Mexico, have also been described (Hayden, 2003; Peterson, 2014; Sunder Rajan, 2017). Through this chapter, we aim to analyze the relationships between pharmaceutical supply—with a strong focus on distribution—and consumers' use of medicines in Benin, Ghana, and Cambodia. We will thus extend recent works carried out in the Global South by pharmaceutical anthropologists on specific health issues, such as mental health in India; sex hormones and menstruation in Brazil, Cambodia, the Philippines, and South or West Africa; as well as AIDS in West Africa (Desclaux & Egrot, 2015; Ecks, 2014; Sanabria, 2016). Our work is centered on the everyday pharmaceuticals used to treat symptoms and acute illnesses.[1] We turned to the pioneering work of Arjun Appadurai and his colleagues (Appadurai, 1986), which focused on material objects and their consumption to highlight the interest in studying the relationships between culture and economics, and conducted an empirical and theoretical investigation on pharmaceuticals pinpointing the intersection between medical anthropology and the social sciences applied to economics (anthropology, sociology, and history).[2] As we will see, the concept of quality appears to be central in our investigation. Economic sociologists, who have increasingly studied this idea since the late 1980s, have shown that this structures the broader market, and ultimately, all types of markets (Steiner, 2005), regardless of what commodities are being considered. However, in these studies, the concept of quality often seems to assume a single tangible meaning, even though it is associated with the complex issue of trust (Karpik, 1989) that we explore later. And yet, we felt it necessary and important to distinguish the objective reality of product quality from its subjective dimensions.

A product's objective quality is measured using technical criteria, which in the case of medicines includes the quantity of active ingredient, the dosage of different compounds, and the degree of impurity established in the product specifications in accordance with its marketing authorization (MA) and one of the internationally recognized pharmacopoeias (Vickers et al. 2018; WHO, 2014). A product's objective quality is defined through certification standards established by organizations, such as the World Health Organization (WHO) or the International Conference on Harmonisation of Technical Requirements for the Registration of Pharmaceuticals for Human Use (ICH),[3] and applied on an international scale for drugs.

Subjective dimensions of product quality—the topic of this chapter—draw on individuals' perceptions of these products, relative to the product's and the manufacturer's reputation. In sociology and anthropology, the concept of perceptions refers to a set of ideas and values that are widely shared by different groups or categories of people. It has become separated from the more ideal concept of "collective representations" (Durkheim, 2007/1895) through the introduction of practices, thus linking the psychological with the somatic (Gélard, 2016). Because perceptions are shared, they reflect back on the subject at hand. The concept of subjectivities, one that extends beyond the methodological register (the researcher's reflexivity in their study site), is relatively recent but increasingly advanced in anthropology, especially when related to health and biomedicine (Derbez, Hamarat, & Marche, 2016; Fainzang & Ouvrier, 2019). For Joao Biehl, Byron Good, and Arthur Kleinman, "subjectivity constitutes the material and the means of contemporary value systems" (2007, p. 5). Regarding issues of social suffering related to health that the authors are exploring in the wake of economic globalization, they highlight that the power issues that come into play at the societal level are largely linked to the subjects' daily experiences and to the significations that they give them. "Capital accumulation and governance occur through the remaking of culture as well as the inner transformations of the human subject" (Biehl, Good, & Kleinman, 2007, p. 5).

Thus, the subjective dimensions of product quality are both specific to the individual and widely shared, as will be shown later. They are also an expression of the temporal evolution of economic powers and trends within countries and, more broadly, global regions. These macrosocial changes and the economic and political actors who try to influence them strongly permeate consumers' subjectivities, as this chapter will illustrate using the example of pharmaceuticals.[4] Hence, we will deconstruct the "imaginaries of consumption"[5] that surround drugs, as with all types of standardized products (the washing machine, wristwatch, car, clothing, food, etc.), in the postcolonial contexts of the three countries where we investigated. How are positive or negative images of the various types of available drugs constructed? What criteria does the purchaser apply to the various products before selecting one? Lastly, what implications might these choices have when dealing with pharmaceuticals—products that beyond being marketed and subjective, are also therapeutic?

## Establishing a typology of pharmaceutical supply and subjective value scales

Our studies led us to conceptualize pharmaceutical supply in the three countries through a typology of available medicines that broadly works for both consumers and distributors.[6] This subjective typology is built on three criteria: the products' supposed geographic origin, their presentation (packaging—individual box, hospital packaging, illustrations, colors, etc.—and dosage form), and their price. This allows us to classify the various available products in the countries using a subjective value scale, ranging from the most to the least valued. By describing the various categories of products, we shall see that this typology is influenced by colonial and more recent history in Benin, Ghana, and Cambodia as well as by the characteristics of local and regional pharmaceutical production in these countries.[7]

### *"French products" and "UK products"*

The first category of medicines illustrates the symbolic weight that the countries' colonial history imposes on individuals' perceptions about medicines. It is the most valued category in terms of drug quality and, in each of the three countries, is described in reference to the former colonial power: France for Benin and Cambodia, the United Kingdom for Ghana. An observation in a pharmacy in Accra illustrates this: "A woman came and asked for 'diclo suppository' and Mark[8] told her he had lofnac [made by an Indian company]. The woman asked 'Don't you have UK?' Mark told her no, and she left without accepting the lofnac. I asked Mark what he thinks about what the woman said. He told me that some people have this perception that low-priced medicines are not efficacious, but it is not always the same" (field diary, October 26, 2016). Observations in places where pharmaceuticals are sold in Ghana revealed that requests such as "a woman just asked for 'Omeprazol UK'" (field diary, May 20, 2015) are not uncommon. As previously described in Benin (Baxerres, 2013), informal sellers refer to them as "French medicines." In Cambodia, they are "*thnam barang*" (*thnam*: medicine, *barang*: French). A woman selling in a pharmaceutical warehouse in Phnom Penh explains that she likes the *thnam barang*. "They have the effect. They're effective. They can cure faster. And it's a little more expensive" (interview on May 5, 2015).

It was revealing to note during our field studies in each of the three countries that the highest quality for medicines was associated with the former colonial power. This is understood as a symbolic register; the coercive power of the former colonial empire is transmitted to products that supposedly originate there. In Ghana, people sometimes mentioned another category, ranked just behind "UK products," of "German products," since Germany was the country's secondary colonial power.[9] From a more pragmatic perspective, it should be recalled that pharmaceutical specialties were introduced in all three countries by the former colonizer, which served as the main supply source for a long time (Monnais & Tousignant, 2006; Pourraz, 2019). This is still the case in Benin (Baxerres, 2013).

This is a subjective category because only some of the products in question actually come from France or the United Kingdom. For example, "French products" are never requested in Ghana, even though from an objective standpoint, French pharmaceutical companies do exist in local markets. More generally, these are drugs manufactured by European and North American multinational pharmaceutical companies, and sometimes by major Indian companies, marketed under a brand name, whether they are innovative, originator products, or generics, and packaged individually for the private sector. In Cambodia, these medicines are recognizable by labeling written in French or more widely in the Roman alphabet.[10] In that country, drugs from South Korea may also be included in the "French products" category. In its role as an Asian economic power, South Korea is universally valued in Cambodia. The two countries maintain university and economic exchanges that help drive this positive image.

As underscored in the previous field excerpts, product price helps establish this highly valued category of medicines. These products are expensive! The relationships between a product's price and its perceived quality, known as the "Veblen effect," named for the economist and sociologist who uncovered this mechanism (Veblen, 2014/1899), are quite evident. Other economists have highlighted that the high price is considered a necessary condition for quality (Wolinsky, 1983). A father of a "middle-class" family in a Beninese semirural area offers this opinion: "The way I see it, the one that is excessively expensive will be effective" (interview on December 8, 2015). Another father of a "poor" family living in Phnom Penh explains: "We really want the *thnam barang*. It is effective and also expensive" (bimonthly monitoring conducted on March 17, 2015).

### *"Local products"*

A second category of products comprises drugs manufactured in the country or possibly in the bordering countries, but with the same type of packaging. In the eyes of consumers and distributors, products in this category are valued significantly less than those in the previous category. Overall, it is common in the three study countries for imports from abroad, especially from Western companies, to be valued more highly than what is produced locally.

In Benin, they are called "pharmaquick drugs," named for the country's only pharmaceutical company—Pharmaquick—that produces generics marketed under an International Nonproprietary Name (INN), usually in hospital packaging (large quantities of loose tablets or most often blister packs in large containers). This subjective category in Benin includes other generics marketed and packaged using the same procedures but manufactured in Togo, Ghana, Nigeria, and China (see figure 11.1 below).

In Ghana and Cambodia, both of which have a relatively developed pharmaceutical industry (36 and 14 companies, respectively), this category primarily includes products actually manufactured in the respective countries. As in Benin, they are either made up of generics marketed under an INN and presented in hospital packaging, or manufactured specifically for the private market and,

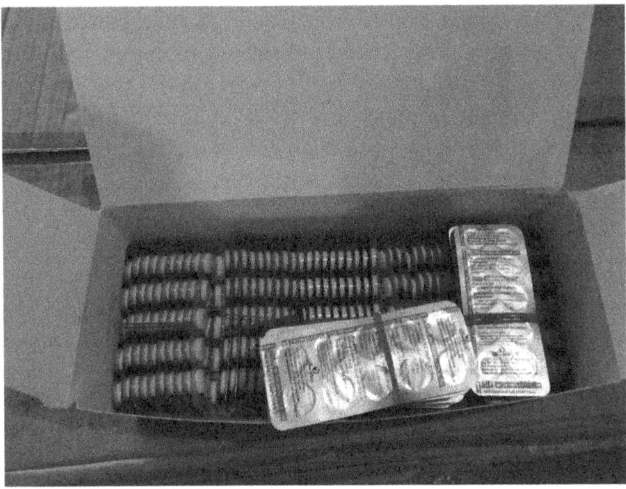

*Figure 11.1* A box of "pharmaquick drugs."

Source: © IRD/Stéphanie Mahamé, Cotonou, March 2019

therefore, marketed under the brand name and packaged in individual boxes. However, other products may also be included within this subjective category. In Cambodia, for example, one of the visible elements of this category is the package insert written in the Khmer language. Thus, even when manufactured in a Western company, a drug that has one of these package inserts can be perceived as "local," which depreciates its potential quality in the eyes of individuals.[11]

As mentioned previously, the price of these "local products" contributes to their lower value when compared with "French" or "UK products." The fact that they are a bargain insinuates poorer quality. A seller in a pharmaceutical warehouse in Phnom Penh points out: "Cambodians don't like to take Cambodian medicines because they believe the quality isn't very good. They prefer French medicines" (interview on March 10, 2015). Another female vendor in a pharmacy explains: "It's true that the cheaper drugs have lower quality" (interview on February 24, 2015). In Ghana, this mother of a "wealthy" family explains: "When I use the foreign paracetamol, its effect, I see... I don't know how to even explain myself. When you use it, from a personal experience, I think that one works much better than the local one" (interview on October 10, 2015). However, these products are not considered to be bad medicines, as this observation conducted in a pharmacy in Accra illustrates: "Another man also came and asked for rubbing alcohol, and Vida told him there was a 'foreign' and 'local' one, and then asked him which one he wanted and the man asked the prices of each and she told him 8 cedis and 10 cedis respectively. The man said he wanted the 8-cedis one"[12] (field diary, March 4, 2017). On the other hand, some people in Ghana and Cambodia also value local manufacturing of pharmaceuticals.[13]

Some companies within the Ghanaian and Cambodian pharmaceutical industry try to elevate their products' image in comparison to other "local products" by emphasizing their connections to the former colonial power or, more broadly, with the West. Their products are sold at a slightly higher price than other "local products." This was the case for one producer in Ghana that was just launching its wholesale activities and primarily imported drugs produced by Western multinationals. This was also the case at a company based in Cambodia, which is said to sell "French products" that it packages in Cambodia.

### *Drugs from neighboring countries*[14]

The category of drugs, perceived as coming from nearby countries, whether from a geographic or historical perspective, is more ambivalent than the two other categories in how it is valued.

In Benin, "drugs from Nigeria and Ghana"—generics marketed under a brand name, imported from Nigeria and/or Ghana and manufactured either there or in Asian countries—are easily recognizable by their colorful packaging with photos or illustrations of the illness that the product is meant to treat (see Figure 11.2). They are inexpensive and, therefore, are perceived as having lower quality than the "French products." But at the same time, some people perceive them as "strong" and effective; we will return to this aspect later.[15]

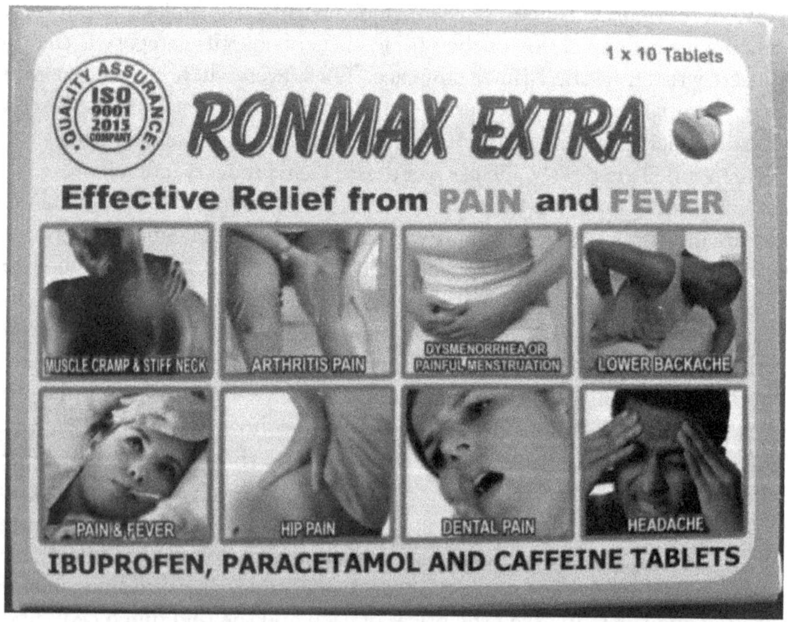


*Figure 11.2* Ronmax Extra® produced in India by Ronak Exim; this pharmaceutical has been renamed "8 illnesses" (in reference to the 8 photos on the box) in Benin and is perceived as a "drug from Nigeria and Ghana" in Benin and as an "Indian product" in Ghana.

Source: © IRD / Aubierge Kpatinvoh, December 2020

In Ghana, "Indian products," also generics marketed under a brand name, are less expensive and thus less valued than "UK products." At the same time, people believe they are effective, hence their popularity, which is further enhanced because they are inexpensive. When talking about the owner of a clinic where she used to work, this mother of a "wealthy family" in Accra said: "Her drugs are not bad but most of the time, these antimalarials that she buys are from India, the majority of them (...). Me, I didn't use to like their medications, but they are not bad (...) so far the ones I have tried, have worked" (interview on March 25, 2015). India is actually a major source of drug supply in Ghana (30% according to Chaudhuri (2016) and the business relations between Ghanaian and Indian pharmaceuticals, particularly within the Commonwealth, are strong. Drugs produced in other Asian countries (such as Indonesia, Pakistan, and China) are incorporated into this subjective category of "Indian products."[16]

In Cambodia, "Vietnamese drugs,"[17] which may be generics marketed under either an INN or a brand name, also fall under ambiguous perceptions. They are poorly perceived, as reflected in the Khmer expression "*thnam yuon*." "*Youn*" derives from Sanskrit "*yavana*," meaning "barbaric." It is a nickname that Cambodians often give to Vietnamese that reflects the political tensions between the two countries.[18] An example of these tensions is a rumor that circulated at the time of our study in Battambang province, claiming that the Vietnamese had sold ampicillin capsules containing hooks to Cambodia to kill Cambodians. This pharmacy vendor explains: "Most people when they see a medicine is from Vietnam, they don't want it. (...). Because they think that is not good, it is not good medicine" (interview in Phnom Penh, April 24, 2015). However, for serious health issues, people in Cambodia who can afford it go to Vietnam for care, where the health system and, by extension, the drugs have a better reputation than in Cambodia.

When applying this value scale to the pharmaceutical supply in these three countries, "drugs from neighboring countries"—despite being especially vulnerable to resentments sometimes between people living in nearby countries due to situations of economic or political domination—fall between the "French" or "UK products" and the "local products." The colorful, eye-catching packaging used for most of these branded generics, unlike INN generic drugs, is clearly a factor in the relatively good value associated with these products.

## "ACTs"

A fourth category of products needs to be introduced: drugs issued from public health programs. We call these "ACTs" in reference to the national malaria programs in the three countries that recommend using artemisinin-based combination therapies (ACTs) to treat uncomplicated malaria. These drugs opened the door to our research on understanding global and local pharmaceutical markets in the context of the Globalmed program. Given the high prevalence of malaria in Benin and Ghana, antimalarial drugs evoke multiple, rich perceptions. By contrast, in Cambodia, malaria is confined to specific geographic areas (mainly in and around forests), and antimalarials, which are not used on a daily basis, are not really an object of popular perceptions.[19] Although we focus on ACTs here, we want to use this category more broadly to discuss the popular perceptions of subsidized drugs introduced into the countries through public health programs with the involvement of so-called transnational actors.[20] These pharmaceuticals have an objective quality, which is certified by the WHO Prequalification of Medicines Programme presented in the introduction of the chapter.

In Benin and Ghana, subsidized ACTs are generics marketed under an INN and sometimes a brand name, usually in specific packaging for public health use and sometimes also in individual boxes (see Figure 11.3 below). These medicines are inexpensive (up to seven times less expensive than unsubsidized ACT; see Chapter 7) and, once again, are valued less than "French drugs" or "UK products." As one assistant in a public health center pharmacy in Cotonou points out: "When you prescribe ACTs[21] for someone here and they take it, 10 days later they come back and say it's not working. You tell them ok, go to the pharmacy and tell them that you have a problem. When they sell them the drugs that they have there, then they're really satisfied" (interview on October 26, 2016).

Nevertheless, people's perceptions of the value of "ACTs" can be improved through State-implemented communication campaigns, so they are perceived as having acceptable "quality." This is especially true in Ghana where the National

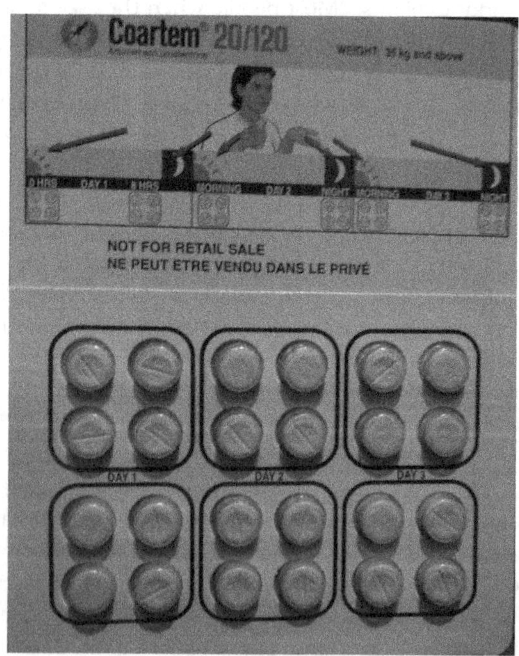


*Figure 11.3* A box of an "ACT," here subsidized Coartem® distributed in Benin.

Source: © IRD/Moïse Djralah, Comè, August 2015

Malaria Control Program developed a very effective communication campaign addressing ACTs, using a green leaf logo representing an artemisinin leaf (see Picture 7.1 in Chapter 7).[22] A mother of a "poor" Ghanaian family, living in a semirural area said: "ACT, isn't it these ones, the yellow tabs? (…). It really helps us in this village. (…). It's very fine. In fact, it's good. (…). That is the best so far…." (interview on February 21, 2015). Despite having acceptable "quality," green leaf "ACTs" in Ghana could still be commonly valued less than "UK products."

Therefore, the countries' available pharmaceutical supply is categorized by consumers and distributors and ranked on a value scale that plays an extremely significant role and is widely shared by individuals. We will now look at the factors that guide consumers when choosing one or another of these categories.

## Subjective quality and the functioning of pharmaceutical markets[23]

What is the impact of these subjective perceptions of pharmaceutical supply and of the quality of locally available drugs on how individuals purchase and use drugs? What do we also learn about how pharmaceutical markets currently function in these countries?

### *Deciding between the subjective quality and objective price of medicines*

Given the subjective typology of medicines presented previously, it is clear that, first and foremost, consumers tend to choose based on the product's price. Thus, people's socioeconomic status guides them toward one drug category or another. Generally speaking, poor people are much more likely to use "local products," "drugs from Nigeria and Ghana," "Indian products," and "ACTs." The most affluent primarily use "French drugs" or "UK products." Also, both in Ghana and Benin, vendors in pharmaceutical distribution locations themselves actually steer people toward one drug category or another, based on their physical appearance, clothing, and how they speak, as explained by this mother of a "poor" family in Accra: "It's the same thing. There is no difference [between the products]. Hmm hmmm but sometimes if you go, they [the sellers] will tell you that this one is from UK. Hmmm hmm and this one too is from Ghana, but it is good" (interview on March 11, 2015). In most cases, poor people have to settle for the lower valued categories, which they justify as best they can. In Benin, for example, people might say that "drugs from Nigeria and Ghana" are very good, that they are effective, but if they could afford it, they would rather go to the pharmacy and purchase "French drugs"; we will discuss the link between the drug category and types of distribution sites in the next section. "What can you do if you can't afford the pharmacy? You have to buy the one that is cheaper than the other one and take care of yourself" (interview with a mother of a "poor" family in Cotonou on December 18, 2014).

However, for a more nuanced investigation, two other factors need to be considered alongside price. First, the specific health goals that the product targets also influence which drug category is selected for purchase. For medicines consumed on a daily basis, for common symptoms such as headache or "fatigue" or even to take care of one's body (vitamins, blood tonics, etc.), "simple" drugs, which people use all the time—"*para and such*," as one hears in Benin—it is not necessarily worth it to find the highest quality product. "Local products," "pharmaquick drugs," and "Indian products" are often sufficient, regardless of the person's socioeconomic status. One customer said, "folic acid will always be folic acid no matter where it is produced" (observation in a pharmacy in Accra on January 11, 2017). A mother of a "wealthy" family living in Cotonou also notes: "I don't usually buy medicines in the market stalls... [...] just '*para*', paracetamol, like when I have a headache and I take *para* right away... for *para*, we know that *para* is just *para*" (interview on December 11, 2014). On the other hand, when a "real" health problem arises and people are concerned enough to consult a health professional, they will try much harder to obtain the prescribed medicines in the highest valued category, depending, of course, on the individual's financial means. The health problem that someone wants to treat can also influence the drug category. "I don't buy malaria drugs for my children in those places [in the homes of neighborhood 'aunties']... Even for myself, I don't buy antimalarials very often from the women; I buy [at the pharmacy]" (interview with a mother of a "wealthy" family in Cotonou on December 23, 2014).

A second important factor to consider alongside price is who exactly is supposed to consume the medicine. "Quality"—and thus, the highest valued drug category—will be more aggressively sought after for children, pregnant women, the most vulnerable, or those who are most cherished. For healthy adults, even the least valued medicines suffice. An observation in a pharmacy in Accra highlights this: "Another old woman came and asked for '*para*, 1 UK and 3 local ones.' The UK brand was for herself, but the local one, according to her, she has visitors and they are many, so it is better to get the local one that is much cheaper to cater to them all. She asked Euget if it works the same as the UK brand and she said yes" (field diary, April 11, 2017). In Benin for example, "drugs from Nigeria and Ghana" are perceived as "strong," very effective drugs, but possibly too strong for "weak" bodies, like children's. Inherent to this second factor is how medicines often become personalized—the fact that a drug may be suitable for one person's body but not another's, even when it is for the same health issue—a situation that must also be considered (Baxerres, 2013; Sarradon-Eck, Blanc, & Faure, 2007; Whyte et al., 2002). Thus, for some people, regardless of their socioeconomic status, an "Indian product," a "drug from Nigeria or Ghana," or a "pharmaquick" will "work" better than a "UK product" or a "French product," for example.

### *Close relationships between drug categories and types of retail structures*

Coupled with product price and the potential customer's socioeconomic status, our study highlights that the different types of pharmaceutical distributors working in Benin and Ghana do not distribute the various drug categories in the same way. Looking at actual pharmaceutical distribution reveals close relationships between the distribution site and the types of drugs offered.

Although they are also available through various means from other retailers, the predominant distribution site for "French drugs" and "UK products" is the private pharmacy, both in Benin and Ghana. This is even more so in Benin where the pharmacist's monopoly is strong (see Chapter 3). Therefore, the "French drugs" category essentially overlaps the other subjective category of "pharmacy drugs" (Baxerres & Le Hesran, 2011). Compared to other pharmaceutical distribution sites in the two countries, the pharmacy has the greatest institutional legitimacy. It is managed or run by a qualified pharmacist. Pharmacies are not equally distributed throughout the country and are mostly located in urban areas. In Accra, they are mostly found in the city's most upscale neighborhoods. In the Ghanaian semirural area that we investigated, there were no pharmacies.

"Local products" are commonly distributed in health centers in both countries, in pharmaceutical warehouses and by informal vendors in Benin, and by OTC medicine sellers in Ghana.[24] Again in Benin, where drug categories and distribution sites are closely linked, "pharmaquick drugs" are also called "hospital drugs," due to their hospital packaging. In Ghana, "local products," marketed in individual packaging for the private sector, are mostly sold by OTC medicine sellers, particularly in rural areas. Commonly using rural outlets for distribution of local drug production in Africa is not a characteristic specific to Ghana. It has also been reported in Tanzania (Chaudhuri, Mackintosh, & Mujinja, 2010).

In Ghana, "Indian products" are also quite commonly sold by OTC medicine sellers. In Benin, "drugs from Nigeria and Ghana" are only available from informal vendors, a category that may include products classified as "local products" or "Indian products" in Ghana. It is interesting to note that products from a specific company located in Ghana are highly valued by informal vendors in the neighboring francophone countries who buy large quantities of them when they go to Ghana for their supply.

"ACTs" are not distributed in the same places in Benin and Ghana, as shown in Chapter 7. In Ghana, they are available from any pharmaceutical distribution actor, both public and private, while in Benin they are only accessible through public health centers and community health workers assigned in rural areas through specific public health programs, such as malaria control.[25]

Therefore, the subjective categorization of drugs also has to do with where they are distributed in the country. The pharmaceutical products available are not the same for everyone but are instead based on the consumer's socioeconomic status and area of residence.

### *Economic "niches" for pharmaceutical companies*

Upstream of distributors, the pharmaceutical companies, in turn, are seeking their market share. According to economic sociologists, in these types of wholesale markets where economic actors engage in ongoing business dealings, unlike the brief encounters in a retail market, "these producers watch each other to define how they want to position themselves into 'niches' that they will occupy on the market in terms of product quality and volume" (Steiner, 2005, p. 41). Hence, in drug markets at play in Benin and Ghana, some companies, such as the abovementioned Ghanaian manufacturer, focus more intensively on the lower class. Their products are inexpensive and are distributed more chiefly through OTC medicine shops and in rural areas. They are also very popular in Beninese informal markets.

Other companies, mainly multinationals from the West, produce brands whose product quality is highly valued. Their packaging is highlighted in such a way as to further emphasize this feature. They are perceived as being "original" products, even long after the drug has entered the public domain or when they were not in fact the originator product. They are expensive and their price further reinforces these perceptions. By comparison, companies that produce locally or in Asian countries are perceived as manufacturing "generics," in the negative sense often associated with these drugs in Ghana and especially in Benin that deviates far from the legal definition.[26] Their low price further reinforces this perception. Nevertheless, the vast majority of people in these countries have relatively low purchasing power. Thus, the market share, in terms of quantity sold, for "local products," "Indian products," or "drugs from Nigeria and Ghana" is significant.[27] These products are widely popular and appreciated by most low-income people. This appreciation increases when the packaging for the private sector is appealing, colorful, and illustrated with photos that show the treatment's expected effects (see Figure 11.2).

Yet, since they also want to be major players in these markets, Western companies develop their generic brands (Chaudhuri, 2016). For example, a new subjective category, playing out among Ghanaian distributors, has emerged in that country: "UK generics." This name designates generic drugs marketed under their INN combined with the name of the company, usually from the West, which cost less than "UK products" but more than "local products" and "Indian products." And these "SuperGenerics" give rise to the paradox articulated by Cori Hayden, namely "the emergence of sameness and similarity as generative forms of distinction and value" (2013, p. 601). However, a middle class is undeniably flourishing in these countries at an annual growth rate greater than in European countries or the United States. As discussed previously, we see that Ghanaian companies position themselves to enter the most highly valued markets.

Drugs for public health programs, the "ACTs," further complicate the hierarchy in these pharmaceutical markets. Although making these products available definitely has public health objectives (in this case to roll back malaria), the producers also manipulate the subjective perceptions of their potential customers. As seen in Chapter 6, they play on both sides of the field, subsidized and unsubsidized markets, using one specific name or using several names for the same molecule, with different packaging and different prices.

## Constructing the subjective quality of drugs and imaginaries of consumption

The biomedical professions and public health actors frequently present drugs as "a commodity unlike any other," for which issues of quality are completely different. We will show that while it has specific features, the drug-as-commodity marketing is constructed like that of many other commodities.[28]

### *Insinuating doubts and urging trust*

As noted previously, the residents of Benin and Ghana who distinguish between the various types of locally available medicines in terms of quality, generally do not perceive the least valued categories ("local products," "Indian products," and "drugs from Nigeria and Ghana") as harmful or toxic. Contrary to what other scholars have pointed out (Hamill et al., 2019; Mackintosh & Mujinja, 2010), in the contexts and on the types of pharmaceuticals that we studied, the medicine's subjective quality does not reflect the issue of drug risks (Fainzang & Ouvrier, 2016; Massé, 2007). Rather, such quality seems to lie much more in a form of "social distinction," in line with Pierre Bourdieu (1984), or even in a "discrimination and prestige mechanism," in line with Jean Baudrillard (1986/1972, p. 9), associated with product consumption. This social distinction enables everyone, regardless of socioeconomic status, to find "their place" in drug market hierarchy; this is rather ironic, since it involves health commodities. This customer, observed in a pharmacy in Accra, rightly points out: "He asked for amlodipine, and Regina brought Wockhardt brand [an Indian company] to him (…). He picked it up, looked at it and said 'What is this you've brought me? I don't want this one.' By then the manager stood by him and told Regina to bring Pfizer's [a US company] brand to him. I asked the guy why he didn't like the Wockhardt brand and (…) he said 'Just like you will not have the money to purchase coca cola and yet go and purchase special cola [a locally produced drink]'" (observation on April 3, 2017).

Of course, economic actors adroitly conflate these two aspects (risk-toxicity and prestige-social distinction). For them, it ultimately means maintaining suspicion around certain products and instilling trust around others (Quet, 2018). Therefore, the idea of subjective effectiveness probably most accurately reflects how consumers assess the different categories of medicines presented previously.[29] The least valued medicines are often perceived not as toxic or harmful, but as less effective than the higher valued ones. "Sometimes when I have some money, I go straight to the pharmacy since pharmacy drugs are more effective. [...]. If you buy at the pharmacy, that works better than if you buy at a house (referring to informal vendors). It works better and it works faster" (interview with a mother of a "poor" family in Mono department in Benin on December 8, 2014). This perceived effectiveness may sometimes lead individuals to consume either twice or half the quantity of certain products.

In economics, price theory alone has long explained market mechanisms, as if only prices regulate economic activity. However, economic sociologists have since shown that an increasing amount of this activity calls for new analysis tools.[30] Based on his research on lawyers in France and highlighting clients' uncertainty when faced with determining the quality of legal services that they are largely unable to assess—as is the case for medicines—Lucien Karpik (1989) emphasizes the ideas of trust and judgment.[31] According to him, uncertainty about the quality of services or products manifests through a distinct mode of regulation that competes with pricing. He therefore differentiates between the "price-market" and the "judgment-market." In the case of pharmaceutical markets, as we have shown previously, price helps shape judgment. It is one of the criteria for constructing subjective perceptions of the quality of products. But it is not the only one.

### *Branding and geographic origin: Creating a reputation and singularity*

Our studies show that a product's subjective quality is only constructed relative to other products of the same type, within economic hierarchies and through competition. The work of economic historians on this topic sheds light on the drivers associated with product quality since the eighteenth century,[32] given the sharp increase in the number of all types of products marketed in the West since that time.

Historians are especially "sensitive to the issue of categorizing [and] have also explored how the various actors' have invested in the agreed-upon forms to produce an order for commodities within which the tension between similarity and singularization is expressed at the foundation of market segmentation and trade dynamics" (Margairaz, 2012, pp. 1–2). These economic historians demonstrate how the concept of product quality, the standards that enable its objectification, and the branding that make it visible have been constructed by the manufacturers themselves in order to ensure their marketing position and to distinguish themselves from their competitors. Philippe Minard proposes an illuminating analysis of the marketing strategies of silversmiths in eighteenth century England, particularly in Birmingham, who wanted to cement their reputation ahead of their competitors in London. They led a "veritable crusade" to create a regulatory assay office in Birmingham, responsible for measuring the quantity of pure silver in a piece and hallmarking it if it met the standard. In this way, the Birmingham manufacturers made "respecting quality standards their warhorse, and ... turned it into a formidable marketing tool," and "their quest to conquer markets led them to advocate for establishing quality controls that they hoped would give them an advantage in terms of reputation and trust" (Minard, 2010, pp. 1136 and 1119). These manufacturers thus began the long process of building a brand image.

Several studies in sociology, economics, and history have investigated labels, certifications, and brands as symbols associated with a product's quality, which strengthen consumer confidence. Whether they view quality based on its objective dimensions (Linnemer & Perrot, 2000), defined in the introduction, or whether they emphasize its subjective dimensions (Boltanski & Esquerre, 2017;

Musselin et al., 2002; Stanziani, 2005), they all show the competitive and commercial aims that, along with strategies, propel these moves to demonstrate quality. According to Luc Boltanski and Arnaud Esquerre, brands began to garner attention at the end of the nineteenth century and then flourished with the rise in marketing (Cochoy, 1999). The authors assert that a dual concern explains the increasing importance placed on brands: "stimulating sales" and "enabling producers to disengage from traders, while ensuring that objects can still be identified in a way that is relatively independent of the identity of the people who sell them." This is about winning customer loyalty, "regardless of where the product is sold" (Boltanski & Esquerre, 2017, pp. 227–228), and building loyalty to a specific product that the customer trusts rather than a single interaction with a vendor. Obviously, advertising accompanies these elements of product singularization, as Sophie Chauveau (2005) has shown with the emergence of pharmaceutical specialties in the eighteenth and nineteenth centuries.

In historical studies, a product's geographic origin appears to play a fundamental role in the singularization and classification of commodities: silver products from Birmingham are distinguishable by the anchor stamped on the pieces, compared to those from London, with its leopard design (Minard, 2010); the white textiles of Holland and those of the East India Company (Margairaz, 2012), and so forth. Therefore, the construction of objective quality often passes through geographic spaces. The protected designation of origin (PDO)—a European legal instrument to create reserved markets (for food products associated with a specific region, or terroir) that is integrated into competition law and economic law and distinct from intellectual property rights because it has no time limit—is proof of this geographic impact. Ultimately, this tool closely resembles trademark law, which "is born with the brand's registration and dies, in theory, with the death of the company that submitted it," but it is more powerful: the PDO "is indissoluble because the land is immortal, immemorial" (Hermitte, 2001, pp. 197–198). Not unlike labels and brands, construction related to geographic spaces also carries undeniable economic advantages. Philippe Minard shows how a geographic space can affect reputation. In the case of silver pieces "made in Birmingham," this involved "building up an attractive reference, a symbol of superior quality" (Minard, 2010, p. 1140). Lynda Dematteo (2016) shows that when confronted with fierce competition from Chinese clothing producers, the Italian textile industry is trying to reposition itself based on high quality and luxury, thus creating a "niche" by emphasizing its "made in Italy" attribute. However, Chinese producers can also play at this game, and Lynda Dematteo notes the case of a Chinese company that uses a brand name that sounds Italian.

We have seen through the example of pharmaceutical supply in Benin, Ghana, and Cambodia that the perceived geographic origin of drugs, linked to national territories (France, United Kingdom, India, Vietnam, Nigeria, and Ghana) is undoubtedly a criterion for "quality" among consumers. This geography of subjective value takes on a specific resonance in the postcolonial contexts of the three study countries. Returning to Mario Biagioli, cited by Cori Hayden (2013, p. 606), it could be said that for Western pharmaceutical companies, the perceptions associated with drugs from the West, in postcolonial contexts, play the role of "intellectual property without intellectual property."

### *Encountering subjectivities, creating attachments*

Economic actors' marketing strategies past and present, which we have attempted to decipher in the previous pages, shape the products that encounter consumers' subjectivity. Some scholars speak of "desires of consumption" (Boltanski & Esquerre, 2017), but this concept is difficult to apply to medicines—a product, first and foremost, of necessity. And yet some vignettes from our ethnographies seem to reflect this. Liliane, mother of a "poor" family living in a Beninese semirural area, exemplifies this. During the 9 months that we monitored her family's pharmaceuticals consumption, she mainly bought "pharmaquick drugs" or "drugs from Nigeria and Ghana" for herself, her husband, and her children from the informal vendors whom she paid between CFA 250 and 500 (between EUR 0.40 and EUR 0.76). One day she bought a box of Parafizz® at CFA 1540 (EUR 2.30) in a pharmacy to treat a headache.[33] It seemed to us that she wanted to "indulge herself" that day, after unexpectedly receiving some money.

Market research conducted by producers and their marketing teams on the drug as an object, especially its packaging, definitely encountered individuals' "imaginaries of consumption" in Ghana, Benin, and Cambodia. Manufacturers employ a variety of factors to construct a product's "subjective quality": using colorful boxes with illustrations and photos showing the drugs' effects; featuring seemingly white-skinned people in the photos on boxes of "Indian products" and "drugs from Nigeria and Ghana"; or using elaborate packaging, complete with a prestigious brand, in contrast to the INN generics sold in hospital packaging, whether "ACTs" or not. As demonstrated by Emilia Sanabria (2016) on the topic of sex hormones, product packaging has an impact on medicines' materiality and, therefore, on the effects that they actually produce, beyond their solely symbolic efficacy.

Producers generate consumer "attachment" to the product through this work on brands and packaging. This idea has been put forward by Michel Callon, Cécile Méadel, and Vololona Rabeharisoa as a second mechanism structuring markets alongside the "singularization" of products. "The consumer is not alone when faced with a product and having to identify its qualities. He is guided and assisted by tangible devices that serve as benchmarks, guide posts, and 'affordances' (allowing and suggesting a course of action) through which information is distributed" (2000, p. 225). In their view, "attachment" occurs at the juncture where an object's characteristics and the symbolic meet—in other words, subjectivities. Other authors discuss the "seduction" that major brands exert on consumers (Stanziani, 2005).

Thus, the object's image combines with price and assumed geographic origin (which is reinforced by the brand name) to complete construction of the drug's "subjective quality." These three criteria appeared to be inherent factors that play an equal role when assigning a value to medicine-as-commodity in postcolonial contexts at the time of our studies. Proving that value is relative depending on the context, era, and commodity concerned, the effect of these three criteria may vary and others may be more influential (rarity, soundness, newness, location, etc.).[34]

This last ethnographic vignette, featuring Indian companies and mass production of low-end products on the one hand, and a former colony and refined, high-quality production inspiring trust on the other, speaks volumes about the "imaginaries of consumption" associated with medicines in the postcolonial contexts that we studied: "Their products are better [referring to products from a European company].... As for Indians, I don't trust them, no, I don't trust them, they are like mass production... like, let me say, emmm, a UK person would do this one, he would take his time, make sure the efficacy, that everything is okay.... But these people they do 'bra, bra, bra' [meaning in a hurry], finish! because they want to produce many, so they wouldn't take their time. When you take a UK product and you take an Indian product, when you look at it closely you would see that there is a difference ... though it's the same active ingredients," (interview with a wholesaler-importer in Accra, August 21, 2014).

## Conclusion

In the three countries where we conducted our studies, a subjective hierarchy of locally available drugs is at play that structures the pharmaceutical markets. This hierarchy is influenced by the countries' colonial and more recent history as well as by the characteristics of local and regional pharmaceutical production. Forms of subjective categorization in pharmaceutical supply are certainly at work in other national contexts, including in the West.[35] Countries' early and recent history, their political conflicts, and the dynamics of global pharmaceutical production all leave their mark, as demonstrated in the examples we have described. One key factor to consider lies in the systems for covering health costs: in countries where medicines are affected by social distinctions when purchased directly by the consumer, as we have highlighted, the standards and reimbursement mechanisms for drugs (and for *which* drugs) are undermined and less effective.

Our research shows a different way to understand the concept of quality when applied to medicines than what is normally advanced in the media and public health actors' discourses (Baxerres, 2014; Hodges & Garnett, 2020; Quet, 2018). The "subjective quality" of medicines, far from their objective certified characteristics—clearly demonstrated by the example of "ACTs"—is, nonetheless, incredibly effective and a key factor in structuring pharmaceutical markets. Subjective quality influences what consumers choose as well as how they use products. It steers the commercial strategies of pharmaceutical companies that position themselves toward different types of clientele (more or less solvent, living in urban or rural areas, rich or poor urban neighborhoods) (see Chapter 9 as well). It also guides which products retailers select to distribute in their pharmacies and shops.

Nevertheless, the drug quality standards discussed in the introduction, while objective, are neither neutral nor immutable. Historians have revealed that how a product's "objective" quality is defined—a transhistorical concept that is assumed to actually exist—evolves and transforms. Their research underscores that "a product's quality is not the same at different times and in different places" (Stanziani, 2005, p. 419). They also demonstrate that "official certification can become a weapon that we must learn how to use and that we can turn against competing manufacturers" (Minard, 2010, p. 1124). Some economists echo this stance when they report "that we sometimes ascribe the goal of supporting producers of good quality to a policy regulating quality" (Linnemer & Perrot, 2000, p. 1399). These historical findings need to be questioned concerning medicines and what might be understood as ever-increasing quality requirements currently incumbent on pharmaceutical production (Pourraz, 2019).

The objective and subjective qualities of drugs ultimately come together in the fact that they both structure economic activity and how markets function, although operating through different processes. It is advisable to be especially vigilant on these issues and to rely on scientific, biomedical, and social science research to inform the "hybrid forums" (Callon, Méadel, & Rabeharisoa, 2000), comprising nongovernmental organizations, transnational actors, economic actors, scientists, and consumers' associations, who never fail to take a stand on the polarizing subject of pharmaceutical drug quality.[36]

## Notes

1. The Globalmed program focused on medicines used to treat malaria. With this as a starting point, our research results primarily concerned common, everyday pharmaceuticals used to treat symptoms and acute illnesses—in short, the most frequently used medicines in the study countries. Our results would have been different if we had begun by focusing our investigation on, for example, medicines to treat chronic diseases.
2. The work of Arjun Appadurai and his colleagues inspired the founding authors of the anthropology of medicines, who used the "social lives of things" as a springboard to propose the study of the "social lives of medicines" (Whyte, Van der Geest, & Hardon, 2002).
3. The WHO certification standard for the quality of medicines is called the WHO Prequalification of Medicines Programme (PQP). It was first applied in 2001 to antiretrovirals for AIDS, then to antimalarials and tuberculosis drugs, and then gradually from 2006 onwards to contraceptives, antivirals for flu, and treatments for acute diarrhea and neglected tropical diseases. The ICH was founded in 1990 and is made up of pharmaceutical regulatory authorities and industry associations from the European Union, the United States, and Japan (Pourraz, 2019).
4. We would like to thank Eve Bureau-Point, head of the study in Cambodia. We are as well grateful to Maurice Cassier, for the scientific discussions we shared on these issues that greatly inspired us while writing this chapter. See the Introduction of the book for more information on the data collection methodology.
5. This concept is advanced by the Vipomar program research team (funded by French National Research Agency—ANR 2014–2018), which addresses "The Political Life of Commodities" in line with seminal anthropological research in consumption (Douglas & Isherwood, 1996), in addition to that of Baczko Bronislaw (1984) on the topic of social imaginaries connected to various political regimes, and of Maurice Godelier (2015), which is more specifically focused on religious imaginaries, as well as games and art.

6. Of course, depending on who is speaking and where they are, some interviewed actors, especially some distributors, might go beyond this categorization and describe more nuanced categories, combining, for example, many more countries where the drugs originate. However, this does not question the operationality of the subjective typology described here.
7. Our previous research, conducted in the city of Cotonou in Benin, already enabled us to demonstrate a subjective typology for drug supply sold in informal markets (Baxerres & Le Hesran, 2011). This study, based on a comparative approach between three countries, extends and enhances the previous research.
8. All first names used in the chapter are pseudonyms.
9. In 1922, part of Togo, colonized by the Germans, was attached to the British "Gold Coast," the former name of present-day Ghana.
10. In Cambodia, the various subjective categories of medicines are partially structured on which alphabet is used on the boxes (Roman, Khmer, Thai, or Vietnamese alphabets).
11. Legally, any drug requesting a Marketing Authorization in Cambodia must include a package insert inside its packaging in the Khmer language. But sometimes a loose sheet of paper added into the box that provides a translation of the package insert in Khmer will suffice. Thus, imported drugs do not always have this insert, whereas drugs manufactured in Cambodia must include a package insert.
12. The Ghanaian currency is the cedi (GHC), and its rate fluctuates regularly. 1 GHC is worth approximately USD 0.20.
13. This valuing factor—locality—operates much more strongly for industrialized herbal medicines (Hardon et al., 2008), as we saw in Chapter 8. Nevertheless, it occasionally affects pharmaceutical specialties as well.
14. No quotation marks have been added to this category, which is etic, unlike the others described in this chapter that are emic. We constructed it so that we would be able to combine categories operating in the three countries where we worked.
15. Some formal drug distributers have a very negative view of drugs that they believe come from Nigeria. People in Benin generally perceive Nigeria as a country that produces low-quality copies of numerous goods (IT equipment, kitchen utensils, automobile parts, etc.). For more information about popular perceptions of "drugs from Nigeria and Ghana," refer to Baxerres (2013).
16. It is interesting to note that medicines included in the "Indian products" category in Ghana fall under the "drugs from Nigeria and Ghana" category in Benin. Also, surprisingly in Benin and Cambodia, popular perceptions do not encompass drugs originating in India, even though India is, in fact, a major source of drug supply in these countries.
17. It would be interesting to also specifically investigate "Thai drugs," which appear to reveal rich perceptions about the pharmaceutical flows between Thailand and Cambodia, as well as relations between the two countries. However, we did not go in depth on this issue during our study.
18. In the 1980s, after bringing an end to the Khmer Rouge regime, the Vietnamese installed the People's Republic of Kampuchea in Cambodia, which was under their control.
19. Malaria continues to be a major public health problem due to antimalarial resistance, which remains prevalent in Southeast Asia, and more specifically, at the border between Cambodia and Thailand (Phyo et al., 2012).
20. The expression "transnational actors" combines different types of extra-national actors currently involved in a country's public health issues: bilateral institutions (the various international aid services) and multilaterals (World Bank, Global Fund), nongovernmental organizations, foundations, and public-private partnerships that are sometimes aligned with the pharmaceutical industry.

21. In Benin, when distribution professionals talk about "ACT," they are referring to subsidized ACT. Sometimes they also use the term "coartem," because the Coartem® brand was overrepresented, if not the only available option, among subsidized ACTs for a long time. Consumers usually say coartem and sometimes ACTs or they describe the medicine. Nonsubsidized ACTs that are sold in pharmacies are known by their trade name, with people using different names depending on their purchasing practices.
22. This campaign was implemented during the launch of the AMFm (Affordable Medicine Facility-malaria), supported by the Global Fund. In Ghana, professional distributors use the term "ACTs" for all ACTs that have the green logo on their packaging; and even if they know that there are different manufacturers, they generally believe that these are the same products. However, consumers talk about "the one taken four-four, the yellow ones," and some also know the term "ACT." As in Benin, unsubsidized ACTs that do not carry the "green leaf" are known by their trade name.
23. The next two, more analytical, sections are based on our studies conducted in Benin and Ghana. The data collected in Cambodia as part of this more exploratory study did not allow for a detailed analysis of the local realities there.
24. For more information on these different actors in pharmaceutical distribution, see Chapter 3. In Ghana, OTC medicine shops are managed by non-pharmacists who are authorized to sell only over-the-counter medicines and some public health program products such as antimalarials or contraceptives. They were numerous in the country (10,424 at the time of our study). Private pharmaceutical warehouses in rural Benin are also held by people who do not have a degree in pharmacy. Owners are authorized to sell essential medicines from a limited list and are under a pharmacist's supervision. Linked to this strict legislation, their number is very few in rural Benin (165 in 2018). Informal vendors in Benin distribute drugs outside of the formal circuits prescribed by the State: in markets, in shops, door to door, at home, on public transport, etc.
25. This reality, which greatly limits individuals' use of "ACTs" in Benin, certainly also has an impact on the low value, noted above, attributed to these drugs in this country.
26. A generic drug is a copy of a proprietary drug whose patent has expired and entered into the public domain and whose therapeutic equivalence, quality, and safety are guaranteed by the drug regulatory agency in force in a territory. In accordance with national laws, generics may be marketed under a brand name or not; the latter are marketed under their INN, sometimes with the name of the manufacturing company or the company's generic division. Generics may be marketed in hospital or individual packaging. In our study contexts, it appears that "generics" are usually associated with drugs sold under an INN in hospital packaging and perceived as having low quality.
27. Medicines manufactured in India account for 30% of the Ghanaian pharmaceutical market. Local production in Ghana covers 30% of the private market in this country (Pourraz, 2019).
28. To define commodity, we have adopted the simple definition recently advanced by Luc Boltanski and Arnaud Esquerre: "anything that entails a price when it changes ownership" (2017, p. 12).
29. The social and symbolic dimensions of drug efficacy have been widely described in anthropology alongside their pharmacological aspects (Garnier & Lévy, 2007; Whyte et al., 2002). More recently, in a literature review that proposes revisiting the anthropology of medicines in line with scientific and technological studies, Anita Hardon and Emilia Sanabria (2017) fall back mainly on the concept of efficacy and its heuristic value. They highlight that this is conditioned by contexts (of the research, Market-State nexus, or regulatory environments) and influenced by the interests, expectations, and practices of both users and economic actors.

30. The neo-classic school of economics has highlighted the subjective theory of value since the so-called marginal revolution (Menger, 1981) (Original work published in 1871). Subsequent economic sociologists further refined an understanding of those realities (Steiner, 2005).
31. Some authors also cite the idea of trust, and its opposite, suspicion, when dealing with medicines (Hamill et al., 2019). However, from our point of view, they do not adequately develop a critical analysis of how these ideas actually play out for economic actors. Refer to Brhlikova et al. (2011) for a more critical use of these notions in the pharmaceuticals field.
32. Since the 1990s, extensive historical research has examined product quality, particularly for food products (bread, wine, milk, meat, etc.), textiles, silversmithing, and luxury items (Béaur, Bonin, & Lemercier, 2017/2006; Minard, 2010; Stanziani, 2005).
33. Parafizz® is manufactured by the Indian company Cipla, but it is a safe bet that since this drug is sold in pharmacies, it passes as a "French drug" in rural Benin.
34. Luc Boltanski and Arnaud Esquerre define value as simply "a system to justify or criticize the price of things" (2017, p. 13).
35. In France, for example, singularization in terms of the quality of various available drugs works largely through the distinction between "generics" and "originator products," with the words "fake" and "real" often being associated with these categories. For various historical and legal reasons, consumer "attachment" to a product, based on its brand name and packaging, does not occur with generics (Nouguez, 2017).
36. On this topic, note the organization of the conference entitled "Medicine Quality and Public Health," the first of its kind held in Oxford in September 2018 and which will be repeated: www.tropicalmedicine.ox.ac.uk/medicinequality2018/, consulted December 16, 2018.

## Reference list

Appadurai, A. (Ed.). (1986). *The social life of things: Commodities in cultural perspective*. Cambridge, UK: Cambridge University Press.

Baudrillard, J. (1986) (Original work published in 1972). *Pour une critique de l'économie politique du signe [For a critique of the political economy of the symbol]*. Paris, France: Gallimard.

Baxerres, C. (2013). *Du médicament informel au médicament libéralisé: Une anthropologie du médicament pharmaceutique au Bénin [From informal to liberalized drugs: An anthropology of pharmaceutical drugs in Benin]*. Paris, France: Les Éditions des Archives Contemporaines.

Baxerres, C. (2014). Faux médicaments, de quoi parle-t-on? Contrefaçons, marché informel, qualité des médicaments… réflexions à partir d'une étude anthropologique conduite au Bénin [Fake drugs, what are we talking about? Counterfeits, informal market, drug quality … thoughts from an anthropological study conducted in Benin]. *Bulletin de la société de pathologie exotique*, *107*, 121–126. https://doi.org/10.1007/s13149-014-0354-9.

Baxerres, C., & Le Hesran, J.-Y. (2011). Where do pharmaceuticals on the market originate? An analysis of the informal drug supply in Cotonou, Benin. *Social Science and Medicine*, *73*(8), 1249–1256.

Béaur, G., Bonin, H., & Lemercier, C. (2006). *Fraude, contrefaçon et contrebande de l'Antiquité à nos jours [Fraud, counterfeiting, and smuggling from Antiquity to the present day]*. Geneva, Switzerland: Droz.

Biehl, J., Good, B., & Kleinman, A. (Eds.). (2007). *Subjectivity: Ethnographic investigations*. Vol. 7. Berkeley, CA: University of California Press.

Boltanski, L., & Esquerre, A. (2017). *Enrichissement: Une critique de la marchandise [Enrichment: A critique of the commodity]*. Paris, France: Gallimard.

Bourdieu, P. (1984). *Distinction. A social critique of the judgement of taste*. R. Nice (Trans.). Cambridge, MA: Harvard University Press. (Original work published in 1979.)

Brhlikova, P., Harper, I., Jeffery, R., Rawal, N., Subedi, M., & Santhosh, M. R. (2011). Trust and the regulation of pharmaceuticals: South Asia in a globalised world. *Globalization and Health*, *7*(10), 2–14.

Bronislaw, B. (1984). *Les imaginaires sociaux: Mémoires et espoirs collectifs [Social imaginaries: Collective memories and hopes]*. Paris, France: Payot.

Callon, M., Méadel, C., & Rabeharisoa, V. (2000). L'économie des qualités [The economics of qualities]. *Politix. Revue des sciences sociales du politique*, *13*(52), 211–239.

Chaudhuri, S. (2016). Can foreign firms promote local production of pharmaceuticals in Africa? In M. Mackintosh, G. Banda, P. Tibandebage, & W. Wamae (Eds.), *Making medicines in Africa: The political economy of industrializing for local health* (pp. 103–121). London, UK: Palgrave Macmillan.

Chaudhuri, S., Mackintosh, M., & Mujinja, P. (2010). Indian generics producers, access to essential medicines and local production in Africa: An argument with reference to Tanzania. *The European Journal of Development Research*, *22*(4), 451–468. https://doi.org/10.1057/ejdr.2010.27.

Chauveau, S. (2005). Marché et publicité des médicaments [Drug market and advertising]. In C. Bonah, & A. Rasmussen (Eds.), *Histoire et médicament aux 19ème et 20ème siècles [History and medication in the 19th and 20th centuries]* (pp. 189–213). Paris, France: Éditions Glyphe.

Cochoy, F. (1999). *Une histoire du marketing: Discipliner l'économie de marché [A history of marketing: Disciplining the market economy]*. Paris, France: La Découverte.

Collin, J., & Otero, M. (2015). Resistance and mutations of non-specificity in the field of anxiety-depressive disorders in Canadian medical journals, 1950–1990. *Social Science & Medicine*, *131*, 228–238.

Dematteo, L. (2016, July). *"Made in Italy" under the hegemony of Chinese textile: Defense of global branding and spilled alienation*. Paper presented at the EASA Conference, Milan, Italy.

Derbez, B., Hamarat, N., & Marche, H. (2016). *La dynamique sociale des subjectivités en cancérologie [The social dynamics of subjectivities in cancerology]*. Paris, France: ERES.

Desclaux, A., & Egrot, M. (Eds.). (2015). *Anthropologie du médicament au Sud. La pharmaceuticalisation à ses marges [Anthropology of medicines in the South. Pharmaceuticalization at its margins]*. Paris, France: L'Harmattan.

Douglas, M., & Isherwood, B. (1996). *The world of goods: Towards an anthropology of consumption*. London, UK: Routledge. (Original work published in 1979.)

Dumit, J. (2012). *Drugs for life. How pharmaceutical companies define our health*. London, UK: Duke University Press.

Durkheim, E. (2007) (Original work published in 1895). *Les règles de la méthode sociologique [The rules of the sociological method]*. Paris, France: Presses universitaires de France.

Ecks, S. (2014). *Eating drugs: Psychopharmaceutical pluralism in India*. New York, NY: New York University Press.

Fainzang, S., & Ouvrier, A. (2016). Mesure des traitements et traitements sur mesure: La gestion du risque médicamenteux par les usagers en France [Treatment measuring and made-to-measure treatments: Management of medicinal risk amongst users in France]. *Terrains & travaux*, *28*(1), 21–40. https://doi.org/10.3917/tt.028.0021.

Fainzang, S., & Ouvrier, A. (Eds.). (2019). Face aux risques médicamenteux [Facing drug risks]. *Anthropologie & Santé, 19*. https://doi.org/10.4000/anthropologiesante.5312.

Garnier, C., & Lévy, J. J. (Eds.). (2007). La chaîne des médicaments. *Perspectives pluridisciplinaires [The drug chain: Multidisciplinary perspectives]*. Quebec, Canada: Presses de l'Université du Québec.

Gélard, M.-L. (2016). L'anthropologie sensorielle en France [Sensory anthropology in France]. *L'Homme, 217*, 91–108.

Godelier, M. (2015). *L'imaginé, l'imaginaire et le symbolique [The imagined, the imaginary, and the symbolic]*. Paris, France: CNRS éditions.

Greffion, J., & Breda, T. (2015). Façonner la prescription, influencer les médecins. Les effets difficilement saisissables du cœur de métier des grandes entreprises pharmaceutiques [Shaping prescriptions, influencing doctors. The hard-to-grasp effects at the heart of large pharmaceutical companies' professions]. *Revue de la régulation. Capitalisme, institutions, pouvoirs, 17*, 1–26.

Hamill, H., Hampshire, K., Mariwah, S., Amoako-Sakyi, D., Kyei, A., & Castelli, M. (2019). Managing uncertainty in medicine quality in Ghana: The cognitive and affective basis of trust in a high-risk, low-regulation context. *Social Science & Medicine, 234*, 112369.

Hardon, A., Desclaux, A., Egrot, M., Simon, E., Micollier, E., & Kyakuwa, M. (2008). Alternative medicines for AIDS in resource-poor settings: Insights from exploratory anthropological studies in Asia and Africa. *Journal of Ethnobiology and Ethnomedicine, 4*(1), 16.

Hardon, A., & Sanabria, E. (2017). Fluid drugs: Revisiting the anthropology of pharmaceuticals. *Annual Review of Anthropology, 46*(1), 117–132.

Hayden, C. (2003). *When nature goes public: The making and unmaking of bioprospecting in Mexico*. Princeton, NJ: Princeton University Press.

Hayden, C. (2013). Distinctively similar: A generic problem. *UC Davis Law Journal, 47*(2), 101–132.

Hermitte, M.-A. (2001). Les appellations d'origine dans la genèse des droits de propriété intellectuelle [Designations of origin in the genesis of intellectual property rights]. *Etudes et Recherches Sur Les Systèmes Agraires et Le Développement, 32*, 195–207.

Hodges, S., & Garnett, E. (2020). The ghost in the data: Evidence gaps and the problem of fake drugs in global health research. *Global Public Health, 15*(8), 1103–1118.

Karpik, L. (1989). L'économie de la qualité [The economics of quality]. *Revue française de sociologie, 30*(2), 187–210.

Linnemer, L., & Perrot, A. (2000). Une analyse économique des 'signes de qualité'. Labels et certification des produits [An economic analysis of "signs of quality." Product labels and certification]. *Revue économique, 51*(6), 1397–1418.

Mackintosh, M., & Mujinja, P. (2010). Markets and policy challenges in access to essential medicines for endemic disease. *Journal of African Economies, 19*(3), 166–200.

Margairaz, D. (2012). Qualité et fiscalité dans l'économie d'Ancien Régime [Quality and taxation in the Ancien Régime economy]. In J. Vögle & R. Salais (Eds.), *Qualitätspolitik. Die Qualität Der Produkte in Historischer Perspektive [Quality policy. The quality of the products from a historical perspective]* (pp. 1–21). Frankfurt am Main, Germany: Campus Verlag.

Massé, R. (2007). Le risque en santé publique : Pistes pour un élargissement de la théorie sociale [Risk in public health: Avenues for broadening social theory]. *Sociologie et sociétés, 39*(1), 13–27.

Menger, C. (1981) (Original work published in 1871). *Principles of economics*. New York, NY: New York University Press.
Minard, P. (2010). Le bureau d'essai de Birmingham, ou la fabrique de la réputation au XVIIIe siècle [The Birmingham Assay Office, or building a reputation in the 18th century]. *Annales. Histoire, Sciences Sociales*, *65*(5), 1117–1146.
Monnais, L., & Tousignant, N. (2006). The colonial life of pharmaceuticals: Accessibility to healthcare, consumption of medicines, and medical pluralism in French Vietnam, 1905–1945. *Journal of Vietnamese Studies*, *1*(1–2), 131–166.
Moynihan, R., Heath, I., & Henry, D. (2002). Selling sickness: The pharmaceutical industry and disease mongering. *British Medical Journal*, *7342*(324), 886–891.
Musselin, C., Paradeise, C., Callon, M., Eymard-Duvernay, F., Gadrey, J., & Karpik, L. (2002). La qualité [Quality]. *Sociologie du Travail*, *44*(2), 255–287.
Nouguez, E. (2017). *Des médicaments à tout prix: Sociologie des génériques en France [Drugs at all costs: Sociology of generics in France]*. Paris, France: Presses de Sciences Po.
Peterson, K. (2014). *Speculative markets: Drug circuits and derivative life in Nigeria*. London, UK: Duke University Press Books.
Phyo, A. P., Nkhoma, S., Stepniewska, K., Ashley, E. A., Nair, S., McGready, R., … Nosten, F. (2012). Emergence of artemisinin-resistant malaria on the western border of Thailand: A longitudinal study. *The Lancet*, *379*(9830), 1960–1966.
Pourraz, J. (2019). *Réguler et produire les médicaments contre le paludisme au Ghana et au Bénin : Une affaire d'Etat ? Politiques pharmaceutiques, normes de qualité et marchés de médicaments [Regulating and producing malaria drugs in Ghana and Benin: A State affair? Pharmaceutical policies, quality standards, and drug markets]*. Doctoral dissertation, Ecole des Hautes Etudes en Sciences Sociales, Paris, France. Retrieved at http://www.theses.fr/2019EHES0014
Quet, M. (2018). *Impostures pharmaceutiques: Médicaments illicites et luttes pour l'accès à la santé [Pharmaceutical deceptions: Illicit drugs and struggles to access health]*. Paris, France: La Découverte.
Sanabria, E. (2016). *Plastic bodies. Sex hormones and menstrual suppression in Brazil*. Durham, NC: Duke University Press.
Sarradon-Eck, A., Blanc, M.-A., & Faure, M. (2007). Des usagers sceptiques face aux médicaments génériques: Une approche anthropologique [Users who are skeptical of generic drugs: An anthropological approach]. *Revue d'Épidémiologie et de Santé Publique*, *55*(3), 179–185.
Stanziani, A. (2005). *Histoire de la qualité alimentaire: XIXe-XXe siècle [History of food quality: 19th-20th century]*. Paris, France: SEUIL Collection Liber.
Steiner, P. (2005). Le marché selon la sociologie économique [The market based on economic sociology]. *Revue européenne des sciences sociales*, *43*(132), 31–64.
Sunder Rajan, K. (2017). *Pharmocracy: Value, politics, and knowledge in global biomedicine*. Durham, NC: Duke University Press.
Van der Geest, S., & Whyte, S. R. (Eds.). (1988). *The context of medicines in developing countries: Studies in pharmaceutical anthropology*. Dordrecht, The Netherlands: Kluwer Academic Publishers.
Veblen, T. (2014) (Original work published in 1899). *Théorie de la classe de loisir [Theory of the leisure class]*. Paris, France: Gallimard.
Vega, A. (2011). Les surprescriptions de médicaments en France : Le vrai méchant loup de l'industrie pharmaceutique [Drug overprescribing in France: The real big bad wolf of the pharmaceutical industry]. *Formindep*. http://www.formindep.org/les-surprescriptions-de.html?debut_memerub=10.

Vickers, S., Bernier, M., Zambrzycki, S., Fernandez, F. M., Newton, P. N., & Caillet. C. (2018). Field detection devices for screening the quality of medicines: A systematic review. *BMJ Global Health*, 3(4), e000725.

WHO. (2014). Model Quality Assurance System for Procurement Agencies, No. 986, Annex 3. *Technical report series*. Geneva, Switzerland: World Health Organization. https://www.who.int/medicines/areas/quality_safety/quality_assurance/TRS986annex3.pdf.

Whyte, R. S., Van der Geest, S., & Hardon, A. (2002). *Social lives of medicines*. New York, NY: Cambridge University Press.

Wolinsky, A. (1983). Prices as signals of product quality. *The Review of Economic Studies*, 50(4), 647–658.

# Conclusion

# Rationalizing drug markets in the Global South

## Re-making medicines essential[1]

*Maurice Cassier and Carine Baxerres*

Ever since medicines began to be considered not only commodities but also essential goods to protect populations, the question has been how to rationalize drug markets in the interest of public health. In this conclusion, we draw on our research and past experience to propose areas for reflection and tools for governing pharmaceutical markets that can be used by public authorities and civil society.

In the history of pharmaceutical policies, the purpose behind the idea of "rational" measures is to introduce therapeutic usefulness criteria to organize the market, reduce the proliferation of pharmaceuticals with no significant medical interest, and rely on evidence-based medicine rather than marketing to decide whether therapies are indispensable or a priority (Halfdan Mahler's report, April 3, 1975).[2] As early as the early 1960s, several governments in so-called developing countries (Ceylon, Peru, Colombia) drafted and applied restricted lists of "basic medicines" to organize accessibility to them and reduce market crowding (Garcia, 2020; Greene, 2016. India and Brazil, two Global South countries that are significant in pharmaceutical geopolitics, changed their industrial property laws in 1970 and 1971, respectively, to authorize the growth of a generics market and to lower drug prices (Cassier, 2008). Several newly independent countries committed to policies of local pharmaceutical production—by private or in some cases public entities—to manufacture copies that cost less than trademarked drugs and to reduce their dependence on the supplies of such products; examples include India, Morocco, Egypt, Ghana, Tanzania, and others. In the late 1970s, the World Health Organization (WHO) developed a model list of essential medicines, which has been revised 20 times since 1977[3]—every 2 years—to help countries establish national lists adapted to their priority health needs. In 1997, the AIDS epidemic spurred South Africa to pass a law promoting the supply and use of generic drugs (Pelletan, 2019). Recent history is not lacking in mechanisms and experiments to develop and regulate pharmaceutical markets, with varying degrees of success and inclusiveness.

Jeremy Greene (2011) draws our attention to the plasticity of the concept of essential medicines and its circulation between the countries of the Global South and North. In our view, the essential nature of therapeutic agents has been redefined by several factors: a new geopolitics of medicines, improvements in the certification of generic drugs, the intervention of patients into intellectual property debates, the creation of regional common markets between Southern countries, the industrialization of traditional remedies, and new convergences between the North and the South on transparency in health product prices. This is evidenced by the geography of the signatories to the draft resolution adopted by the World Health Assembly in May 2019, entitled "Improving the transparency of markets for medicines, vaccines, and other health products," between the "Pharmerging" countries (South Africa, Brazil, India, Kenya, Egypt), and the countries of Southern and Eastern Europe (Italy, Spain, Greece, Portugal, Russian Federation) among others.[4]

What follows is a summary of seven areas of reflection on policies and tools for regulating drug markets.

## Using essential drug lists

Short lists of "basic medicines" or "essential medicines" were designed as tools to rationalize pharmaceutical markets and drug use in a way that is beneficial to public health. It is useful to recall the WHO Director General's objectives before the 28th General Assembly of Health on April 3, 1975. One was for developing countries to boost the efficiency of their medicine expenditures, burdened by excessively high prices, to avoid selling medications that have been withdrawn from the market in their country of origin because they are dangerous or lack efficacy, or something many of us have since forgotten, "the export of expired products to developing countries not in a position to perform quality control." Other objectives were ensuring the availability of treatments, the production of which was halted because they were not considered sufficiently profitable, and ensuring that the essential drugs selected are available at "reasonable prices" (Halfdan Mahler's report, cited earlier).

The criteria for selecting medicines for inclusion in the Essential Medicines List (EML) are crucial here to govern the pharmaceutical market to benefit public health in terms of safety, therapeutic usefulness, and product accessibility. EMLs must be formulated using International Nonproprietary Names (INNs), provoking the wrath of the International Federation of Pharmaceutical Manufacturers Associations (IFPMA), which views this as a declaration of war against its brands. The principle of a limited list of 220 products in 1977—all in the public domain due to expired patents—is also denounced by industry actors who argue for the dynamics of markets and innovation.

For the WHO, the development and implementation of an EML adapted to health needs assumes that countries have a national pharmaceutical policy as well as the tools, institutions, and experts to select, import, potentially locally produce, and distribute these medicines. The WHO adopted an Action Programme on Essential Medicines in the late 1970s to assist countries with this task, and in 1978 that organization deployed a specific action in the "African region" that proposed African countries subscribe to the WHO quality system, train prescribers, and draft an initial list of 40 medicines to encourage pooled purchasing for the countries of the region (report of March 26, 1979, WHO archives).[5] In the 1990s, WHO economists would disseminate guidelines proposing centralized procurement, financing options for essential medicine purchasing either by creating an international fund or through the marketplace using the cost recovery system,[6] and conditions for local production (Dumoulin, Kaddar, & Velasquez, 1991).

African states generally adopted the EML in the 1980s, in the context of the economic crisis, the introduction of the Bamako Initiative's cost recovery system in 1987 (Blaise, Dujardin, de Béthune, & Vandenbergh, 1998), and contraction in public health expenditures (see Figure C.1). As Cassandra Klimeck and Georges Peters (1995), economists focused on pharmaceutical policy in Africa, have noted, "for this reason, the [essential medicines] system has become a symbol of scarcity for health care providers and inhabitants in some countries" (p. 49). EMLs then began to target obtaining cheaper supplies by using generic drugs. Ghana and Benin, like many African countries, established EMLs in the late 1980s: 1987 in Benin and 1988 in Ghana. In the French-speaking countries of Africa, central purchasing offices for essential medicines were set up to obtain supplies of generics,[7] at which point we see the use of the category of "Essential Generic Medicines" (EGM) (Crozier, 2017). In these francophone countries, the devaluation of the CFA franc in 1994 accelerated the use of EGMs.

Comparative studies of EMLs reveal variations from the WHO list. We find that essential medicines are selected in consideration of the country's current

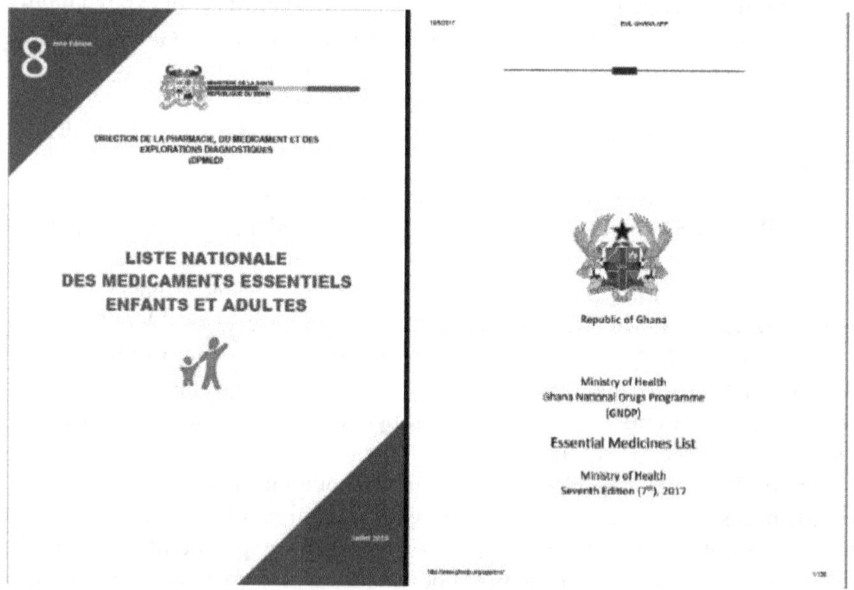


*Figure C.1* Benin and Ghana Essential Medicines List.

Source: Available for free on the Benin and Ghana Web sites for pharmaceuticals

prescription practices, and that drugs recently added to the WHO EML (e.g., new hepatitis C antivirals) are adopted by fewer countries than those that had been on the list previously. Countries with lower national wealth also tend to omit more of the essential medicines on the WHO list (Persaud et al., 2019). A major change that occurred in the early 2000s in the WHO's selection of essential medicines is the listing of new patented therapies, including antiretrovirals (ARVs) for HIV/AIDS, which Médecins Sans Frontières (MSF) had been demanding. To what extent are EMLs in middle- and low-income countries likely to incorporate these patented essential medicines, with their much higher prices?

With regard to the registration of new therapeutic classes in the WHO EML, we found that Ghana and Benin have included almost all ARVs for HIV/AIDS and artemisinin-based combination therapies (ACTs) for malaria. However, the same is not true for the new molecules that have arrived since 2012 to fight drug-resistant tuberculosis: while Benin's list includes bedaquiline, it does not include delamanid; Ghana's list does not include either one. Only a few of the new hepatitis C antivirals that have come on the market since 2014 and were quickly registered on the WHO EML appear on Benin's 2017 EML (two generics for sofosbuvir), but all are absent from Ghana's 2017 EML. Finally, new cancer compounds included on the WHO list are underrepresented in both countries. These departures from the WHO list are partly explained by the funding options for these therapeutic classes: ARVs and ACTs (with ACT prices much lower than those of ARVs) are largely funded by the global donor market (Global Fund), while the new hepatitis C antivirals and new anticancer drugs are patented compounds that fall outside these markets and are thus largely inaccessible. The share of donor funding is lower for anti-TB drugs than it is for AIDS and malaria drugs, hence the greater price sensitivity of governments to these new molecules. Ghana's EML reminds us of the selection criteria it adopted: in addition to product safety and usefulness, it includes two economic criteria relating to cost: "the drug with the lowest cost, calculated on the basis of the whole course of treatment"; and local production, "the drug for which economically convenient manufacturing is available in the country."[8] EMLs are thus clearly embedded in countries' economies.

We report several limitations to the application of EMLs. Although creating such lists can help determine which drugs may be reimbursed by health coverage, their application is hampered by the limitations of such health coverage in low-income countries, even one like Ghana that has rolled out universal health coverage (Antwi, 2019). The share of government health spending is lower than direct household payments and has tended to stagnate or even decrease in recent years. Households account for 40% of health spending in Ghana and 45% in Benin.[9]

In African countries, although cost recovery has reduced shortages (Dumoulin & Kaddar, 1993), economists and public health specialists have nonetheless pointed out the impact of this mechanism on social inequalities in health and the difficulty poor populations have accessing treatments (Klimeck & Peters, 1995; Ridde, 2005). The market logic that underpins cost recovery may also hinder the adoption of a limited list of essential drugs, since sellers prefer a wider range of products and those with higher margins (Dumoulin & Kaddar, 1993). High drug prices, especially for the new patented molecules on the WHO EML, are major barriers for populations. Even though sofosbuvir is listed on Benin's EML to treat hepatitis C, its price is still quite high despite the fact that the country is eligible to receive generics from the licenses distributed by Gilead to generics manufacturers for low-income countries.[10] In Ghana, experts are encouraging the government to procure generic versions of the drug (Tachi, 2018).

Under such conditions, specific intellectual property arrangements appear necessary so that generic forms of innovative essential medicines can be made available, while simultaneously extending international and national public funding and universal health coverage to acquire these products. For health coverage to be viable, action must be taken on drug prices.

## Promoting local production

Local production has been an aspect of essential drug policy since the 1970s (Velasquez, 1991). A meeting between the WHO and the African region in Brazzaville in 1980 concerning local production recommended intercountry or regional initiatives to avoid market fragmentation.[11] The creation of quality control laboratories was discussed in conjunction with local production, and a few countries, such as Burundi, Zaire, and Rwanda, requested technical assistance. The WHO handbook on the economics of essential drugs published in 1991 by Jérôme Dumoulin, Miloud Kaddar, and Germán Velasquez points out that although the impact on prices is unclear, local production will ensure a secure supply; however, they note that the establishment of such production must take into account the uncertainties of obtaining raw materials and machinery (1991). The international pharmaceutical industry was very reticent about these initiatives to promote local industry: recall that it withdrew its investments from the African region in the 1990s in the context of structural adjustment policies that reduced markets (Peterson, 2014).

In this book, we studied the local production policy in Ghana immediately after independence that established manufacturing plants, turning to direct investment from foreign firms and negotiating technology transfer agreements (Pourraz, 2019). Some African States encouraged the establishment of a pharmaceutical industry using the public or private sector (Chorev, 2020; Mackintosh, Banda, Tibandebage, & Wamae, 2016). Through a study of the emergence of pharmaceutical production in three East African states—Kenya, Tanzania, and Uganda—Nitsan Chorev demonstrates that international development aid cannot replace State intervention to support markets (by reducing taxes on imports of raw materials, allowing a certain higher price margin for locally produced medicines in tenders, encouraging local manufacturers to produce essential drug kits) and to promote technological training and gradually raise manufacturing standards. International aid and government pharmaceutical policy must complement each other to create markets and organize technology transfer. Conversely, Jessica Pourraz (2019) described the failure of a dozen industrial projects in Benin due to the lack of a national policy geared toward local production. International aid can also produce adverse effects if local producers are unable to compete with Global Fund-subsidized drugs, as in the case of Ghanaian firms that produced ACTs in the early 2010s.

There is a debate about the value and viability of producing drugs locally versus importing them from the large manufacturing countries in the Global North or Asia that largely dominate the market. Economists and political actors alike[12] point to the high cost of capital in Africa (Chaudhuri, Mackintosh, & Mujinja, 2010), the shortage of industrial pharmacists, the near absence of bioequivalence laboratories to test generic drugs, the problem of harmonizing standards for drug certification and registration, and the fragmentation of markets. The COVID-19 crisis has revived discussions on local production in a context marked by disruptions in the supply of active ingredients and drugs from China and India.

Here we list five important elements to be considered in this debate.

First, in order to combine industrial policy and public health interests, prioritizing investments in the manufacture of medicines on the essential drug lists is key.[13]

Second, a viable pharmaceutical industry cannot be constructed without both a technological and a regulatory infrastructure. The priority must be on training a sufficient number of industrial pharmacists, creating bioequivalence laboratories for the region, and strengthening the staff and equipment of regulatory authorities.

Third, it is essential not only to create investment funds to finance the industry, as proposed in the Abidjan Declaration in 2019, but to drastically reduce the cost of capital to the extent of offering zero or even negative interest rate loans to encourage industrial investment (Cassier, 2018).

Fourth, West African countries do not seem to be taking advantage of the flexibilities offered by the World Trade Organization (WTO) to the least-developed countries to copy new therapies free of charge and free of patents. If these flexibilities were applied, by revising the Bangui agreements[14] for example, a window would open for local African production; note that Indian manufacturers have had to comply with pharmaceutical patents since 2005.

And finally, it is important to recall that the WHO's essential medicines policy included the use of traditional pharmacopoeia. The policies for certifying herbal mixtures as well as R&D projects to isolate new active substances should be extended (see Chapter 8 on Ghana's policy in this area).

## Crafting standards for "essential" quality

The issue of substandard or falsified medicines (per the categories adopted by the WHO), or "counterfeit" and "fake medicines," has polarized public debate and the political scene since the early 2000s (Baxerres, 2015; Quet, 2018). Benin has been a singular site for this debate since the Call of Cotonou issued by ex-French President Jacques Chirac in 2009. In her research on pharmaceutical markets in Nigeria, Kristin Peterson (2014) analyzed the abrupt change that took place under structural adjustment policies in the 1990s, namely, the shift from a market dominated by trademarked drugs, sometimes produced by multinational firms that had set up shop locally, to a market dominated by generic drugs "of varying and often low quality" (p. 5), some of which the author states are sold on "unofficial" markets. Nitsan Chorev (2020) also notes that the liberalization of markets with structural adjustment policies has further enabled the arrival of "substandard" drugs. She reminds us that multinationals also used to sell substandard drugs in Africa.[15]

At the same time, Nitsan Chorev observes the implementation of more restrictive regulations in both manufacturing and importing countries. India's major pharmaceutical companies are using the WHO prequalification system (see Chapter 6) to guarantee the quality of the generic drugs they make to treat AIDS and malaria, raise their production standards, and dominate the global donor market.[16] "Second-tier" Indian firms are also improving their standards as those of importing countries rise. African manufacturers are benefiting from technology assistance programs to raise their production standards, and some firms, for example, in Kenya, are succeeding in getting their ARVs prequalified. Others, such as Danadams in Ghana (Pourraz, 2019), may not be able to pursue the prequalification process to its conclusion, but even so are raising their manufacturing standards. Ghana's Food and Drugs Authority (FDA) decided in 2012 to establish a program to help local firms apply Good Manufacturing Practices (GMP) (see Chapter 1).

This raising of standards creates a hierarchy of firms and markets, with firms that achieve prequalification and thus access to the global donor market, i.e., the large Indian manufacturers, in one tier, and most African firms that have only national certifications so are confined to national or regional markets in another. As we saw in the first section of this book, there are also significant disparities between the regulatory means in African countries, e.g., between Ghana's FDA with 50 pharmacists in 2016, and the Directorate of Medicines of Benin, which had only 6, including 2 civil servants and 4 contract workers (Pourraz, 2019). Africa also has very few laboratories authorized to conduct bioequivalence testing, so firms must subcontract this work to the Middle East or India.

Improving the safety of generic drugs requires the widespread use of GMP and control testing for pharmaceutical equivalence and bioequivalence in drug copies. Bioequivalence has gradually become a "gold standard" in Mexico (Hayden, 2013) and Brazil (Correa, Cassier, & Loyola, 2019); Morocco, which targets exporting to sub-Saharan Africa, established its own laboratory in 2016. However, the cost to access this standard, in terms of clinical trials, represents a barrier for most African laboratories.[17] International technical assistance programs should be combined with national programs to help firms manage this transition. While a few firms are likely to obtain WHO prequalification to access an international market, the majority will supply domestic and regional health needs. In this context, gradual compliance with GMP and certification of pharmaceutical equivalence as bioequivalence tests become more broadly used seems to be an acceptable route, particularly for generics included in the EMLs. Regional integration initiatives could facilitate this process.[18]

It is also appropriate to question the notion of "over-quality" raised by some experts. A pharmacist from a French company specializing in the preparation of drug registration dossiers in the United States and Europe and involved for several years in a WHO prequalification request for a factory in Tanzania wondered about this: "It is true that we sometimes have slightly divergent interpretations of the guidelines, and I am less accustomed to WHO prerequisites than the consultant who is a specialist in that, so we worked in tandem to be sure not to create over-quality in an African laboratory, because that is not the goal; the goal is for them to manufacture a drug, risk-free, but we don't want to create over-quality as we sometimes do in Europe; we must do something rational, but not be more royalist than the king, either" (interview, Bordeaux, July 2016). It therefore seems wise to question what is a "rational" or "essential" quality standard that improves the safety of essential generic drugs at a manageable cost.

Keep in mind that the over-quality mentioned by this expert is a strategy to create a barrier to market entry, one that benefits the most powerful firms and excludes manufacturers who cannot advance the required investments, as noted in the conclusion of Chapter 11.

## Common markets and regional institutions

The regional dimension appears in the WHO essential medicines program as early as the beginning of the 1980s. At a meeting of the WHO African region, there was talk of creating quality control laboratories at the regional or subregional level.[19] In 2013, after analyzing the flow of drugs between Ghana, Nigeria, and Benin, we envisaged a reform of pharmaceutical regulation to harmonize marketing authorizations on a regional scale (Baxerres, 2013 ; Baxerres & Marquis, 2018). Beginning in 2014, the Economic Community of West African States (ECOWAS) launched a Regional Pharmaceutical Plan (the ECOWAS Regional Pharmaceutical Plan or ERPP) that provides for the harmonization of pharmaceutical regulations, measures to support local production, and the creation of a regional bioequivalence center to be located in Ghana (Pourraz, 2019). In 2015, ECOWAS joined an initiative funded by the World Bank, the Gates and Clinton Foundations, and NEPAD (New Partnership for Africa's Development), which is being rolled out across eight African Economic Communities and was initially implemented in East Africa. NEPAD aims to harmonize drug regulatory practices through the African Medicines Regulatory Harmonization (AMRH) initiative, in particular the adoption of the autonomous agency model. Jessica Pourraz noted several difficulties involved in this harmonization process: between French- and English-speaking countries, between manufacturing and importing countries, and between the drug agency model and the Ministry of Health Pharmacy Directorate model, used until recently in Benin and Côte d'Ivoire (see Chapter 1). Francophone countries fear that the AMRH initiative will eclipse their own efforts at harmonization, under way since the mid-2000s within the West African Economic and Monetary Union (UEOMA).[20]

The ECOWAS harmonization initiative is based primarily on the use of a Common Technical Document (CTD) to register medicines in the region's 15 countries. ECOWAS plans to establish its own certification system to promote adoption of the new standard by firms in the region. This system, approved by the WHO, is aligned with international standards for manufacturing (GMP) and bioequivalence. The establishment of a regional regulation should boost industrial investment.

It should be noted that while proximity between assessors and industry is likely to promote the application of these standards, the cost of industrial and quality control investments to access them implies that a specific economic program be implemented to equip companies in order to overcome the standards barrier faced thus far by regional firms in terms of WHO prequalification. The number of companies that will be able to access regional and international markets, and the number that will be limited to certifications and strictly national markets, will depend on this support effort.

There is yet another difficulty: this process of harmonizing rules tends to favor countries with the most extensive regulatory mechanisms and the most modern firms and highlights interregional disparities. The harmonization of regional market rules presupposes concomitant cooperation projects to determine the distribution of manufacturing or quality control and bioequivalence laboratories between countries, so as to create a degree of convergence between them. There is also the issue of distinguishing between a regional agency and the national registration bodies. These are classic problems faced by common or single markets. Boris Hauray's work on the process of harmonizing standards and procedures for marketing medicines in Europe prior to the creation of the European Medicines Agency, from the mid-1960s to the mid-1990s, showed the ambivalence and fluctuations in the positions of both States and firms regarding whether to stay with national agencies or to adopt more or less unified and centralized forms of registration procedures at the regional level (Hauray, 2007).

## Pharmaceutical distribution: A dynamic balance of market offerings and professional control

Our research on pharmaceutical distribution in Benin and Ghana highlighted the asymmetry of market supply between the two countries. In Benin, there were 243 community pharmacies in 2015 operating under the pharmacist-owner system, and 165 private pharmaceutical depots under non-pharmacist ownership but under the authority of a pharmacist. In Ghana, there were 2175 community pharmacies, where the managing pharmacist is not necessarily the owner, along with 10,424 over-the-counter (OTC) medicine shops, which are owned and managed by non-pharmacists who must attend post-registration training sessions (see Chapter 3). The asymmetry of supply is also very pronounced in the private wholesaler trade. Even accounting for the population and national wealth differences between the two countries, the disparity in pharmaceutical distribution is unmistakable and explains the proliferation of the informal market in Benin.

The asymmetry is attributable to the differences in pharmaceutical legislation: Benin applies the principle of the pharmacist's monopoly, part of its legal heritage from France, which requires the pharmacist to be the owner of the community dispensary or wholesale company, which itself has public service obligations (a pharmacist must still closely supervise private pharmaceutical warehouses), whereas in Ghana, community pharmacies and private wholesalers are open to capital investment, consistent with that country's heritage of British law, a practice moderated by pharmacist control in the sale of prescription drugs in pharmacies and by the theoretically compulsory presence of a pharmacist at private wholesalers. The freedom to raise and mobilize capital for distribution in the two regimes is quite different.

At the end of our analysis of these issues, we consider solutions put forward by local actors to correct the imbalances that arise in each system. In Ghana, this would involve limiting market excesses in both the retail and wholesale sectors: OTC licensees or pharmacists in wholesale companies are present in a wide variety of sectors, despite inspections by regulatory authorities. The proposals aim to strengthen professional control, in particular by associating it with participation in the ownership of wholesale companies. In Benin, the aim would be just the opposite: to liberalize retail distribution in order to attract more candidates to open pharmaceutical depots, the numbers of which have been declining, and thus shift the boundary between the formal and the informal (the multitude of vendors). We believe liberalization of retail distribution—like what we find in Ghana—combined with a closer supervision of wholesale distribution—as is the case in Benin—would be an appealing prospect for taking advantage of the economic dynamics generated by the market while governing them to meet public health needs and local realities. This is not the path that was adopted in Cambodia, where the inverse is true: retail distribution is under a pharmacist's monopoly and wholesale distribution is liberalized.

The goal of these solutions is to offset market dynamics with management by the profession. Balancing the two is a delicate task. Requiring pharmacists to hold the majority of shares in a wholesale company, if not all of them, fortifies professional control but reduces sources of capital. In the first section of the book, we saw how pharmacists in some francophone countries (Benin, Côte d'Ivoire) have tried to get around this issue by organizing themselves into public limited liability companies or cooperatives. Note that in the 1960s French law also invented the figure of the "responsible pharmacist" in distribution and production companies in order to dissociate capital formation from professional control.[21]

Liberalizing the creation of private pharmaceutical depots in Benin in order to broaden supply in the countryside necessarily implies some form of oversight by regulatory authorities, which are sorely lacking in pharmacists. The State could also create incentives to encourage the establishment of pharmacies in rural areas. Other forms of regulation and education of informal vendors could also be considered, such as that attempted in Cambodia (see Chapter 4). We propose further strengthening the role of the health professions to counteract self-medication, which is significant in both countries' markets (Chapter 10).

## Making room for consumers and civil society in pharmaceutical market regulation

Although this book analyzes the power of consumers through self-medication—Chapter 10 refers to "essential" management of health events by families—patients as civil society actors are not very present in our work. This is because we did not investigate HIV/AIDS drugs but focused on antimalarial drugs, and malaria patients are less organized as civil society actors on the drug policy scene, despite some recent initiatives (Impact Santé Afrique, Civil Society for Malaria Elimination, AIDS Watch Africa).[22]

This is unlike the late 1990s, when patient associations played a major role in structuring the ARV market, and especially in promoting access to generics (Eboko & Mandjem, 2011; Pelletan, 2019). This was particularly the case in South Africa, Uganda, Kenya, and Côte d'Ivoire. Fred Eboko and Yves Paul Mandjem have characterized a plurality of associative models, self-organized by patients or created through initiatives by medical staff or international organizations. Their actions ranged from prevention and patient assistance, to medical staff support (Soriat, 2014), to demands for access to treatment. The South African association "Treatment Access Campaign" (TAC), created in South Africa in 1998, mobilized legal pressure to defend the South African law promoting generics in court, against multinational pharmaceutical companies and alongside the government, and then brought a lawsuit against the South African government that was slowing down the ARV deployment (Heywood, 2009). In the end, TAC obtained voluntary licenses from multinational firms for patented molecules that allowed the manufacture of generics. Patient associations are potential partners in drug policy. In her dissertation on the pharmaceutical industry in South Africa, Charlotte Pelletan (2019) described a "health coalition" that involved the Ministry of Health, the generics industry, and patient associations.

In addition to their action on market dynamics and "logistics regimes," to use the expression of Mathieu Quet and his colleagues (2018), who discuss them (see Chapters 4, 7, 8, 10, and 11),[23] patient associations are likely to get engaged in access to essential medicines, pricing, and intellectual property.[24] They may be involved in the management of essential drug purchasing offices and national and international drug supply programs to monitor supply disruptions, similar to the South African associations that never hesitate to take legal action.

Recent initiatives aim to federate patient associations at the regional level, such as the Civil Society Institute for HIV and Health in West and Central Africa, created in 2018, which combines 81 associations.[25] This initiative is supported by the French public agency for technical cooperation, the 5% Initiative. It is a civil society organization mobilized by Global Health actions in support of the Global Fund. At the same time, federated patient associations may also be inclined to involvement in therapeutic activism to demand access to treatment.

Finally, associative movements are a place where the Global North and the South converge for access to treatment. ACT UP has cooperated with many associations in Africa (Broqua, 2018).

## Commons and pharmaceutical markets

In 2016, the chief economist of the French Development Agency (AFD), Gaël Giraud, raised the concept of the commons to apply it to development economics: "A commons is a natural or cultural resource shared by a group, with precise rules of distribution, preservation, and promotion."[26] In the health sector, he mentions the drug pipeline for neglected diseases developed by the Drugs for Neglected Diseases initiative (DND*i*) Foundation (see Chapter 5).

If we apply the perspective of commons to medicines, they should be made into accessible, nonexclusive goods, the technology of which must be shared in a collective framework, governed by well-defined communities of actors who ensure that they are extensively distributed, and if necessary, preserved from opportunistic appropriation (Cassier, 2017). They could be distributed free of charge through a public economy or by humanitarian nongovernmental organizations (NGOs), or on a nonexclusive market, at affordable prices and supported by mechanisms for pooling health expenditures that lead to universal access. Here we come back to four conditions that could support the "commons" features of medicines.

In one way, the criteria for selecting essential medicines take the chosen drugs out of the classic commodity framework. The priority is not the profit margin per treatment unit and unlimited market expansion through brands, marketing, and so forth, but rather the cost savings with an associated guarantee of safety and therapeutic efficacy. And this occurs in the context of a designation that, unlike a brand name, is not an exclusive intellectual right but instead and intentionally a common name. Recall that the essential medicines policy recommends caution with regard to pharmaceuticalization:[27] it is not about fostering unlimited growth in the market and consumption, merely introducing some order through limited lists.

We saw earlier that there is a barrier to the dissemination of essential drugs when they are patented (see the new therapies for AIDS, tuberculosis, cancer, hepatitis C, etc. that are listed in the WHO EML). In such cases, the WHO or NGOs propose sharing the patents and authorizing the production of generic drugs for low- and middle-income countries.[28] They also propose using the flexibilities of the WTO's TRIPS (Trade-Related Aspects of Intellectual Property Rights) agreements to suspend these patents temporarily (the "compulsory license").

Chapter 5 returns to the notion of common property in relation to the invention and dissemination of ACTs. It concludes that putting the basic ACT molecules and the formulations developed by DND*i* (ASAQ, ASMQ)[29] in the common domain has helped overcome monopolies, allowed production to become dispersed, and resulted in affordable prices. That chapter also shows how technology sharing requires specific transfer investments to acquire the necessary industrial capacities.

The dissemination of medicines as common goods, accessible by and affordable for the population, also presupposes the extension of various forms of health expenditure pooling mechanisms: markets subsidized by global donors, public spending by States, universal health coverage, mutual health organizations, distribution by humanitarian NGOs, and so on.

Finally, we come back to a previous point: patient associations and humanitarian organizations can play a key role in defining and managing medicines as common goods, by demanding modifications to intellectual property rights, promoting the use of essential medicines (MSF), and participating in the actual conception of a drug's therapeutic use value, following the example of MSF and DND*i*. These, too, are actions toward drug market transparency as promoted by the WHO Declaration of May 2019, mentioned at the beginning of this conclusion, and conveyed by associations in the Global North, such as the Observatoire de la Transparence des Politiques du Médicament [Drug Policy Transparency Monitoring Center] in France (Londeix & Martin, 2019), and in the Global South, such as the ABIA Association in Brazil or I-MAK in the United States and India.[30]

The seven regulatory tools and powers that we have just laid out are largely interdependent. Drawing up a list of essential medicines can guide a policy of local production and serve as a basis for setting up health coverage; strengthening drug agencies and quality control laboratories strengthens local production and monitoring of pharmaceutical supply and distribution networks; and intervention by consumers and citizens is likely to promote the expansion of health coverage and price vigilance to make treatments accessible. These technical, financial, and political instruments and mechanisms could create market governance that is more favorable to public health, patients, and the populations to be protected,

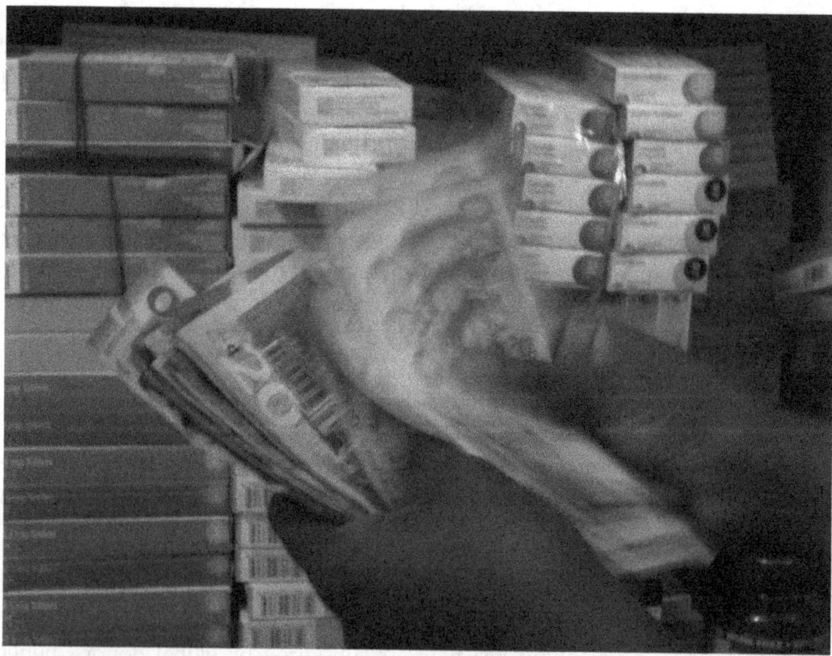

*Figure C.2* Pharmaceutical business in the Global South.

Source: © IRD/Carine Baxerres, Accra, May 2015

and a better balance between the drug's therapeutic use value and the market value. This contrasts with the waves of "commodification" that have occurred since the origin of the pharmaceutical industry, extensively explored in this book at currently at work today.

## Notes

1. The second part of the title is inspired by the work of Jeremy Greene (2011), discussed in this chapter.
2. WHO Archives Essential Drugs A28-11: Reports 1975–1990.
3. "The selection of Essential Drugs," report from a WHO expert committee, 1977, 40 p. See https://apps.who.int/iris/handle/10665/41272?show=full, accessed November 2020.
4. "Improving the transparency of markets for medicines, vaccines, and other health products." Draft resolution proposed by Andorra, Brazil, Egypt, Eswatini, Greece, India, Italy, Kenya, Luxembourg, Malaysia, Malta, Portugal, Russian Federation, Serbia, Slovenia, South Africa, Spain, Sri Lanka, and Uganda. See https://apps.who.int/gb/ebwha/pdf_files/WHA72/A72_ACONF2Rev1-en.pdf, accessed November 2020.
5. WHO Archives E19 445 3F J1 1979.
6. The 1987 Bamako Initiative imposed user fees in sub-Saharan Africa to compensate for the lack of government funding (Dumoulin & Kaddar 1993; Ridde, 2005).
7. The first purchasing centers were created in francophone countries (Benin, Burkina Faso, Chad, Mali, Niger, and Senegal). In 1996, they joined forces through the African Association of Central Medicine Stores for Generic Essential Drugs (ACAME), which today comprises 22 countries throughout West and Central Africa, the Indian Ocean, and the Maghreb, and whose number continues to grow (there were 19 members in 2010). They are still overwhelmingly French-speaking. See http://www.acame.net, accessed December 2020.
8. EML, Ghana, seventh edition, 2017: https://www.moh.gov.gh/wp-content/uploads/2020/07/GHANA-EML-2017.pdf, accessed September 2020.
9. WHO Global Health Expenditure Database: https://apps.who.int/nha/database, accessed September 2020.
10. Chronic hepatitis C treatment expansion. Generic manufacturing for developing countries, Gilead Sciences, 2014: https://www.gilead.com/~/media/Files/pdfs/other/HCV%20Generic%20Agreement%20Fast%20Facts%20102214.pdf, accessed in September 2020.
11. WHO archives E19 445 3F J1 1979.
12. For example, see the "Abidjan Call for the Industrialization of West Africa into Poles of Excellence," in February 2019: http://lists.healthnet.org/archive/html/e-med/2019-02/msg00020.html, accessed September 2020.
13. Here we may draw inspiration from the Product Development Partnerships encouraged by Brazil's Ministry of Health to produce a list of "strategic" drugs (Cassier & Correa, 2019).
14. See the recommendations of the International Treatment Preparedness Coalition (ITPC): "Intellectual Property and Access to Medicines in Côte d'Ivoire, Senegal, and Nigeria," March 2019, Pauline Londeix and Fouad Boutamak, 60 pages. See http://itpcwa.org/uploads/fr/ressources/brochures/5cc2ff434f6ce.pdf, accessed November 2020.
15. Cassandra Y. Klimeck and Georges Peters (1995) show that French firms sold medicines in Africa in the 1970s with fanciful and possibly dangerous indications.
16. Indian companies account for two-thirds of WHO-prequalified drugs (Lantenois & Coriat, 2014).

17. The Head of the Diseases Control and Prevention Departments of the Kenya Ministry of Health and Public Sanitation, Dr Willis Akhwale, stated "Kenya is also a country which grows and produces Artemisia and artemisinin but, due to the stringent WHO prequalification standards, is precluded from local manufacturer of 'pre-qualified' ACTs," Artemisinin Conference, 2013, Nairobi, Kenya.
18. Brazil has successfully gone down this path over a period of about 15 years by gradually harmonizing the standards for "similar" and "generic" products: in 1999, only generics had to show bioequivalence, through clinical trials (in vivo trials), while "similars" had to pass pharmaceutical equivalence tests in the laboratory (in vitro testing) to establish the structural similarity of the molecules and guarantee a qualitative and quantitative composition of active ingredient equivalent to that of the reference drug. In 2014, both types of copies had to satisfy bioequivalence tests (Correa, Cassier, & Loyola, 2019). The certified generic copies are under an INN in Brazil, while the similar ones have a trademark.
19. WHO Archives, E19 445 3F J1 1979 Africa.
20. It should be noted that ECOWAS is made up of both anglophone and francophone countries (Ghana, Guinea, Liberia, Nigeria, Sierra Leone, Cape Verde, and The Gambia), which do not have the same industrial capacity and therefore carry different weight in the policies advocated, whereas UEOMA is overwhelmingly made up of francophone countries (Benin, Burkina Faso, Côte d'Ivoire, Mali, Niger, Senegal, Togo, and Guinea-Bissau).
21. The concept of "responsible pharmacist" appeared in France through statutes and decrees between 1961 and 1969, with Decree 69-13 of January 2, 1969, clearly establishing a dissociation of capital ownership and pharmaceutical responsibility (Fillion, 2013; Ruffat, 1996).
22. See these organizations' websites: https://impactsante.org/; https://cs4me.org/; https://aidswatchafrica.net/strengthening-youth-leadership-and-engagement-in-the-fight-against-malaria-in-africa/, accessed November 2020.
23. Mathieu Quet and his colleagues give the example of Southeast Asian patients who go to other countries, via "suitcase" imports, to find products that they cannot get at home because of national or international legislation (hepatitis C treatments, contraceptive or abortive pills).
24. As an example see Médecins du Monde's campaign "Le prix de la vie [The price of life]": https://leprixdelavie.medecinsdumonde.org/fr-FR/ and the White Paper "Médicaments et progrès thérapeutique : Garantir l'accès, maîtriser les prix [Medicines and therapeutic progress: Guaranteeing access, controlling prices]": https://www.leslivresblancs.fr/livre/sante-medecine/medicaments/medicaments-et-progres-therapeutique-garantir-lacces-maitriser-les.
25. See https://www.enda-sante.org/fr/content/expertise-france-sengage-aupres-de-linstitut-de-la-societe-civile-pour-le-vih-et-la-sante-en, accessed November 2020.
26. "Les communs, un concept-clé pour l'avenir du développement [The commons, a key concept for the future of development]" Paris, October 25, 2016. See https://ideas4development.org/communs-developpement/, accessed November 2020.
27. See the Introduction, where this concept is explained.
28. See for example the Medicines Patent Pool created in 2010: https://medicinespatentpool.org, accessed November 2020.
29. ASAQ stands for the combination artesunate-amodiaquine and ASMQ for artesunate-mefloquine.
30. ABIA, or Brazilian Interdisciplinary AIDS Association: http://gapwatch.org/; and I-Mak, Initiative for Medicine Access & Knowledge: https://www.i-mak.org/2018/04/26/tahir-amin-transparency-drug-pricing/.

## Reference list

Antwi, A. A. (2019). *The pathway of achieving the universal health coverage in Ghana: The role of social determinants of health and "health in all policies."* Doctoral dissertation. University of Lille. France. Retrieved at http://www.theses.fr/2019LIL1A002.

Baxerres, C. (2013). *Du médicament informel au médicament libéralisé: Une anthropologie du médicament pharmaceutique au Bénin [From informal to liberalized drugs: An anthropology of pharmaceutical drugs in Benin]*. Paris, France: Les Éditions des Archives Contemporaines.

Baxerres, C. (2015). Contrefaçon pharmaceutique: La construction sociale d'un problème de santé publique [Pharmaceutical counterfeiting: The social construction of a public health problem]. In A. Desclaux, & M. Egrot (Eds.), *Anthropologie du médicament au Sud. La pharmaceuticalisation à ses marges [Anthropology of medicines in the South. Pharmaceuticalization at its margins]* (pp. 129–146). Paris, France: L'Harmattan.

Baxerres, C., & Marquis, C. (Eds.). (2018). *Regulations, markets, health: Questioning current stakes of pharmaceuticals in Africa.* (Conference proceedings). HAL, Ouidah, Benin. https://hal.archives-ouvertes.fr/hal-01988227

Blaise, P., Dujardin, B., de Béthune, X., & Vandenbergh, D. (1998). Les Centrales d'Achat de Médicaments Essentiels : Une priorité pour les systèmes de santé des pays en développement [Central Purchasing Offices for Essential Medicines: A priority for health systems in developing countries]. *Cahiers Santé*, 8, 217–226.

Broqua, C. (Ed.). (2018). Se mobiliser contre le sida en Afrique: Sous la santé globale, les luttes associatives [Mobilizing against AIDS in Africa: Association battles under global health]. *Collection Anthropologies et Médecines*. Paris, France: L'Harmattan.

Cassier, M. (2008). Une nouvelle géopolitique du médicament (1980–2005) [A new geopolitics of medicine (1980–2005)]. In A. Flahaut, & P. Zylberman (Eds.), *Des epidémies et des hommes [Epidemics and humans]* (pp. 101–109). Paris, France: La Martinière.

Cassier, M. (2017). Médicaments et communs [Drugs and commons]. In M. Cornu, F. Orsi, & J. Rochfled (Eds.), *Dictionnaire Des Biens Communs [Dictionary of common goods]* (pp. 792–794). Paris, France: Presses Universitaires de France.

Cassier, M. (2018). Concluding Remarks. In C. Baxerres, & C. Marquis (Eds.), *Regulations, markets, health: Questioning current stakes of pharmaceuticals in Africa* (pp. 30–40). (Conference proceedings). HAL, Ouidah, Benin. https://hal.archives-ouvertes.fr/hal-01988227.

Cassier, M., & Correa, M. (Eds.). (2019). *Health innovation and social justice in Brazil.* Cham, Switzerland: Palgrave Macmillan.

Chaudhuri, S., Mackintosh, M., & Mujinja, P. (2010). Indian generics producers, access to essential medicines and local production in Africa: An argument with reference to Tanzania. *The European Journal of Development Research*, 22(4), 451–468. https://doi.org/10.1057/ejdr.2010.27.

Chorev, N. (2020). *Give and take: Developmental foreign aid and the pharmaceutical industry in East Africa.* Princeton, NJ: Princeton University Press.

Correa, M., Cassier, M., & Loyola, M. A. (2019). Regulating the copy drug market in Brazil: Testing generics and similar medicines (1999 to 2015). In M. Cassier, & M. Correa (Eds.), *Health innovation and social justice in Brazil* (pp. 241–276). Cham, Switzerland: Palgrave Macmillan.

Crozier, P. (2017, September). *L'ACAME et les Centrales nationales d'achats de médicaments essentiels au cœur du développement sanitaire [The ACAME and Central Purchasing Offices of Essential Medicines at the heart of health development]*. Paper presented at the Journée des opérateurs français de la santé au Burkina Faso [French Health Operators Day in Burkina Faso]. Ouagadougou.

Dumoulin, J., & Kaddar, M. (1993). Le paiement des soins par les usagers dans les pays d'Afrique francophone. Rationalité économique et autres questions subséquentes [Payment for care by users in French-speaking African countries. Economic rationality and other subsequent issues]. *Sciences Sociales et Santé, 11*(2), 81–119.

Dumoulin, J., Kaddar, M., & Velasquez, G. (1991). *Access to drugs and finance. Basic economic and financial analysis WHO*. Geneva, Switzerland: WHO. https://apps.who.int/iris/handle/10665/61475?show=full.

Eboko, F., & Mandjem, Y.-P. (2011). ONG et associations de luttes contre le sida en Afrique. Incitations transnationales et ruptures locales au Cameroun [NGOs and associations that fight AIDS in Africa. Transnational incentives and local ruptures in Cameroon]. In F. Eboko, F. Bourdier, & C. Broqua (Eds.), *Les Suds face au sida. Quand la société civile se mobilise [The South confronted with AIDS. When civil society mobilizes]* (pp. 205–230). Marseille, France: Éditions de l'IRD.

Fillion, M. (2013). *La responsabilité du pharmacien responsable au sein de l'entreprise pharmaceutique : Etat des lieux en 2013 et impact des évolutions règlementaires [Responsibility of the head pharmacist within the pharmaceutical company: State of play in 2013 and impact of regulatory changes]*. Unpublished State dissertation [Thèse d'Etat], Université de Lorraine, Vandœuvre lès Nancy, France.

Garcia, V. (2020). La construction et la régulation de l'industrie et du marché de médicaments en Colombie (1914–1971). Contribution à une histoire de la mondialisation du médicament [The construction and regulation of the drug industry and market in Colombia (1914–1971). Contribution to a history of the globalization of medicines]. Unpublished doctoral dissertation, Ecole des Hautes Etudes en Sciences Sociales, Paris, France.

Greene, J. A. (2011). Making medicines essential. *Biosocieties*, 6(1), 10–33.

Greene, Jeremy A. 2016. " 'Pharmaceutical Geographies. Mapping the Boundaries of the Therapeutic Revolution', in *Therapeutic Revolutions: Pharmaceuticals and Social Change in the Twentieth Century*, Edited by Jeremy A. Greene, Flurin Condrau and Elisabeth Siegel Watkins, The University of Chicago Press, p 150–185.

Hauray, B. (2007). Les laboratoires pharmaceutiques et la construction d'une Europe des médicaments [Pharmaceutical laboratories and the construction of a Europe of medicines]. *Revue Française Des Affaires Sociales*, 3–4, 233–256.

Hayden, C. (2013). Distinctively similar: A generic problem. *UC Davis Law Journal, 47*(2), 101–132.

Heywood, M. (2009). South Africa's Treatment Action Campaign: Combining law and social mobilization to realize the right to health. *Journal of Human Rights Practice, 1*(1), 14–36.

Klimeck, C. Y., & Peters, G. (1995). Une politique du médicament pour l'Afrique. *Contraintes et choix [A drug policy for Africa. Constraints and choices]*. Paris, France: Karthala.

Lantenois, C., & Coriat, B. (2014). La « préqualification » OMS: Origines, déploiement et impacts sur la disponibilité des antirétroviraux dans les pays du Sud [WHO "prequalification": Origins, deployment, and impacts on antiretroviral availability in Southern countries]. *Sciences Sociales et Santé, 32*(1), 71–99.

Londeix, P., & Martin, J. (2019). Prix du médicament. Dans l'arène du débat [Drug prices: In the debate arena]. *Vacarme*, 3(88), 60–67.

Mackintosh, M., Banda, G., Tibandebage, P., & Wamae, W. (Eds.). (2016). *Making medicines in Africa: The political economy of industrializing for local health*. London, UK: Palgrave Macmillan.

Pelletan, C. (2019). *Le médicament, l'Etat et les marchés : La co-construction de l'industrie pharmaceutique et de l'Etat en Afrique du Sud [Medicines, the State, and markets: The co-construction of the pharmaceutical industry and the State in South Africa]*. Doctoral dissertation, Université de Bordeaux, France. Retrieved from http://www.theses.fr/2019BORD0099.

Persaud, N., Jiang, M., Shaikh, R., Bali, A., Oronsaye, E., Woods, H., ... Heneghanb, C. (2019). Comparison of essential medicines lists in 137 countries. *Bulletin of the World Health Organization*, 97(6), 394–404C. https://www.who.int/bulletin/volumes/97/6/18-222448.pdf.

Peterson, K. (2014). *Speculative markets: Drug circuits and derivative life in Nigeria*. London, UK: Duke University Press Books.

Pourraz, J. (2019). *Réguler et produire les médicaments contre le paludisme au Ghana et au Bénin : Une affaire d'Etat ? Politiques pharmaceutiques, normes de qualité et marchés de médicaments [Regulating and producing malaria drugs in Ghana and Benin: A State affair? Pharmaceutical policies, quality standards, and drug markets]*. Doctoral dissertation, Ecole des Hautes Etudes en Sciences Sociales, Paris, France. Retrieved at http://www.theses.fr/2019EHES0014.

Quet, M. (2018). *Impostures pharmaceutiques: Médicaments illicites et luttes pour l'accès à la santé [Pharmaceutical deceptions: Illicit drugs and struggles to access health]*. Paris, France: La Découverte.

Quet, M., Pordié, L., Bochaton, A., Chantavanich, S., Kiatying-Angsulee, N., Lamy, M., & Vungsiriphisal, P. (2018). Regulation multiple: Pharmaceutical trajectories and modes of control in the ASEAN. *Science, Technology and Society*, *23*(3), 485–503. https://doi.org/10.1177/0971721818762935.

Ridde, V. (2005). *Politiques publiques de santé et équité en Afrique de l'ouest. Le cas de l'Initiative de Bamako Au Burkina Faso [Public policies for health and equity in West Africa. The case of the Bamako Initiative in Burkina Faso]*. Doctoral dissertation, Université Laval, Quebec, Canada. Retrieved from http://hdl.handle.net/20.500.11794/18117.

Ruffat, M. (1996). *175 ans d'industrie pharmaceutique française. Histoire de Synthélabo [175 years of French pharmaceutical industry. History of Synthélabo]*. Paris, France: La Découverte.

Soriat, C. (2014). *Les acteurs associatifs contre le sida au Bénin: De la professionnalisation au gouvernement des corps [AIDS association actors in Benin: From professionalization to government bodies]*. Doctoral dissertation. University of Lille. France. Retrieved at http://www.theses.fr/2014LIL20016.

Tachi, K. (2018). Hepatitis C virus infection in Ghana: Time for action is now. *Ghana Medical Journal*, 1(52), 1–2. http://dx.doi.org/10.4314/gmj.v52i1.1.

Velasquez, G. (1991). Origine et évolution du concept de médicament essentiel promu par l'OMS [Origin and development of the essential drug concept promoted by WHO]. *Tiers Monde*, 32(127), 673–680.

# Index